T0195101

Clinical Applications of
3D PRINTING IN FOOT AND ANKLE SURGERY

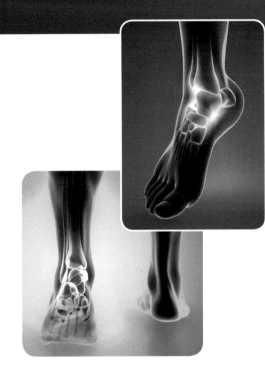

Edited by

PETER D. HIGHLANDER, DPM, MS

Director
Foot & Ankle Surgery
The Reconstruction Institute
The Bellevue Hospital, Bellevue
Ohio
United States

ELSEVIER

Elsevier
1600 John F. Kennedy Blvd.
Ste 1800
Philadelphia, PA 19103-2899

Senior Content Development Manager: Somodatta Roy Choudhury
Executive Content Strategist: Belinda Kuhn
Senior Content Development Specialist: Malvika Shah
Publishing Services Manager: Shereen Jameel
Project Manager: Vishnu T. Jiji
Senior Designer: Renee Duenow

Printed in India

Last digit is the print number: 9 8 7 6 5 4 3 2 1

Working together
to grow libraries in
developing countries

www.elsevier.com • www.bookaid.org

To Lindsey, the places we have been, the footsteps and handprints
For tomorrow, the next one to follow and all that is to come
To all of our dreams we have yet to apprehend

Contributors

Bijan Masood Abar, MHSc
Mechanical Engineering and Materials Science
Duke University, Durham
North Carolina
United States

Nicholas B. Allen, BS
PhD Student
Department of Orthopaedic Surgery
Duke University, Durham
North Carolina
United States

Emilio Bachtiar, BEng, MSE
PhD Student
Mechanical Engineering and Materials Science
Duke University, Durham
North Carolina
United States

Patrick R. Burns, DPM
Assistant Professor
Orthopaedic Surgery
University of Pittsburgh School of Medicine, Pittsburgh
Pennsylvania
United States

Alan Catanzariti, DPM
Director of Residency Training
The Foot and Ankle Residency Program at West Penn Hospital
Allegheny Health Network, Pittsburgh
Pennsylvania
United States

Aman Chopra, BA
Research Fellow
Department of Orthopaedic Surgery
Duke University, Durham
North Carolina
United States

Coleman Oliver Clougherty, DPM, MA
Orthopaedic & Rheumatology Institute
Cleveland Clinic, Cleveland
Ohio
United States

James M. Cottom, DPM, FACFAS
Fellowship Director
Orthopaedics
Florida Orthopaedic Foot & Ankle Center, Sarasota
Florida
United States

Gerard J. Cush Jr., MD
Director
Foot and Ankle Surgery
Evangelical Community Hospital, Lewisburg
Pennsylvania
United States

J. Kent Ellington, MD, MS, FAAOS
Orthopaedic Surgeon
Foot and Ankle
OrthoCarolina Foot & Ankle Institute, Charlotte
North Carolina
United States

Ken Gall, PhD
Professor
Mechanical Engineering and Materials Science
Duke University, Durham
North Carolina
United States

Amar R. Gulati, DPM
Attending Physician
Progressive Feet
Carlin Springs Road, Arlington
Virginia
United States

Peter D. Highlander, DPM, MS
Director
Foot & Ankle Surgery
The Reconstruction Institute
The Bellevue Hospital, Bellevue
Ohio
United States

Lee M. Hlad, DPM, FACFAS
Fellowship Director
Deformity Correction & Advanced Surgical Skills
    Fellowship;
Medical Director
Institute for Corrective Surgery;
Partner
Ankle & Foot Associates, Waycross
Georgia
United States

Lance Johnson, DPM
Foot & Ankle Surgeon
Blanchard Valley Orthopaedics and Sports Medicine
Blanchard Valley Health System, Findlay
Ohio
United States

Cambre Kelly, PhD
Vice President of Research
Department of Research
restor3d, Durham
North Carolina
United States

Alina Kirillova, PhD
Assistant Professor
Department of Materials Science & Engineering
Iowa State University, Ames
Iowa
United States

Paul R. Leatham, DPM, MA
Podiatry
Christus Trinity Clinic
Christus Mother Frances Hospital, Tyler
Texas
United States

Ryan J. Lerch, DPM
Surgical Fellow
The Reconstruction Institute
The Bellevue Hospital, Bellevue
Ohio
United States

Naji S. Madi, MD
Foot and Ankle Surgery Fellow
Department of Orthopaedic Surgery
Duke University, Durham
North Carolina
United States

Jeffrey E. McAlister, DPM
Founder
Foot and Ankle
Phoenix Foot and Ankle Institute, Scottsdale
Arizona
United States

Sarah Messina, DPM
Detroit Medical Center, Detroit
Michigan
United States

Jason Nowak, DPM, FACFAS
Physician
Foot & Ankle Surgery
Shasta Orthopaedics & Sports Medicine, Redding;
Fellowship Director
Northern California Reconstructive Foot & Ankle
    Fellowship;
Shasta Orthopaedics & Sports Medicine, Redding;
Founder
Shasta Ortho Foot & Ankle Institute
Shasta Orthopaedics & Sports Medicine, Redding
California
United States

Selene G. Parekh, MD, MBA
Professor of Orthopaedic Surgery
Orthopaedic Surgery
Duke University, Durham
North Carolina
United States

Sham J. Persaud, DPM, MS
Attending Physician WPFAS
Advanced Orthopaedics and Rehabilitation, Washington
Pennsylvania
United States

Mark Razzante, DPM
Assistant Professor
California School of Podiatric Medicine at Samuel Merritt
    University
California
United States

Charles A. Sisovsky, DPM, AACFAS
Foot and Ankle Surgery
Orthopaedic Associates, Evansville
Indiana
United States

Eric So, DPM
Foot and Ankle Surgery
Bryan Health, Lincoln
Nebraska
United States

Garret Strand, DPM, AACFAS
Foot and Ankle Surgery
Shasta Foot and Ankle Institute, Redding
California
United States

Daniel J. Torino, MD
Chief Resident
Orthopaedic Surgery
Geisinger, Danville
Pennsylvania
United States

David Vier, MD
Orthopaedic Surgery
Baylor University Medical Center at Dallas, Dallas
Texas
United States

Benjamin R. Wagner, MD
Orthopaedic Foot and Ankle Surgery
Geisinger Medical Center, Danville
Pennsylvania
United States

Benjamin Wesorick, BS
Senior Design Engineer
restor3d, Durham
North Carolina
United States

Joseph R. Wolf, DPM, AACFAS
Foot and Ankle Surgeon
Florida Orthopaedic Foot and Ankle Center, Sarasota
Florida
United States

Hui Zhang, MD
Orthopaedic Surgery
Foot and Ankle Surgery
Aurora Health Care, Milwaukee
Wisconsin
United States

Foreword

I have been in foot and ankle education for over two decades—writing, teaching, and lecturing—and I have had the opportunity to instruct and guide dozens of students and residents over the years. As anyone in my position would tell you, watching someone you have mentored grow the seeds of their education is one of the greatest gifts. I have had that satisfaction with many of my residents, which has given me a profound sense of pride and fulfillment. But any educator would also be lying if they said they did not learn just as much from their students. Being surrounded by active minds and youthful energy helps promote discussion and advances in our understanding.

I have known Pete Highlander for a decade and had the honor of signing his surgical residency training certificate as his residency director during his time at the University of Pittsburgh. I initially met Pete as a medical student and noticed his passion for knowledge. He was excited about his future and had a desire for a residency that would expose him to impassioned leaders and front-line treatments. We were lucky enough to have Pete join us in Pittsburgh for his surgical training where his talents found a home and an environment to grow. Pete was an exceptional resident, showing his work ethic and enthusiasm for his profession, and becoming a role model in his senior year for the underclasses. During our teaching sessions, Pete engaged his co-residents, students, and faculty with meaningful questions, and you could sense that he had a healthy curiosity about the next step. I watched Pete put in the time and effort, showing a strong and capable individual destined to continue his journey after graduation.

Since leaving Pittsburgh to start his practice and career, I have stayed in close contact with Pete. While lecturing at a conference together several years ago, I again saw an excitement in his eye, his new passion involving patient-specific custom implants. He has been a pioneer, being one of the first to bring these ideas to the mainstream of foot and ankle surgery. Pete put his mind to learning the science and making inroads with industry, making this innovative technology more established and available. His passion and now years of experience have provided alternatives for those of us dealing with complicated foot and ankle pathology. I have learned from Pete Highlander, and this "first-of-its-kind" textbook is a prime example of his passion, hard work, knowledge, and skill. As someone involved in Pete's education and professional journey, I could not be prouder.

The text begins with three chapters of the science and background that all foot and ankle surgeons should become familiar with 3D-printed technology. The chapters that follow are step-by-step techniques and examples from well-experienced surgeons. These chapters cover many topics including the use of 3D-printed implants for difficult revisions such as first metatarsal phalangeal joint and ankle replacement failure, as well as management of talar pathology, solutions for revision fusions of the foot and ankle, and wedge-printed technology to address angular deformities. These chapters reveal design rationales from well-known surgeons who are helping lead the way with this technology, as well as their expert opinion and tips to help the reader in their decision-making process when confronted with a similar pathology.

Foot and ankle treatments and surgical procedures have grown significantly over the past few decades. The hardware available and the procedures offered have allowed all of us treating complicated pathology to expand our indications and offerings. This textbook adds to our understanding and knowledge of advanced foot and ankle surgery, and will be the building block for future 3D-printed patient-specific technology.

Pete Highlander has been at the forefront of this emerging foot and ankle surgery technology. His passion has spread through his lectures and discussions with colleagues and now with this text. I had the honor of being part of Pete's education, but I have also learned from him and appreciate the guidance he has given me over the years. Let us all continue to learn from each other.

Patrick R. Burns, DPM
Assistant Professor of Orthopaedic Surgery
University of Pittsburgh School of Medicine

Preface

The human foot is a masterpiece of engineering and a work of art.

LEONARDO DA VINCI

My first experience using 3D printing technology involved a young, active patient with advanced avascular necrosis following a talar neck fracture years prior to seeing me. The patient declined several previous opinions for fusion or amputation. Essentially, this motivated patient was looking for any other option. I presented the possibility of a total talus replacement, although I admittedly had no experience performing the procedure. After weeks of consideration and reading, the patient and I were confident this was the best path forward. As I immersed myself preparing for the surgery, I became increasingly inspired to learn more about the science and engineering involved with 3D printing technology and its utility in medicine. Nonetheless, the ankle was reconstructed, pain was reduced, and much of the lost function was restored. In the years to follow, I utilized 3D printing technology to reconstruct a myriad of foot and ankle conditions and I have witnessed the overwhelming impact it has had on so many people's lives.

For its use in medicine and surgery, 3D printing has been described as a disruptive technology, which may be valid in several ways. Personally, 3D printing has been "disruptive" to how I approach and manage the most challenging and complicated foot and ankle pathologies. Over the last several years, I realized many other surgeons were having similar observations and attitudes toward the technology. 3D printing technology may represent a paradigm shift in foot and ankle surgery because of the ability customize implants and instrumentation, thus permitting patient-specific surgery. 3D printing technology also provides an opportunity for academic cross-pollination, especially between physicians and engineers. Working with numerous engineers has been one of the most rewarding collaborations I have had professionally. Optimistically, I believe that interdisciplinary collaborations will expedite the development of practical and revolutionary medical innovations.

The goals of creating this text were multifactorial. First, to enhance awareness and understanding of 3D printing technology I intended to unite like-minded physician-scientists, surgeons, and engineers dedicated to reconstructive foot and ankle surgery. Further, I desired to gather expert opinions regarding patient selection, implant design considerations, and technical pearls and pitfalls from thoughtful and innovated surgeons. Ultimately, I hope this text will provide a rich and robust knowledge base for engineers and surgeons with an interest in 3D printing technology. I hope all readers gain a better understanding of the power of 3D technology to enhance our patients' lives.

While writing and editing this text I realized several truths. This project is not close to completion or comprehensive, therefore I hope subsequent editions, dedicated courses, platforms, and conferences are to follow. I am optimistic that this textbook is a step closer to a better understanding of 3D printing technology and its uses in foot and ankle surgery. Presently, 3D printing in foot and ankle surgery can be utilized efficaciously for surgical planning, creation of patient (or surgeon)-specific guides and instrumentation, as well as customized implants for osseous pathologies; however, applications in soft tissue repair have yet to be realized. In other words, we have yet to realize the full capacity and power the technology likely possesses. Nevertheless, it is my honor and privilege to present the first textbook dedicated to 3D printing technology in foot and ankle surgery.

Peter D. Highlander

Acknowledgments

A daunting task such as this textbook would not have been possible without many great people around me. I would like to acknowledge the extraordinary debt I owe to all of the authors for their affable contributions. In fact, I am confident I learned far more compiling and editing their work than I ever expected. During the bulk of time spent preparing this textbook, I was also mentoring Lance Johnson, DPM and Paul Leatham, DPM as part of their fellowship training. I am particularly appreciative of their contributions to the textbook and for thought-provoking discussions we shared regarding 3D printing. Their diligence, thoughtfulness, and willingness to help others was impactful and contagious to our entire staff.

The mentorship I have received enhanced my trajectory professionally and without it I would not have had the ability nor the opportunity to work on projects like this textbook. I would like to acknowledge in particular, Christopher VanOrman, PhD who as my undergraduate research advisor taught me the fundamentals of scientific writing and observation. As a graduate student, Graham Shaw, PhD provided me with several invaluable opportunities, such as editing his biochemistry textbook and publishing peer-reviewed research. I must also acknowledge my most influential mentor, Patrick R. Burns, DPM, who continues to encourage my growth as a surgeon and educator far beyond my formal surgical training.

To the administration and staff at The Bellevue Hospital and The Reconstruction Institute, I am truly blessed to have a team as dedicated and passionate as they are in providing the highest quality of care for our patients. Their trust permitted me to become an early adopter of 3D printing and their continued support has allowed me to gain experience and perspective.

I would not be who I am without my parents, Rhonda and Charlie Weyer, who taught me that hard work and perseverance coupled with faith is the framework to recognizing and fulfilling my life's purpose. Finally, my children, Henry, Samuel, Ann, and Grace, who recognized the importance of this project and patiently tolerated my absence.

Peter D. Highlander

Contents

Engineering and Historical Perspectives

1

Historical Perspectives on 3D Printing

BIJAN MASOOD ABAR, CAMBRE KELLY, NICHOLAS B. ALLEN, KEN GALL

Introduction

3D printing has changed the landscape of medical devices by accelerating innovation and expanding what is possible to make. Ideas that used to be too expensive or not possible can now be easily 3D printed. Today 3D printing is used for several applications, ranging from toys to complex surgical implants. While 3D printing has been applied to many disciplines, this chapter will focus on concepts relevant to orthopedic surgery. This chapter will provide a framework for understanding 3D printing concepts that can be used to take a deep dive and apply principles in more specific topics in subsequent chapters. The chapter will start by introducing the advantages of 3D printing and outlining the historical development of 3D printing, before introducing the various methods of 3D printing and explaining how 3D printing technology is regulated by the US Food and Drug Administration (FDA).

Advantages of Additive Manufacturing

Additive manufacturing (AM) is an overarching term to describe a process of selectively joining material to create a 3D object. In contrast, traditional manufacturing methods, such as subtractive manufacturing, involve selectively removing parts of the starting material to create the final object. AM is commonly referred to as "3D printing," and the two terms are often used interchangeably. Despite AM technology being relatively new, it has revolutionized manufacturing since its inception in the 1980s. The rapid adoption of AM is due to the many advantages AM has over traditional manufacturing, which are important to keep in mind when deciding if AM is the correct approach for a specific application.[1]

Economically Produce Custom Items

The production of custom items without AM techniques is time and cost prohibitive. Creating custom metal parts is a prime example. Technical expertise is needed to accurately machine metal parts to the desired specifications. With AM, a new 3D model can be created using computer-aided design (CAD) and fabricated with a 3D printer. Most manufacturing methods follow the economy of scale, where the unit cost decreases as the total number of units increases. However, with 3D printing the cost per unit does not change significantly between 1 and 100 units. The ability to practically produce custom parts has been leveraged in orthopedic device development to use a patient's imaging to create a device that matches to the patient's unique anatomy.

Rapid Prototyping

The ability to easily create custom objects has accelerated innovation. Before the advent of AM, prototyping was expensive, and it took a long time to create the prototype. This bottleneck would limit the number of prototypes designers would choose to create. Using AM, developers can now quickly and cheaply iterate through several designs. They can quickly test what works well and what does not, therefore increasing the speed to market and quality of devices.

Complex Structures

AM allows for the fabrication of structures that are either not practical or not possible using traditional manufacturing methods. For example, curved structures that are expensive to create by machining are just as easy to create as straight structures when using AM. AM also allows engineers to precisely introduce and control internal structures like porosity. In comparison, conventional methods to create porous structures, such as salt leaching, do not allow precise control of the size and distribution of the pores. The ability to create porous structures has been used to create implantable devices where the surrounding tissue, such as bone, can grow into the device and effectively integrate the device into the body.

Less Wasted Material

AM processes generally use fewer materials than subtractive manufacturing methods. Subtractive manufacturing methods involve starting with a block of material larger than the final part and removing the excess material. The excess materials can either be expensive to reuse (e.g., metal scraps in machining), or not possible to reuse (e.g., wood shavings in carpentry). In contrast, some AM methods only deposit material that is used for the final part, while other AM methods allow for excess material to be reused. The reduction in wasted materials can reduce the cost and environmental impact of AM parts.

Historical Perspective of 3D Printing

The development of 3D printing has rapidly expanded since the 1980s. Early versions of 3D printers were limited to specific materials and prohibitively expensive. Today's 3D printers are used by everyone from hobbyists making toys to medical manufacturers creating implants. The following section will outline key milestones in 3D printing. A historical perspective on 3D printing will highlight the pace and scope of past innovation and establish the trajectory for the future.

Foundation of 3D Printing Techniques

The underlying process for the first 3D printer was proposed in 1977 when Swainson and Kramer outlined a process to create 3D structures by using light to selectively polymerize photoactive resin. This process would later become known as stereolithography (SLA). Three years later, Hideo Kodama filed a provisional patent for a light-based 3D printing process, but he did not file the full application in time to be granted a full patent. Hideo Kodama's contributions to the development of 3D printing were documented in 1981 when he published the first article demonstrating 3D printing entitled "Automatic Method for Fabricating a Three-Dimensional Plastic Model With Photo-Hardening Polymer"[2] (Fig. 1.1).

The first full patent for an SLA printer was issued to Chuck Hall in 1986. In his patent application, he described the printer as:

A system for generating three-dimensional objects by creating a cross-sectional pattern of the object to be formed at a

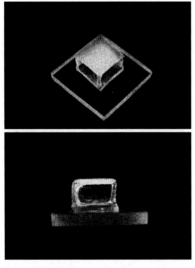

• **Fig. 1.1** The first published 3D-printed object, as shown in Hideo Kodama's 1981 manuscript "Automatic method for fabricating a three-dimensional plastic model with photo-hardening polymer." (Reproduced from Hideo Kodama, Automatic method for fabricating a three-dimensional plastic model with photo-hardening polymer, Review of Scientific Instruments 52, 1770 (1981), https://aip.scitation.org/doi/10.1063/1.1136492 with the permission of AIP Publishing.)

selected surface of a fluid medium capable of altering its physical state in response to appropriate synergistic stimulation by impinging radiation, particle bombardment or chemical reaction, successive adjacent laminae, representing corresponding successive adjacent cross-sections of the object, being automatically formed and integrated together to provide a step-wise laminar buildup of the desired object, whereby a three-dimensional object is formed and drawn from a substantially planar surface of the fluid medium during the forming process.[3]

In other words, Chuck Hall described a method whereby a liquid starting material is turned into a 3D object by selectively exposing the liquid to radiation or a specific reactant to solidify a 2D plane, one layer at a time. He went on to cofound 3D Systems, which brought the first commercial SLA printer to market in 1988. 3D Systems continues to be an important contributor in the 3D printing space to date. For his work on SLA, the STL (STereoLithograph) format commonly used for 3D files, and 3D Systems, Chuck Hall is considered by many to be the father of 3D printing.

The development of SLA printing inspired the invention of other 3D printing methods that are commonplace today. Carl Deckard at the University of Texas applied for the first patent describing selective laser sintering (SLS) in 1986 and was granted the full patent in 1989. The patent described SLS as:

An apparatus for selectively sintering a layer of powder to produce a part made from a plurality of sintered layers.[4]

In SLS, powder particles are selectively fused together to form the final 3D object, and SLS was the first example of powder bed fusion (PBF). That same year, Scott Crump applied for a patent for an:

apparatus incorporating a movable dispensing head provided with a supply of material which solidifies at a predetermined temperature, and a base member, which are moved relative to each other along "X," "Y," and "Z" axes in a predetermined pattern to create three-dimensional objects by building up material discharged from the dispensing head onto the base member at a controlled rate.[5]

He described a method where a material is melted and extruded out of a nozzle that can move in the three spatial directions (x, y, and z), where it solidifies into a 3D object. The process described by the patent is the foundation for fused deposition modeling (FDM), the form of 3D printing most familiar to people today. Scott Crump went on to cofound Stratasys, which remains a key player in the 3D printing market today. Also occurring in 1989, Emanual Sachs at MIT submitted a patent for:

A process for making a component by depositing a first layer of a fluent porous material, such as a powder, in a confined region and then depositing a binder material to selected regions of the layer of powder material to produce a layer of bonded powder material at the selected regions.[6]

In the new printing process, a binder solution is selectively deposited onto a powder bed to produce a 3D object. Sachs' publication of the new printing method marked the beginning of the term "3D printing" being used to describe AM and was the foundation for binder jet printing. Z Corporation commercialized binder printing in 1993 and was later acquired by 3D Systems in 2012. Shortly after binder printing was commercialized, a new kind of printing was induced when Heisley Cooperation received a patent in 1999 for a new method of 3D printing invented by Michael Feygin for:

A laminated object manufacturing (LOM) system for forming a plurality of laminations into a stack to create a three-dimensional object.[7]

By stacking and laminating cut-out sheets of materials, a 3D object can be formed relatively quickly.

The early pioneers of 3D printing described here the laid the foundation for the field. Thanks to their work, 3D printing was poised to rapidly evolve to meet the needs of diverse fields. The choice of materials, scale, speed, precision, and cost of 3D printing quickly improved throughout the 21st century and allowed for the applications of 3D printing to quickly expand beyond research labs.

3D Printing in Medicine

The newfound ability to fabricate patient-specific parts rapidly and cheaply led to 3D printing quickly establishing its foothold in medicine. Scientists have continued to apply 3D printing techniques to develop educational models, surgical guides, prosthetics, implants, and artificial organs. Early adoption of medical 3D printing was led by dentistry, orthopedic surgery, and urology. As early as 1994, 3D printing was reported to be used to plan reconstructive craniofacial surgery.[8,9]

3D-Printed Implants

The ability to 3D print high-strength biocompatible materials opened the door to printed weight-bearing structures. An early example occurred in 2008 with the first 3D-printed leg prosthetics. Shortly afterward, the world saw the first reported upper extremity prosthetic: in 2015, a carpenter lost his fingers in an accident and his treatment spurred a global collaboration led by Ivan Owen, a mechanical special effects artist.[10]

The 2010s saw a wave of FDA-cleared orthopedic implants (Fig. 1.2). In contrast to prosthetics, implantable devices require more rigorous evaluation and control processes to be utilized. In 2010 Exactech received FDA clearance for the first 3D-printed orthopedic implant. The Novation Crown Cup with InteGrip is an acetabular cup with a porous surface created with AM techniques[11] (Fig. 1.3). The vast majority of the approved printed devices

(79%) from 2000 to 2016 were made of metal.[12] The first polymer implant was not approved until 2013 when Oxford Performance Material developed OsteoFab Patient-Specific Facial Device (OPSFD), a patient-specific cranial implant printed using poly-ether-ketone-ketone (PEKK)[13] (Fig. 1.4). Oxford Performance Material expanded on their printing technology to develop the SpineFab Vertebral Body Replacement (VBR) System, the first polymeric spinal implant approved by the FDA in 2015[14] (Fig. 1.5).

Bioprinting

Bioprinting is holistically defined as fabrication using "computer-aided transfer processes for patterning and assembling living and nonliving materials with a prescribed 2D or 3D organization in order to produce bioengineered structures serving in regenerative medicine, pharmacokinetic, and basic cell biology studies."[15,16] Bioprinting technologies are commonly grouped into three distinctive categories relative to their fabrication methods and similar modalities. These groups include extrusion-based bioprinting, droplet-based bioprinting, and energy-based bioprinting (Fig. 1.6). Early iterations of 3D printers were limited in material selection, resolution, and speed. As the technology evolved, scientists inched closer to being able to print fully functional tissues or organs. A critical breakthrough came in 2000 when Thomas Boland, a bioengineer at the University of Texas, introduced the field of bioprinting.[17] He modified an HP inkjet printer to lay down a bioink composed of living cells suspended in culture media. Since then, tissue engineers have worked on improving bioprinting techniques to fabricate bone or cartilage constructs. By printing large segments of tissues with a patient's own cells, providers can treat large defects without the drawbacks of autografts or allografts, including limited supply, donor site morbidity, need for intraoperative modifications, risk of immune rejection, and long-term mechanical failure.[18] Bioprinted bone and cartilage constructs have been successful in cell and animals studies, but they are not commercially available to date.[19] Limitations for the clinical application of bioprinting include small size of bioprinted constructs, limited number and diversity of cells in the construct, lack of robust vascular networks to support cell growth, relatively poor mechanical properties that are insufficient to withstand physiological loads, and a lack of clear regulatory guidance from the FDA specific to bioprinting.[20,21]

Introduction to 3D Printing Technologies

Since the early establishment of SLA 3D printing, many AM methods have been developed (Fig. 1.7). Each method has its pros and cons when it comes to material selection, resolution, speed, cost, mechanical properties, and the technical skills needed to operate the machine. The various methods are characterized into seven general groups according to the ASTM F2792 standard.[1] Each method has its own advantages and disadvantages, which are important to understand to determine appropriate methods for specific

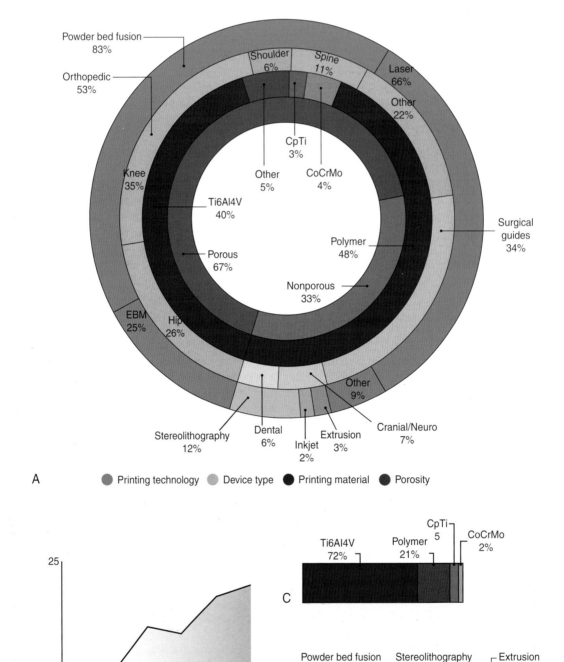

• **Fig. 1.2** An overview of additive manufacturing (AM) devices cleared by the Food and Drug Administration through the 510(k) pathway from January 2000 to April 2016. (A) Concentric pic charts breaking down the method of printing, clinical application, printed material, and porosity of 3D-printed devices. (B) The number of cleared AM devices each year from 2010 to 2015. (C) The materials used to print porous printed devices. (D) The printing method used to create porous printed devices. *EBM*, Electron beam melting. (Source: Ricles LM, Coburn JC, Di Prima M, Oh SS. Regulating 3D-printed medical products. *Sci Translat Med.* 2018;10(461):eaan6521. doi: 10.1126/scitranslmed.aan6521. Reprinted with permission from AAAS.)

applications[22] (Table 1.1). The following section will outline and provide a brief introduction to the seven groups.

Vat Photopolymerization

Vat photopolymerization (VP) is the oldest form of 3D printing, first introduced by Hideo Kodama and Charles Hall. In VP, a basin of liquid photopolymer resin is selectively exposed to a light energy source to polymerize the resin into a solid 2D layer. The build tray is then moved in the z direction. The steps are repeated in a layer-wise pattern until the part is complete (Fig. 1.8). The energy source can be placed above or below the vat of photopolymer to

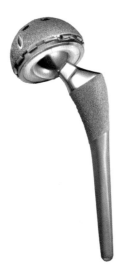

• **Fig. 1.3** The Novation Crown Cup with InteGrip by Exactech was the first orthopedic implant to be approved by the Food and Drug Administration. (Source: https://www.exac.com/hip/novation-crown-cup/.)

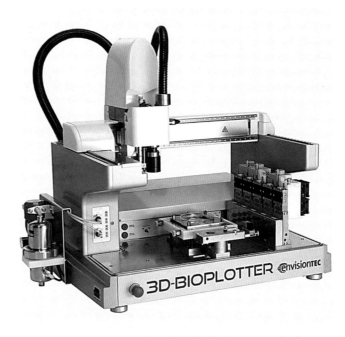

• **Fig. 1.6** The 3D-Bioplotter from EnvisionTec is an example of a commercial extrusion-based bioprinter available today. (Source: https://envisiontec.com/3d-printers/3d-bioplotter/manufacturer-series/.)

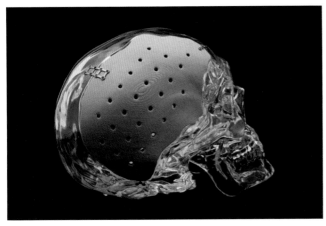

• **Fig. 1.4** In 2013, OsteoFab, a Patient-Specific Cranial Device, was the first 3D-printed polymer implant cleared by the Food and Drug Administration. This device replaces bony voids in the skull. (Source: https://oxfordpm.com/osteofab-medical-devices.)

construct the printed part from the top-down or bottom-up, respectively. VP allows users to print parts with a fine resolution and smooth surface finish. However, material selection is limited to resins that can undergo photopolymerization. Within VP, there are subgroups of printing techniques based on the specific photopolymerization method. SLA utilizes a focused laser to polymerize the resin point by point. Digital light processing (DLP) uses a digital projector to expose the resin to the entire 2D projection of the printed layer at the same time, thereby increasing the print speed. The first DLP printers used UV projectors. More recently, LED projectors have been implemented to bring down the cost of the printers. Continuous liquid interface production (CLIP) has emerged as the fastest method of VP. While most VP methods require the part to be removed from resin in-between each layer to reform the resin-part interface, CLIP uses an oxygen-permeable membrane at the base of the resin reservoir to create a persistent liquid reservoir interface where the part can be continuously printed.

Powder Bed Fusion

In PBF, a uniform layer of powder is rolled onto the print bed. An energy source is used to fuse the powder into a 2D projection of the printed part. A new layer of powder is then rolled over the part in progress and the existing powder and the process is repeated in a layer-by-layer fashion. In the end, the final printed part is encased in a bed of unfused powder that can be reused for future prints (Fig. 1.9). Unlike other printing methods, support structures do not need to be printed as the unfused powder provides support during the printing process. PBF is commonly used to print metal parts with excellent mechanical properties, such as titanium and

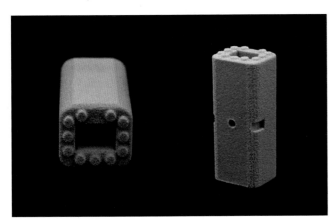

• **Fig. 1.5** SpineFab is the first polymeric 3D-printed spinal device used to replace damaged vertebral bodies in the thoracolumbar spine. (Source: https://oxfordpm.com/osteofab-medical-devices.)

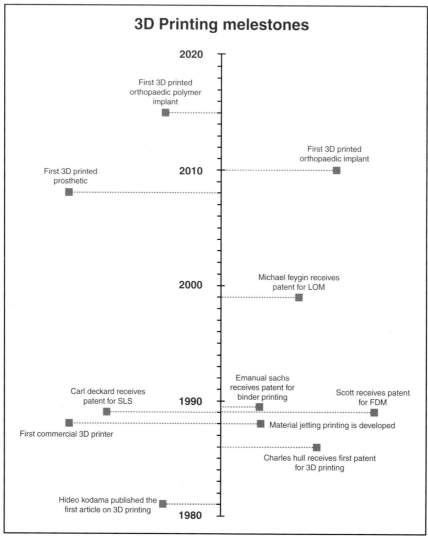

• **Fig. 1.7** A timeline of the significant milestones in 3D-printed orthopedic devices. *FDM*, Fused deposition modeling; *LOM*, laminated object manufacturing; *SLS*, selective laser sintering.

TABLE 1.1 **A Comparison of the Seven General Categories of 3D-Printing Methods**

Methods of 3D Printing	Principle	Subgroups	Common Materials	Advantages	Limitations
Vat photopoly-merization	A basin of a liquid photopolymer is selectively exposed to light to solidify an object layer by layer	SLA DLP CLIP	Photopolymers (e.g., methacrylates)	• Fine resolution • Smooth surface finish	• Limited material selection • Poor mechanical properties • Requires curing step
Powder bed fusion	For each layer, a uniform layer of powder is added to the print bed. An energy source is used to selectively fuse powder to form a solid object	SLS SLM EBM DMLS	Metals (e.g., Ti, CoCr) Polymers (e.g., nylon)	• Can produce high-strength parts • Powder provides support for overhanging structures • Fine resolution	• Slow print speeds • Poor surface finish • Relatively expensive • Technical expertise needed to operate
Extrusion	The starting filament is heated and extruded through a nozzle that moves in the x, y, or z direction	FDM/FFF	Thermoplastic polymers (e.g., PLA, ABS, PCL, PCU)	• Easy to use • Cheap • Can print with multiple material and colors	• Relatively poor accuracy • Support material attached to object • Slow print speed • Relatively thick layers

TABLE 1.1	A Comparison of the Seven General categories of 3D-Printing Methods—cont'd				
Methods of 3D Printing	**Principle**	**Subgroups**	**Common Materials**	**Advantages**	**Limitations**
Binder jet	For each layer, a uniform layer of powder is added to the print bed and a liquid binder is selectively added to form a solid object		• Polymers • Stainless steel • Glass • Sand	• Fast print speed • Prints at low temperatures • Large print volumes • Can recycle unused powder	• Need to clean printed part • Poor mechanical properties
Sheet lamination	A thin sheet of material is cut into a specified shape and fused to adjacent layers	LOM UC	• Paper sheets • Plastic sheets • Metal sheets	• Fast print speed • Low cost • Large print volumes	• Limited material • Layer height is fixed • Waste unused materials
Material jetting	Analogous to a 2D inkjet printer, material is jetted onto a build plate in a layer-wise fashion	Polyjetting	Photopolymers Wax	• High resolution • Print with multiple materials	• Only print polymer and wax
Direct energy deposition	An energy source directly fuses material coming out of a nozzle that can move in the x, y, or z direction	DMD LENS EBAM	Metals that can be welded (e.g., Ti, CoCr)	Fast print speed • Can produce high-strength parts • Large print volumes	• Expensive printer • Poor resolution • Poor surface finish • No removable support structures

ABS, Acrylonitrile butadiene styrene; *CLIP*, continuous liquid interface production; *CoCr*, cobalt chrome; *DLP*, digital light processing; *DMD*, direct metal deposition; *DMLS*, direct metal laser sintering; *EBAM*, electron beam additive manufacturing; *EBM*, electron beam melting; *FDM*, fused deposition modeling; *FFF*, fused filament fabrication; *LENS*, laser-engineered net shaping; *LOM*, laminated object manufacturing; *PCL*, polycaprolactone; *PCU*, polycarbonate urethane; *PLA*, polylactic acid; *SLA*, stereolithography; *SLM*, selective laser melting; *SLS*, selective laser sintering; *Ti*, titanium; *UC*, ultrasonic consolidation.

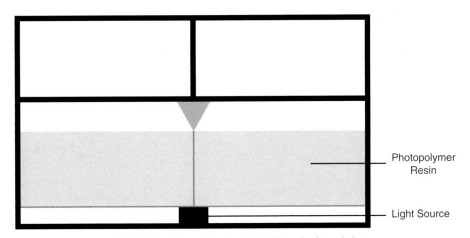

• **Fig. 1.8** A schematic of vat photopolymerization printing.

cobalt chrome alloys, allowing for the creation of high-strength structures used in orthopedic implants. Compared to other printing methods, PBF is slower. The fused powder particles result in a rough surface finish or unwanted porosity that often has to undergo postprocessing steps, such as polishing or hot isostatic pressing (HIP). The subtypes of PBF are determined by the method to fuse the powder particles. SLS uses a laser to sinter or fuse powder particles of metals or polymers, such as nylon. In contrast, selective laser melting (SLM) uses a laser to completely melt the powder. Electron beam melting (EBM) utilizes an electron beam, instead of laser, to completely melt the powder. PBF is the most common form of printing orthopedic devices, making up 86% of FDA-approved devices.[12]

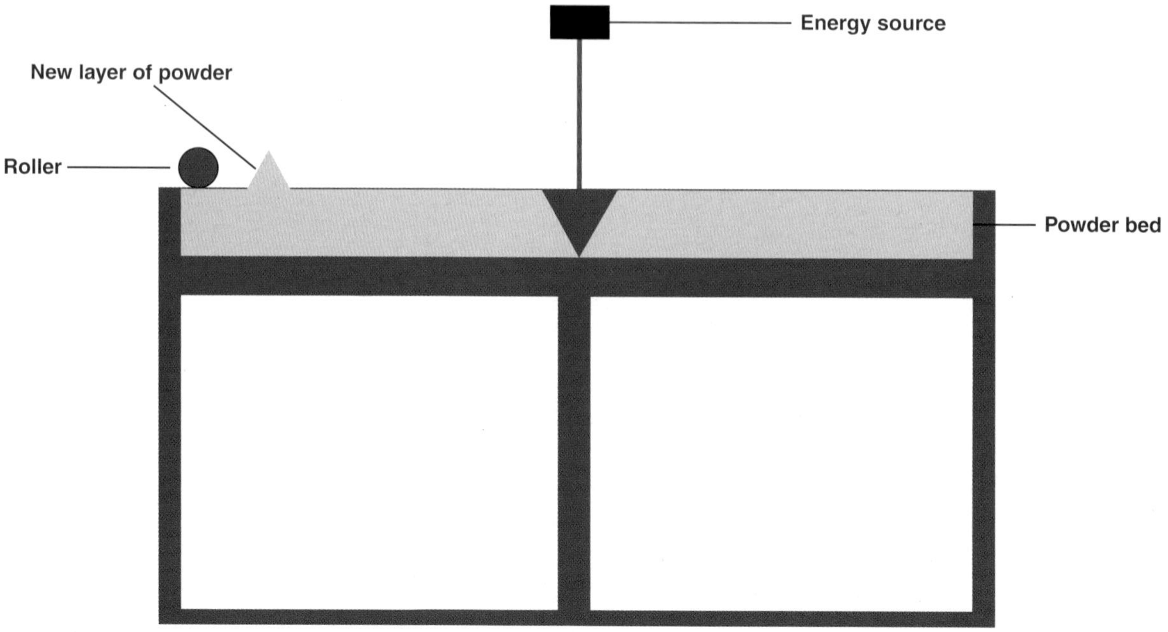

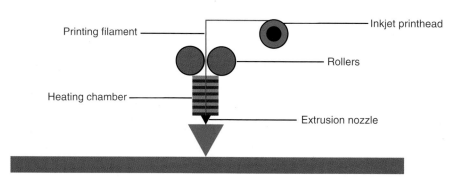

• **Fig. 1.9** A schematic of powder bed fusion printing.

• **Fig. 1.10** A schematic of extrusion printing.

Extrusion

Extrusion printing is what is most commonly envisioned as 3D printing. It is commonly referred to as FDM or fused filament fabrication (FFF). The print material is extruded or forced through a small nozzle that deposits the material to form a 2D projection of the final part. The nozzle or the bed is then positioned before the next layer is printed (Fig. 1.10). FDM is most commonly used to print thermoplastics, where a spool of thermoplastic filament is fed into the print head with rollers. The filament is heated into a liquid in the print head and extruded out of the nozzle, where it solidifies as it cools. FDM printers are generally the cheapest and easiest to use printers. However, comparatively, FDM has poor resolution, requires postprocessing to remove support material, and is not well suited to printing overhanging structures. Extrusion printing also includes common bioprinting methods where a bioink composed of cells and a support matrix is extruded onto a print bed using a syringe or pneumatic pump.

Binder Jet

Binder jet printing is very similar to PBF. A layer of powder made up of the desired material is uniformly placed on the print bed. Instead of using a laser or high-energy heat source, a binder solution is selectively deposited onto the powder layer. The binder forms a solid part once added to the powder. The process is repeated in a layer-by-layer fashion until the solid part is completed and encased in powder (Fig. 1.11). The solid part often requires a curing step in the powder before it can be removed. The unused powder is then removed and can be recycled. Binder jet printing is relatively fast and can be used to print large parts. Like PBF, the powder provides support while printing, so support structures are not needed. In contrast to PBF, a high-energy laser is not needed, so binder jet printing requires fewer safety precautions. However, the final parts generally have poor mechanical properties.

Sheet Lamination

Sheet lamination describes a method where a sheet of material is cut and layered to form a final part. The process begins with a material being rolled over the print bed. The material is cut into a 2D layer of the desired part with a laser or knife. The cut material is fused to the previous layers and the excess material is removed (Fig. 1.12). The two most common

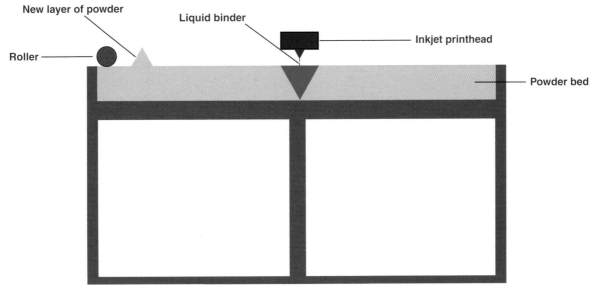

• **Fig. 1.11** A schematic of binder jet printing.

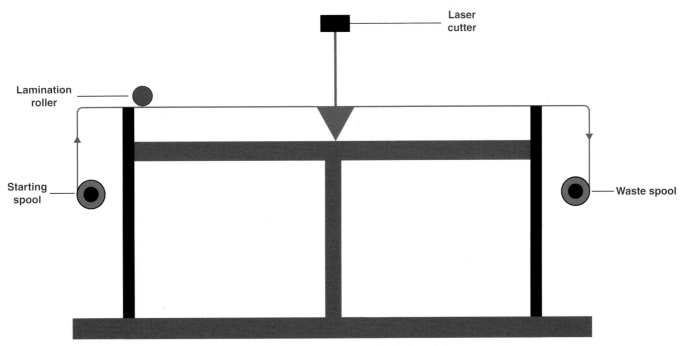

• **Fig. 1.12** A schematic of sheet lamination printing.

forms of sheet lamination are ultrasonic additive manufacturing (UAM) and laminated object manufacturing (LOM). These methods differ in the process used to fuse the layers together. UAM utilizes ultrasonic welding to fuse sheets of metal. On the other hand, LOM utilizes an adhesive to bond layers of paper. Sheet lamination is a relatively fast process and uses common materials, making it relatively inexpensive. However, the layer height of the object is determined by the thickness of the starting sheet and the process only can be applied to a limited selection of materials.

Material Jetting

Material jetting is a printing process most similar to a standard 2D inkjet printer. A print head jets various materials onto the print bed, followed by a light that solidifies the photopolymer material. The process is repeated layer by layer until the final part is complete (Fig. 1.13). Material jetting can print with very fine resolutions and allows multiple colors and materials to be printed at the same time. This type of printing is used extensively to print accurate anatomical models. The printed object does need to undergo a curing process like other methods. However, similar to FDM, support materials need to be printed as there is no powder bed.

Direct Energy Deposition

Direct energy deposition (DED) is a combination of PBF and extrusion printing. Metal powder or metal wire is fed through

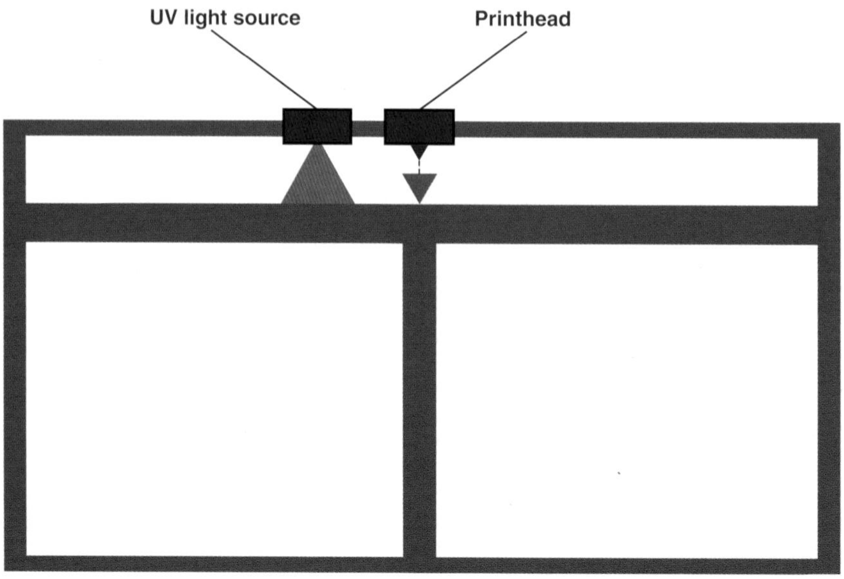

UV light source   Printhead

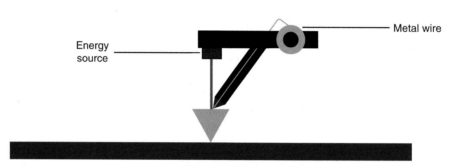

• **Fig. 1.13** A schematic of material jetting.

Energy source   Metal wire

• **Fig. 1.14** A schematic of direct energy deposition printing.

a nozzle and is immediately melted by a focused energy source. The nozzle and energy source move in x, y, and z directions relative to the print bed to deposit and fuse metal in a layer-by-layer fashion (Fig. 1.14). DED can also be referred to as direct metal deposition (DMD). The energy source can be a laser in laser-engineered net shaping (LENS), an electron beam in electron beam additive manufacturing (EBAM), or a plasma arc in wire arc additive manufacturing (WAAM). Compared with other forms of metal printing (e.g., PDF), DED has fast print speeds. DED can create large parts that can support large loads. The feed stock for DED can be easily changed to print with a new material. The direct welding of metals onto the parts makes DED a useful method for adding components to or repairing existing parts. Like all methods of AM, DED has some limitations. Compared with other methods, DED machines are relatively expensive. Objects printed by DED have relatively poor resolution and a poor surface finish. Unlike PBF, there is no easily removable support structure, making features such as overhangs difficult or impractical to print.

Regulation of Additive Manufacturing

All the AM processes described here provide the manufacturers with several inputs that can be used to finely tune

their product. However, this flexibility can be a double-edged sword. The increased number of design parameters means there are more places for errors to occur and more variables that must be optimized. Due to the high level of accuracy and precision required for medical implants, the FDA has published guidance for manufacturers to ensure patient safety. The following section first establishes the nuance between a patient-matched device (PMD) and a "custom" device. The second section will walk through a typical workflow to produce an AM device and highlight the steps the FDA recommends for specific consideration. As all devices require FDA approval, a comprehensive understanding of the regulatory landscape can aid in the product design and decrease the time it takes for a device to reach the market, in turn improving the lives of patients.

Patient-Matched Devices

AM methods allow engineers to economically produce small product quantities with complex geometries. This advantage has been extensively leveraged to manufacture PMDs. Various methods of medical imaging can be used to create a 3D model of the patient's anatomy and create a device specific to the individual patient and their anatomy. A common misconception is that PMDs are "custom" devices and therefore are exempt from certain FDA recruitments. In order to qualify as a custom device, the device must be created under the direction of a physician or dentist, and the potential to produce multiple units of the device types must not exceed five units per year.[23] The potential to produce multiple devices is defined by the number times the specific indication occurs where the proposed device or an alternative device can be used. If an alternative device is legally marketed and is domestically available for the same indication as a proposed device, the proposed device could not be classified as a custom device. The FDA provides several examples of custom devices, such as a surgeon ordering screws for a toddler requiring a C2 posterior cervical fusion after a car accident. Since there are no approved screws that are the correct size for this pediatric case, and the scenario is too infrequent to support a clinical trial, a custom screw can be manufactured under the custom device exemption. Commercial PMDs are designed for a special case but must fall within a defined design or performance envelope. The performance envelope describes the upper and lower limits for each dimension, the acceptable mechanical properties, and any other clinically relevant factors.

FDA Guidelines for Additive Manufactured Devices

Due to the rapid adoption of 3D printing technology, the overall market grew to $9.9 billion in 2018 and is expected to reach $34.8 billion in 2024.[9] The explosion of AM devices entering the market in the last decade has led the FDA to publish a report entitled "Technical Considerations for Additive Manufactured Medical Devices" to provide general guidance to industry partners.[23] The report emphasizes that AM devices will generally have the same expectations and regulations as their non-AM counterparts.

There are specific steps unique to the processing of an AM device that the FDA highlights as needing additional consideration. The production of AM devices involves multiple steps including imaging anatomic features, designing a 3D model, slicing the model with appropriate software, validating materials used for printing, printing the device, postprocessing of the device, and final testing of the print. Characterization of each step in the printing process should be documented and include a description of the process, identification of process parameters that demonstrate the tradeoff in optimizing one parameter at the cost of another, output specification, and how each parameter can affect future steps.

Acquiring Imaging Data

All printed PMDs depend on accurate imaging. Manufacturers need to take into account the minimum feature quality each of the imaging modalities can produce and any smoothing or image processing that is used. Furthermore, the anatomical features imaged before the PMD is produced can change over time with progression of the underlying pathophysiology. Therefore, the maximum amount of time that can pass from when the imaging was completed to the implantation of the device should be reflected in the expiration date of the device.

Designing the 3D Model

The 3D models for PMD are typically made by modifying standard device models to match the imaging of the patient's anatomy with various software. The FDA recommends that any software used to create the final 3D model undergoes internal checks to ensure that the final device falls within the prespecified performance envelope. Specialized software is also used to produce support materials. Certain methods of printing, such as extrusion or vat polymerization, require support structures to be printed in order to fabricate overhangs or internal voids. Too many support structures can result in excessive surface marks or extra residue left after removing the support. Too little support can result in the collapse of a printed structure, leading to a failed print. The device master record for an AM device should include a complete description of the support geometry and protocol for removing the support.

Slicing the 3D Model

Before a device can be printed, the 3D model needs to be sliced to create a 2D projection that can be fabricated in a layer-by-layer printing process. The choice of layer thickness affects the resolution of the printed device and print speed. However, layer thickness is constrained by the limitations of the specific printing method and starting material properties. The optimal layer thickness used for production should be documented and reflect a balance between quality, accuracy, and print speed that is possible for the specific AM method. The orientation of the slices can also have a significant effect on the quality of the device. The orientation of the printed layers introduces inherent anisotropy in the mechanical properties and, therefore, can affect the performance of the device.

Printing Materials

The form of the printing material used in AM is a significant factor in the quality of the printed device, whether it's powder, monomers, or filament. To ensure the quality and consistency of the printing materials, the FDA recommends that each component of the printing material, including any additive or crosslinkers, should be thoroughly documented and include the identity of the material, the material supplier, and the certificate of analysis. Furthermore, the properties of the materials can change throughout the printing process. For example, the melting and extrusion of the thermoplastic in FDM can change the material properties. These changes should be understood and documented by the manufacturer. Additionally, certain AM processes reuse unused printing materials in subsequent batches, which adds another layer of complexity. As an example, the FDA cites the ratio of virgin powder to reused powder in PBF. The ratio can change the energy needed to fuse the metal powder and in turn affect the final mechanical properties of the device. The FDA recommends that any material reuse process be documented and that manufacturers should provide justification that material reuse does not adversely affect the quality of the printed device.

Printing Process

There are many variables in the printing process that need to be considered when fabricating an AM device, including but not limited to energy input, location on the build plate, and build path. Energy input is specific for each printing method. For PBF or VP, laser energy is used to fuse the powder or polymerize the resin. The amount of energy determines the thickness of each layer and how well the layers adhere to each other. In extrusion printing, the energy used to heat up the nozzle determines how well the material can flow through the nozzle. The placement of printed objects within the print bed and the density of other parts on the printed bed can impact the quality of the final device. For example, placing parts too close to each other or placing a part at the edge of the plate have been shown to produce poor prints. Various placements within the build volume should be tested to determine the optimal placements of printed devices. The build path, which is the order energy or the material is released on the build plate, can affect the quality of the printed device. For example, if the laser in PBF sweeps from left to right in a pass and then right to left on a subsequent pass, one side of that layer has more time to cool. Therefore, the FDA recommends that manufacturers test if different build paths affect the final device. Each build path should be documented and the optimal path should be consistently utilized for each print.

Postprocessing

Many AM processes require some degree of postprocessing before the device can be used. Postprocessing steps can include removing support material, curing photopolymer in UV light, surface polishing, or exposing metal to HIP. These processes can impact the performance of the device and therefore must be documented, and the effects must be understood. Manufacturers should establish procedures to monitor and control each process. Some of the postprocessing procedures can have negative effects. The FDA uses HIP as an example. HIP is used to reduce porosity and improve fatigue properties of metal devices, but it can also reduce the modulus or yield strength of the material. Manufacturers should describe methods implemented to mitigate any adverse effects of postprocessing.

Testing and Validation

The fabrication of an AM device involves the optimal configuration of numerous variables at every step in the process. The tradeoffs made by each decision should be understood and documented. The device development process should include extensive testing to evaluate mechanical properties such as modulus, yield strength, ultimate strength, viscoelasticity, fatigue or wear resistance, dimensions and surface topography of the device, and material chemistry of the final device. The FDA recommends that manufacturers also test the worst-case combination of dimensions and features to better understand how input variables could impact the final performance. Even after all the input variables are optimized and appropriate control processes are in place, it is possible for errors to occur in device production that could lead to an adverse event. To mitigate any errors, the FDA recommends that manufacturers print test samples known as test coupons with every print batch. The test coupons should include a description explaining why it is representative of the final printed device. The test coupon can then be used for destructive testing that is capable of exposing errors in the manufacturing process that are not evident by visual inspection.

Conclusion

Since the inception of 3D printing in the 1970s, 3D printing has rapidly expanded into multiple fields and has become a household word. The early work of scientists such as Kodama, Hall, Deckard, and Sachs established the fundamental printing techniques. The early methods have since evolved into numerous specific methods with their own advantages and disadvantages, and the methods are generally classified into one of seven overarching groups. The quick adoption of 3D printing in orthopedic surgery is due to the ability of 3D printing to economically produce high-strength devices with patient-specific geometries and porous internal structures. Currently, 3D printing is used for educational models, surgical guides, prosthetics, and implants. The increased degrees of freedom come at a small cost. Manufacturers need to work with the FDA to justify the numerous design decisions that need to be made and place appropriate control and validation procedures to ensure the safety and efficacy of printed devices.

AM devices will become more common in orthopedic surgery as the technology becomes more refined and more accessible. The practice of placing trial devices with standard sizes may be replaced by printed devices engineered for patients' anatomy and biomechanical needs. Advances will be made to improve both the mechanical properties, including strength and fatigue behavior, as well as improve biological properties, including resistance to infections and consistent osseous integration. The overwhelming majority of printed implants are made from metal and are used to replace bone. As the ability to print soft materials improves, printed implants will be used to replace more soft tissues, including tendons, ligaments, and cartilage. While synthetic implants made from metal or polymers can quickly provide mechanical support and improve the quality of life for patients, the ultimate goal is to print natural structures using a patient's own cells that can integrate seamlessly with the surrounding tissues. The trajectory of advances in 3D printing suggests that there will continue to be breakthroughs in the years to come.

References

1. Designation: F2792—12a. Standard terminology for additive manufacturing technologies. ASTM International. doi:10.1520/F2792-12A. https://web.mit.edu/2.810/www/files/readings/AdditiveManufacturing-Terminology.pdf. Accessed June 16, 2022.

2. Kodama H. Automatic method for fabricating a three-dimensional plastic model with photo-hardening polymer. *Rev Sci Instrum.* 1981;52:1770.

3. *US4929402A*—Method for production of three-dimensional objects by stereolithography. Google Patents. https://patents.google.com/patent/US4929402A/en. Accessed January 27, 2021.

4. *US5597589A*—Apparatus for producing parts by selective sintering. Google Patents. https://patents.google.com/patent/US5597589A/en. Accessed January 27, 2021.

5. *US5121329A*—Apparatus and method for creating three-dimensional objects. Google Patents. https://patents.google.com/patent/US5121329A/en. Accessed January 27, 2021.

6. *US5204055A*—Three-dimensional printing techniques. Google Patents. https://patents.google.com/patent/US5204055A/en. Accessed February 4, 2021.

7. *US5730817A*—Laminated object manufacturing system. Google Patents. https://patents.google.com/patent/US5730817A/en. Accessed February 4, 2021.

8. Dittmann W, Bill J, Wittenberg G, Reuther J, Roosen K. Stereolithographie als neue methode in der rekonstruktiven operationsplanung bei komplexen knochernen defekten der schadelbasis. *Zentralbl Neurochir.* 1994;55:209-211.

9. Fan D, Li Y, Wang X, et al. Progressive 3D printing technology and its application in medical materials. *Front Pharmacol.* 2020;11:122.

10. Manero A, Smith P, Sparkman J, et al. Implementation of 3D printing technology in the field of prosthetics: past, present, and future. *Int J Environ Res Public Health.* 2019;16:1641.

11. FDA. 510(k) Premarket Notification. https://www.accessdata.fda.gov/scripts/cdrh/cfdocs/cfpmn/pmn.cfm?ID=K102975. Accessed January 3, 2021.

12. Ricles LM, Coburn JC, Di Prima M, Oh SS. Regulating 3D-printed medical products. *Sci Transl Med.* 2018;10:6521.

13. FDA. 510(k) Premarket Notification. https://www.accessdata.fda.gov/scripts/cdrh/cfdocs/cfpmn/pmn.cfm?ID=K121818. Accessed January 4, 2021.

14. FDA. 510(k) Premarket Notification. https://www.accessdata.fda.gov/scripts/cdrh/cfdocs/cfPMN/pmn.cfm?ID=K142005. Accessed January 4, 2021.

15. Groll J, Boland T, Blunk T, et al. Biofabrication: reappraising the definition of an evolving field. *Biofabrication.* 2016;8:013001.

16. Guillemot F, Mironov V, Nakamura M. Bioprinting is coming of age: report from the International Conference on Bioprinting and Biofabrication in Bordeaux (3B'09). *Biofabrication.* 2010;2:010201.

17. Patel P. The path to printed body parts. *ACS Cent Sci.* 2016;2:581-583.

18. De Long WG, Einhorn TA, Koval K, et al. Bone grafts and bone graft substitutes in orthopaedic trauma surgery. *J Bone Jt Surg.* 2007;89:649-658.

19. Matai I, Kaur G, Seyedsalehi A, McClinton A, Laurencin CT. Progress in 3D bioprinting technology for tissue/organ regenerative engineering. *Biomaterials.* 2020;226:119536.

20. Murphy SV, De Coppi P, Atala A. Opportunities and challenges of translational 3D bioprinting. *Nat Biomed Eng.* 2020;4:370-380.

21. Mason J, Visintini S, Quay T. *An Overview of Clinical Applications of 3-D Printing and Bioprinting. CADTH Issues in Emerging Health Technologies.* Ottawa ON: Canadian Agency for Drugs and Technologies in Health; 2016.

22. Aimar A, Palermo A, Innocenti B. The role of 3D printing in medical applications: a state of the art. *J Health Eng.* 2019;2019:5340616.

23. Custom Device Exemption—Guidance for Industry and Food and Drug Administration Staff CDRH. 2014. https://www.fda.gov/media/89897/download.

2

CT to Software and Other Considerations

BENJAMIN WESORICK, CAMBRE KELLY, KEN GALL

Introduction

To design implants that are personalized to the patient's anatomy and a specific surgical plan, engineers rely on medical imaging to create accurate anatomical reconstructions. CT image data is commonly required in orthopedic applications due to the volumetric dataset presented and clear contrast of bone, but MRI and X-ray data can also be used in unique cases. There are numerous commercially available software packages that use a similar process to convert a series of 2D medical images into 3D models. However, the focus of this chapter will be specifically on CT scanning (and its most common file format, DICOM), as it is commonly the ideal modality for most orthopedic applications.

Software Workflow

Segmentation

To better explain the relevant CT scan parameters, it is useful to understand the software steps used to convert medical imaging into a 3D model. Once imported into an image viewer, DICOMs are segmented to model each bone as a separate entity. Images are viewed slice by slice and the contours of each bone are isolated through a combination of manual and automated processes. Hounsfield units, which describe radiodensity, are converted into grayscale values that allow for simple image processing. Thresholds are applied to the entire image stack to filter only the Hounsfield units of interest. Metal, bone, and soft tissue can quickly be separated from one another provided that the contrast remains uniform throughout the image. Any pixel in the scan volume that falls within the selected threshold is included and added to a binary mask. When all the pixels in a given mask are viewed in 3D space, the rough shape of the segmented anatomy can be visualized (Fig. 2.1). Once thresholding is complete and bone has been isolated, it is still critical to separate the different regions of bony anatomy from one another. While some implants could be designed

without the manual segmentation of each individual bone, it is often essential to visualize anatomical corrections.

Separating anatomy with similar Hounsfield units (such as separating different bones) is typically the most complicated part of segmentation. When joint spacing is ideal, region-growing algorithms can be used to separate one bone from another. Region-growing algorithms separate regions with similar contrast by "growing" out from one pixel and moving to a surrounding pixel if there is any connectivity to another pixel in the mask.[1] Accordingly, if two bones are in adjacent pixels at any point of the joint, a region-growing algorithm will connect the two bones. When region growing is not possible, the contours of the bones are manually traced to separate bony regions. Depending on the quality of the CT scan, this tracing must be done on each individual slice (Fig. 2.2).

Converting 2D to 3D

Once each bone has a corresponding mask that contains all the pixels of anatomy, it is converted into a 3D model using the pixel size and slice thickness of the CT scan. It is important to note that because bone masks are binary, there is no way to count partial pixels. To create the 3D models, the pixels in each bone mask are converted into a 3D cloud which is then used to generate a uniform, connected surface mesh for manipulation within a 3D modeling software package. This happens in multiple steps. Due to the nature of contrast in CT scans, the raw 3D point cloud from the bone mask will not be uniform, meaning that it will typically have holes, extraneous shells, and an inconsistent surface that does not match the bone. To convert this point cloud into a usable model, pixels that are not connected to the main shell are removed and the anatomy is often "wrapped" with a mesh that closes all the gaps in the model (Fig. 2.3). The result is a uniform single surface that can be manipulated in a computer-aided design (CAD) software package. Surprisingly, the mesh surface that results from segmentation is surprisingly consistent, even between different software packages. When analyzing nine different commercially available segmentation

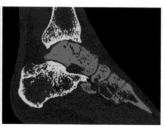
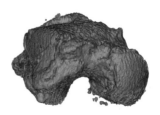

• **Fig. 2.1** Overall bone mask separating the bone from the surrounding tissues in a foot and ankle CT scan *(left)*. Representative segmentation showing the separation of bony anatomy *(middle)*. 3D visualization of pixels in one bone mask *(right)*. (Images courtesy of Restor3d, Inc, Durham, NC.)

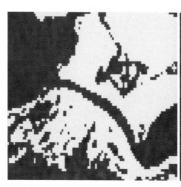
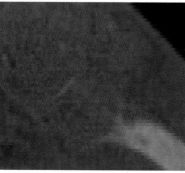

• **Fig. 2.2** Binary mask with clear joint spacing that allows for region-growing algorithms *(left)*. Slice showing different bones in adjacent pixels, requiring manual segmentation to separate bones *(right)*. (Images courtesy of Restor3d, Inc, Durham, NC.)

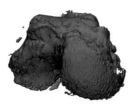
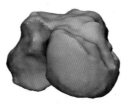
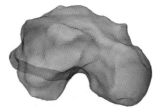

• **Fig. 2.3** Pixels for one bone mask visualized in 3D. Extraneous shells and gaps in the outer surface of the model can be easily visualized *(left)*. The result of wrapping (closing gaps under 3 mm) for the binary mask, converting the point cloud into a surface mesh *(middle)*. The same mesh shown with transparency to highlight the uniform surface with no internal lesions *(right)*. (Images courtesy of Restor3d, Inc, Durham, NC.)

software packages, the mean error in the triangle shape between the final meshes was 0.11 mm.[2]

It is essential to convert the anatomy into meshes for several reasons. First, in medical applications 3D printers use mesh or triangle-based file formats (e.g., STLs) as their input files.[3] To print anatomical models, all anatomy must be converted into meshes. Second, because patient-specific implants are designed directly from the surrounding anatomy, the models must be able to be manipulated freely in the design suite. In the case of a total talus, the starting point for design is the surface mesh of the contralateral talus. Once all relevant anatomy has been converted into a mesh that accurately represents the anatomy, implant design can begin (Fig. 2.4).

CT Scan Considerations

Because binary masks from segmentation are directly used in design, there are several important considerations for CT images that make them suitable for preoperative planning and implant design. Both the specific scan parameters and scanning instructions used make a difference in the final quality of the devices designed.

Scanning Parameters

Recommended CT scan parameters are provided by the implant manufacturer before 3D printing (Fig. 2.5). In general, all recommendations are designed to minimize the

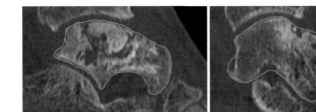
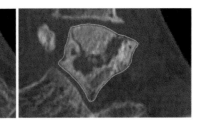

• **Fig. 2.4** Representative CT slices showing the outer contour of a surface mesh overlaid on the original CT scan. Despite removing extraneous shells and gap closing, the contours typically match the initial anatomy closely. (Images courtesy of Restor3d, Inc, Durham, NC.)

Pixel Spacing	≤ 0.5 mm
Slice Thickness	≤ 1.25 mm
kVp	120
MA	*Determined by scanner software*
File Type	*Uncompressed DICOM*

• **Fig. 2.5** Recommended scan parameters for implant design and 3D printing. (Image courtesy of Restor3d, Inc, Durham, NC.)

size of each voxel, the smallest 3D volume element in a CT scan.[4] In particular, it is ideal to minimize voxel size relative to the surrounding anatomy and maximize contrast per voxel.

Pixel Spacing and Slice Thickness

Pixel spacing and slice thickness both define the smallest 3D volume or voxel size in a CT scan.[5] Both parameters are defined in the scan protocol and can be readily extracted in the DICOM tags. Pixel spacing refers to the width of each pixel in the XY plane.[5] Because clinical CT scans are taken

axially, the pixel spacing always corresponds to the width of the pixels in the axial plane. Typically, this number does not need to be altered and is under 0.4 mm for most CT protocols. Slice thickness, or the distance between axial CT slices, is the second parameter that contributes to the smallest volumetric element in a scan and varies by CT protocol. Slice thickness typically ranges from 0.37 mm to 2.5 mm depending on the protocol used. Importantly, because this quantity is not the same as pixel spacing, CT images are rarely isometric, meaning that axial pixilation is visible in the initial surface models that are created from the CT scan (Fig. 2.6). The difference in the reconstructed anatomy for a large-thickness scan is noticeable and impacts the final design. In some cases, a high slice thickness can make it almost the engineer's best guess to model the outer contours of the implant (Fig. 2.7).

On the other hand, DICOMs with extremely low slice thickness, or slice thickness that is equal to the pixel spacing, are extremely conducive to implant design. In these cases, engineers can preserve exact surfaces from the mirrored contralateral, particularly in articulating regions with uniform curvatures, allowing the implant to exactly mimic

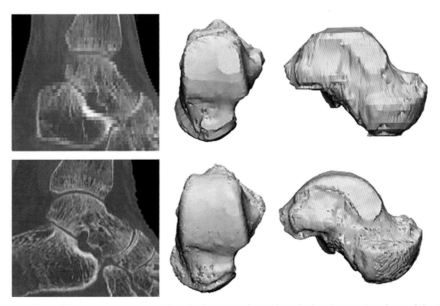

• **Fig. 2.6** *(Top)* CT scan with 2.5 mm slice thickness and resulting pixelated reconstructions of the talus that have a low level of detail and make design of the custom 3D-printed implant difficult. *(Bottom)* CT scan with 0.625 mm slice thickness and resulting volumetric reconstructions of the talus which provide a high level of detail for design of the custom 3D-printed implant. (Images courtesy of Restor3d, Inc, Durham, NC.)

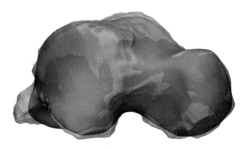
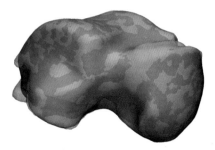

• **Fig. 2.7** Comparison between implant body *(gray)* and the mirrored contralateral talus model (bone color) from which it was designed. *(Left)* The input DICOM has a 3.0 mm slice thickness. *(Right)* The input DICOM has a slice thickness of 0.37 mm, equal to pixel spacing. (Images courtesy of Restor3d, Inc, Durham, NC.)

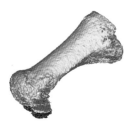
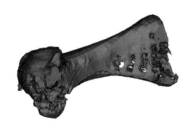

• **Fig. 2.8** Comparison of initial 3D point cloud from the same patient before (*Left*, slice thickness = 0.37 mm) and after *(right)* downsampling of the CT scan (*Right*, slice thickness = 1.50 mm). (Images courtesy of Restor3d, Inc, Durham, NC.)

natural anatomy (Fig. 2.8). This improves the quality of the final implant by reducing the amount of guesswork in design and helps to ensure the function of the final device by allowing the implant to perfectly match surrounding anatomy.

Image Compression or Downsampling

During the process of exporting DICOM files, scans with low slice thickness, and conversely a high total number of slices, may be compressed, effectively removing slices from the image stack (see Fig. 2.8). While this does shrink the file size, by increasing the usable slice thickness it reduces the quality of scans from a design perspective. It is important to have the uncompressed scans for 3D printing.

Tube Voltage and Current

The CT tube voltage and current are reported as kVp and mA, respectively. Although decreasing the tube voltage has significant effects on lowering the patient radiation dose, it also leads to unpredictable increases in image noise as the max attenuation of bone does not match the expected value. This increase in image noise can be offset with an increase in the tube current. Because the resulting increase in the tube current causes the patient dose to increase, a set voltage potential of kVp is recommended for printing applications as image noise greatly effects the thresholding and segmentation process; 120 kVp is an accepted safe amount of radiation for a foot and ankle CT scan.[6] Although tube voltage can be modulated individually, in most cases it is automatically set to 100 mA based on the tube voltage.[7]

Scanning Instructions

In addition to the specific scanning parameters used, there are several other important instructions, such as field of view (FoV) and patient positioning, that effect the usability of a scan for 3D design. Instructions for scanning are also provided by the implant manufacturer (Fig. 2.9).

Patient Positioning

Patient positioning during the CT scan plays a large role in implant design, especially in foot and ankle applications. In almost all cases, one of the first steps in preoperative planning is to reposition the anatomy to a weight-bearing position. This is crucial for several reasons. In fusion cases, the anatomy must be in an ideal position before the device can be designed, particularly if it is registering directly to anatomical surfaces. In these cases, the device sets the fixation trajectories, meaning the fusion would be on an incorrect trajectory if the anatomy was in the as-scanned position. Similarly, in total ankle replacement cases, the positioning of the talar dome relative to the talar body is based on the relationship of the tibia and talus in all three anatomical planes. To correctly set the axial rotation of the talar dome and the varus/valgus orientation of the hindfoot, the foot must be in a neutral position (foot positioned at 90 degrees to the leg). In design, engineers much match the surgical technique by digitally repositioning the foot to mimic a surgeon holding the foot at neutral before cutting the talus.

With these considerations in mind, the positioning of the patient's foot in a CT scanner plays a large role in device design. Although the bones of the foot and ankle can be freely repositioned in the design software, it is challenging to know whether corrections made in the 3D modeling software are both accurate for a specific patient or attainable in the operating room with soft tissue constraints. To remedy that, the ideal CT scan positions the foot as close to neutral or even weight bearing as possible. This can be attained several ways. When available, weight-bearing CT scans provide the most information for preoperative planning and implant design, as little to no repositioning of the anatomy is required. For patients with varus/valgus deformities, weight-bearing scans are the gold standard to ensure that the deformity can be adequately measured and corrected. If a weight-bearing CT scan

Acquisition Mode	Helical, axial, and cone beam CT modes are acceptable.
Kernel	Moderate or soft tissue reconstruction algorithm.
Field of View	Captures entire required bone region. Recommended field of view ≤40 cm, however a larger FoV may be necessary in some cases.
Contralateral Scan	Contralateral scan is preferred in all cases. It is required in many cases.
Positioning	Weight-bearing scan preferred (if applicable). If weight-bearing is not an option in a foot & ankle scan, the foot should be placed such that the transverse plane is parallel to the gantry.
Bilateral Scans	Bilateral scans may be taken in single CT acquisition if there is no pre-existing hardware. If taking bilateral scan, the FoV may need to be larger (30 cm).
Scan Date	Scan older than 6 months cannot be used for design, unless otherwise previously discussed.
Reformatting	No reformatting into coronal or sagittal planes is needed.

• **Fig. 2.9** Recommended scan instructions for implant design and 3D printing. *FoV*, Field of view. (Image courtesy of Restor3d, Inc, Durham, NC.)

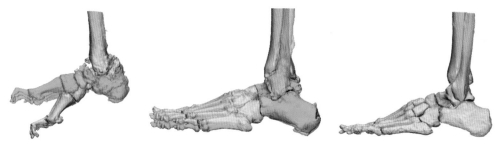

• **Fig. 2.10** Anatomy repositioned at neutral by engineers *(green)* in comparison to as-scanned anatomy *(bone color)* to show the difference in corrections required. *(Left)* The foot was not scanned in a neutral position. *(Middle)* The foot was held at neutral during scanning. *(Right)* The foot scanned in a weight-bearing CT scanner with little to no repositioning required. (Images courtesy of Restor3d, Inc, Durham, NC.)

is not an option, scanning protocols require that the patient's foot be positioned at 90 degrees to the leg using either a boot or a block to hold the foot during the scan.[8] In these situations, although the true weight-bearing position of the foot is not known, the required repositioning is typically minimal and the tibial–talar relationship can be determined. In cases where a past CT is used and the foot is not at neutral, implants can still be designed but special care should be given to the ensure that the anatomical corrections required will be attainable in the operating room (Fig. 2.10). In these situations, weight-bearing radiographs can often help engineers to use that specific patient's anatomy to guide corrections.

Field of View

The field of view (FoV) measures the amount of bony anatomy in the CT image acquisition field. Because there is a set number of pixels in each image, the FoV is directly related to the spatial resolution, or smallest voxel size.[9] Accordingly, it is ideal to have as small a FoV possible, decreasing the pixel spacing, provided that all affected anatomy is included in the scan. For this reason, for foot and ankle scans, a maximum FoV of 40 cm is recommended by several different manufactures of 3D-printed implants.

While this is much larger than would be ideal to minimize pixel spacing, there are several other considerations that affect this recommendation.

As previously shown, including the full foot from the calcaneus through the metatarsals is recommended to help visualize anatomical corrections. The foot can be positioned with a ground plane between the calcaneus, 5th metatarsal, and sesamoids. Similarly, including as much of the tibia as possible allows for better visualization of the tibial canal. With these considerations in mind, it is ideal to keep the FoV as small as possible while capturing the entire foot.

Scan to Surgery Timeline

To avoid changes in bony anatomy due to further deformity or growing pathology, only CT scans that were taken within the last 6 months should be used. This requirement is especially crucial in cases where cutting guides are designed to closely register to the anatomy.

Other Considerations

Metal Artifacts

In many cases that require preoperative planning and implant design, there is preoperative hardware that can cause

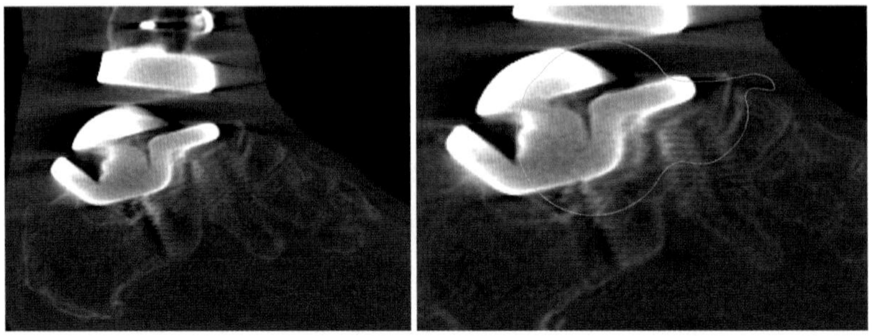

• **Fig. 2.11** *(Left)* Sagittal CT slice of a total ankle prosthesis causing significant scattering and metal artifacts that disrupt the contours of the calc. *(Right)* Proposed implant *(blue)*, which uses a reamed calcaneal surface rather than relying on anatomical contours. (Images courtesy of Restor3d, Inc, Durham, NC.)

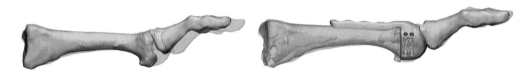

• **Fig. 2.12** *(Left)* Preoperative anatomy *(bone color)* compared with mirrored contralateral anatomy *(green)* for a patient with loss of length in their second metatarsal after a previous surgery. *(Right)* The designed implant uses the contralateral as a reference and exactly adds back the missing length, restoring the native positioning of the phalanges. (Images courtesy of Restor3d, Inc, Durham, NC.)

significant beam hardening and metal artifacts that affect diagnostic evaluation, disrupt anatomical contours, and add significant challenges to implant design.[10] When possible, hardware attenuation algorithms should be used in the CT protocol in order to help minimize any scatter in the scan and aid in the design workflow. Despite these algorithms, in many cases the artifacts caused by preoperative hardware are unavoidable, and the added unreliability of the surface contours of the anatomy should be noted and factored into design decisions. In cases with extreme artifacts, implants with more generalized bone preparation should be considered (Fig. 2.11). Instead of having the 3D-printed implant directly register to the preoperative contours of the anatomy, the preoperative plan could include a planned cut or reaming diameter that the implant would be designed to match.

Contralateral Anatomy

Although the contralateral anatomy is only required in some cases, it is always helpful in design, providing more information on the distinction between unique patient anatomy and deformity. There are several considerations for when a contralateral scan would be a necessity for design. First, if the implant is designed to articulate against native cartilage. In the case of a total talus, or any hemiarthroplasty device, using the contralateral articular surface allows for the best possible match between implant and cartilage. While it is possible to design this surface from the opposite side of the joint, the contralateral allows true restoration of healthy anatomy without requiring the engineer to guess the joint spacing, concavity, and cartilage thickness. Second, in cases where the affected anatomy is significantly collapsed or shortened, the contralateral anatomy allows better restoration of length to match healthy anatomy

(Fig. 2.12). Third, in rare cases of large bony defects or trauma, the contralateral anatomy can be used to rebuild features that might be completely missing from the affected side.

With these considerations in mind, when possible bilateral scans are recommended if a contralateral scan is required. When the unaffected side has metal hardware, it is important to position the contralateral limb on a different axial plane such that the scatter from one side will not affect the scan results from the other.

Other Modalities

MRI

The uses of MRIs in preoperative planning and design work are limited due to the generally high slice thickness. Despite the clear spatial resolution of MRIs in one plane, because slice thicknesses are generally higher than CT scans, they do not provide enough spatial information in all three planes to create meshes for implant design (Fig. 2.13). Additionally, because soft tissues and bony anatomy have similar grayscale values, separating different regions of anatomy is often a completely manual process that relies on individually tracing the contour of interest in every slice. With these two considerations in mind, MRI can be used as an alternative way to verify the fit of a device within the anatomy, rather than as a starting point for design.

X-ray

Due to the lack of 3D information, X-rays, much like MRIs, are only useful in some cases. As already mentioned,

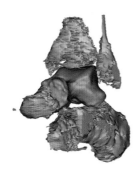
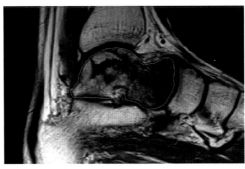

• **Fig. 2.13** *(Left)* Surface meshes of the tibia, fibula, navicular, cuboid, and calcaneus *(bone color)* segmented from an MRI with a slice thickness of 3.0 mm shown compared to the talus segmented from a CT scan with a slice thickness of 1.25 mm. *(Right)* A contour of the total talus implant shown on an MRI slice to verify the anatomical fit. (Images courtesy of Restor3d, Inc, Durham, NC.)

weight-bearing X-rays can help supplement a non–weight-bearing CT scan, particularly in foot and ankle applications. Additionally, in cases of a long bone deformity, linear X-ray measurements can be used to determine the amount of length correction that is required.

References

1. Anshad PYM, Kumar SS, Shahudheen S. Segmentation of chondroblastoma from medical images using modified region growing algorithm. *Cluster Comput.* 2019;22(suppl 6):13437-13444. doi:10.1007/s10586-018-1954-0.

2. Kamio T, Suzuki M, Asaumi R, Kawai T. DICOM segmentation and STL creation for 3D printing: a process and software package comparison for osseous anatomy. *3D Print Med.* 2020;6(1):1-12. doi:10.1186/s41205-020-00069-2.

3. Di Prima M, Coburn J, Hwang D, Kelly J, Khairuzzaman A, Ricles L. Additively manufactured medical products—the FDA perspective. *3D Print Med.* 2016;2(1):4-9. doi:10.1186/s41205-016-0005-9.

4. Yiit Özer S. Detection of vertical root fractures by using cone beam computed tomography with variable voxel sizes in an in vitro model. *J Endod.* 2011;37(1):75-79. doi:10.1016/j.joen.2010.04.021.

5. Shafiq-Ul-Hassan M, Zhang GG, Latifi K, et al. Intrinsic dependencies of CT radiomic features on voxel size and number of gray levels. *Med Phys.* 2017;44(3):1050-1062. doi:10.1002/mp.12123.

6. Koivisto J, Kiljunen T, Kadesjö N, Shi XQ, Wolff J. Effective radiation dose of a MSCT, two CBCT and one conventional radiography device in the ankle region. *J Foot Ankle Res.* 2015;8:8. doi:10.1186/s13047-015-0067-8.

7. Raman SP, Mahesh M, Blasko RV, Fishman EK. CT scan parameters and radiation dose: practical advice for radiologists. *J Am Coll Radiol.* 2013;10(11):840-846. doi:10.1016/j.jacr.2013.05.032.

8. Giardini P, Di Benedetto P, Mercurio D, et al. Infinity ankle arthroplasty with traditional instrumentation and PSI prophecy system: preliminary results. *Acta Biomed.* 2020;91(18):1-18. doi:10.23750/abm.v91i14-S.10989.

9. Miyata T, Yanagawa M, Hata A, et al. Influence of field of view size on image quality: ultra-high-resolution CT vs. conventional high-resolution CT. *Eur Radiol.* 2020;30(6):3324-3333. doi:10.1007/s00330-020-06704-0.

10. Marcus RP, Morris JM, Matsumoto JM, et al. Implementation of iterative metal artifact reduction in the pre-planning-procedure of three-dimensional physical modeling. *3D Print Med.* 2017;3(1):5. doi:10.1186/s41205-017-0013-4.

3

Material Science for 3D Printing in Medicine

CAMBRE KELLY, ALINA KIRILLOVA, EMILIO BACHTIAR, KEN GALL

Introduction

Materials Science and 3D Printing

As discussed in Chapter 1, materials for 3D printing include polymers, ceramics, metals, and composites. The materials used to fabricate a 3D part are dependent on the performance, or the "requirements" of the final part for its application. Material selection is also dependent on the 3D-printing technology used, as not all materials can be manufactured using all available 3D-printing methods. Thus, the intersection of material science with 3D printing has grown into a vast and popular field since the 2000s. Continued work in this field will produce a better understanding of materials, manufacturing, and their use in medical applications.

Processing-Structure-Property-Performance Relationships

In material science, processing-structure-property-performance relationships define the correlation between the way a part is made and the resulting behavior and application of the part. Processing refers to the steps a raw material undergoes during the manufacture of a final part. This can include both primary and secondary processing steps. For a 3D-printed part, additive manufacturing is typically the primary processing step in which a raw material in the form of a filament, resin, powder, or other type, is converted to a 3D part. Secondary processing of the part may include heat treatment, surface treatment, or other additional steps to achieve the desired structure and therefore properties. The performance, or function, of the part is dependent on its various properties. In orthopedic applications, performance is typically driven by a tradeoff between the mechanical and surface properties of a given application. For example, a hemiarthroplasty implant must be high strength and fatigue resistant, as well as have a bearing surface with a low coefficient of friction to minimize wear. These relationships help material scientists and engineers to select materials for a given application, as well as to discover new materials.

Materials Selection

As described earlier, processing of a material defines its structure, and thus the resulting material properties. In load-bearing orthopedic applications, mechanical (structural) performance is typically a priority when designing an implant. In additive manufacturing, due to the wide selection of materials and processing technologies, a top-down strategy can be employed to first define the desired properties of a part for a given application. For example, for a tibial tray of a total ankle prosthesis, engineering requirements may prescribe a minimum strength before failure, as well as a coefficient of friction of the surface interfacing with the polyethylene insert, amongst other requirements. These properties and their interrelationships must be considered in order to define the appropriate processing steps to achieve the end goal.

Most importantly, these properties help to define the materials that can be used for the part. Material selection charts, also often called Ashby plots, are often used in these cases to identify materials that can meet defined the specifications for a given application (Fig. 3.1). The following sections give an overview of the current state of the art for materials produced by 3D printing for medical applications and biomedical research.

Aside from selecting the type of material (metals, polymers, ceramics, or composites thereof), there are other important material and final implant characteristics that need to be addressed for the successful fabrication of a 3D-printed orthopedic device (Fig. 3.2).

Metals

From the perspective of orthopedic implant applications, the first 3D-printed implants were metallic. Given the historical

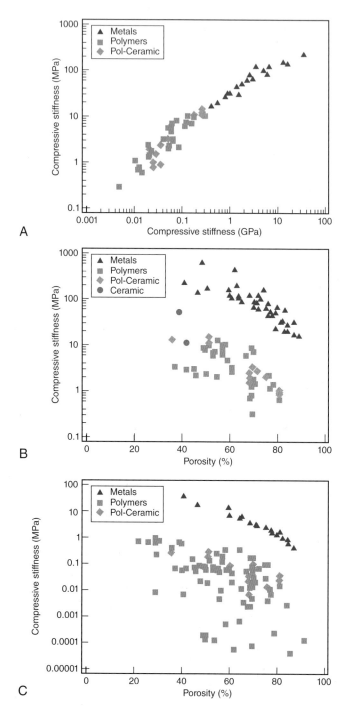

• **Fig. 3.1** Materials selection charts of compressive properties of 3D-printed synthetic porous materials. (A) Compressive strength versus compressive stiffness. (B) Compressive strength versus porosity. (C) Compressive stiffness versus porosity for 3D-printed biomaterials of all architectures for various material types. (Source: Kelly CN, Miller AT, Hollister SJ, Guldberg RE, Gall K. Design and structure-function characterization of 3D printed synthetic porous biomaterials for tissue engineering. *Adv Healthcare Mat.* 2018;7:1701095.)

devices cleared by the United States Food and Drug Administration (FDA) between 2010 and 2015.[1] Implants fabricated from commercially pure (unalloyed) titanium and cobalt chromium (CoCrMo) alloy have also been developed and cleared, albeit to a far smaller degree.

Titanium and Titanium Alloys

Titanium, both commercially pure (CP) and the most common alloy, Ti6Al4V, have long been used in the human body for various load-bearing and nonloaded applications.[2] In fact, the first 3D-printed implant cleared for use by the FDA was a titanium alloy acetabular hip cup manufactured by Exactech, Inc. Due to its high strength and fatigue resistance, Ti6Al4V is the standard choice for load-bearing orthopedic implants. The manufacture of porous implants with complex, interconnected lattices has been a primary use case for additive manufacturing in implants. Of the devices produced by additive manufacturing (AM) with a porous lattice, 72% are Ti6Al4V. These include devices such as spinal fusion cages, osteotomy wedges, and arthroplasty components, where osseointegration of the implant is critical to a successful clinical outcome.[1] Thus, research efforts at the intersection of AM and the biomedical field are focused on optimization of porous lattices to improve the efficacy of such implants. This includes investigation of the tradeoff between design and manufacturing, the mechanical properties of porous scaffolds, and the associated in vivo performance.[2,3]

Nickel titanium (NiTi) is another alloy used in medical device applications. To date, no additively manufactured implants fabricated from NiTi have been cleared by the FDA. However, there many research efforts have been dedicated to overcoming the challenges related to additive manufacturing of the alloy.[4-6] AM has also led to the development of new alloys that are designed with compositions that are well suited for the additive process. One such example is titanium niobium (TiNb) alloys, which have received increasing research attention due to their ability to reduce the bulk material modulus while maintaining high strength similar to Ti6Al4V.[7,8] Challenges in the 3D printing of titanium and its alloys include the sensitivity to oxidation, which is discussed further here. This is a particular challenge for NiTi, where even small changes in atomic composition drastically effect the material's properties, and the ability to achieve super elasticity.

Cobalt Alloys

Cobalt chromium ($Co_{28}Cr_6Mo$) is a high-strength alloy with a low coefficient of friction, which facilitates its use in articulating applications where reduction of wear is critical (Fig. 3.3). While its adoption into the additive manufacture of implants has lagged behind titanium alloys, there are an increasing number of implants that use this alloy, including the talar implant for a total ankle arthroplasty system (Wright Medical Infinity TAR). Similar to titanium, CoCrMo alloy

use of titanium and its alloys for skeletal reconstruction, the development of these materials was at the forefront of the adoption of additive manufacturing technologies in the orthopedics industry. The adoption of 3D printing has been dominated by titanium alloy, with 40% of such medical

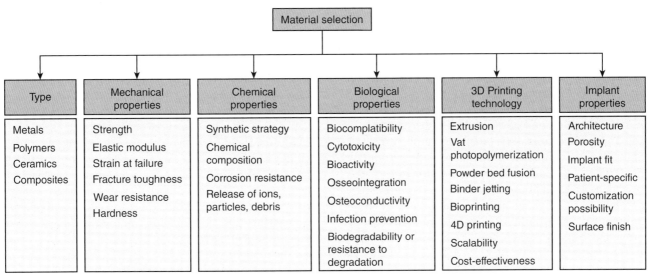

Material selection					
Type	**Mechanical properties**	**Chemical properties**	**Biological properties**	**3D Printing technology**	**Implant properties**
Metals Polymers Ceramics Composites	Strength Elastic modulus Strain at failure Fracture toughness Wear resistance Hardness	Synthetic strategy Chemical composition Corrosion resistance Release of ions, particles, debris	Biocomplatibility Cytotoxicity Bioactivity Osseointegration Osteoconductivity Infection prevention Biodegradability or resistance to degradation	Extrusion Vat photopolymerization Powder bed fusion Binder jetting Bioprinting 4D printing Scalability Cost-effectiveness	Architecture Porosity Implant fit Patient-specific Customization possibility Surface finish

• **Fig. 3.2** Requirements for appropriate material selection of 3D-printed orthopedic implants.

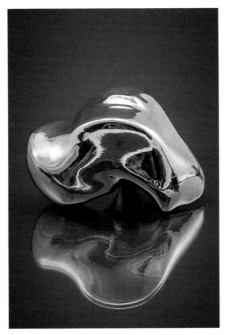

• **Fig. 3.3** A total talus replacement prosthesis produced by laser powder bed fusion of cobalt chromium. (Image provided by Restor3d, Inc, Durham, NC.)

forms a spontaneous oxide layer. Thus, similar solutions to allow high-temperature processing with oxidation of the surface are employed. Additionally, the resulting surface of as-printed parts requires significant postprocessing to reduce the roughness to within the specifications defined for articulating arthroplasty components (<0.05 μm per ASTM 2033).

Other Metals

Stainless steels, including 17-4 and 316L, are commonly used in surgical applications for both implants and instruments.

The use of powder bed fusion (PBF) for producing stainless steel implants has been less widely adopted than for titanium alloys.[1] However, opportunity exists to use 3D printing for the production of stainless steel plates or other orthopedic applications.

3D printing of precious metals has also been demonstrated in the scientific literature; for example, pure silver bone scaffolds which exhibit antibacterial properties.[9] Other work has investigated the addition of copper (Cu) or gold (Au) to traditional alloy systems to impart antimicrobial properties to the implant.[10] These additions to the alloy system also have an effect on the mechanical properties of the materials, which needs ongoing research to be better understood.

A number of bulk metallic glass systems have also been under investigation for the AM of implants, including $Ti_{47}Cu_{38}Zr_{7.5}Fe_{2.5}Sn_2Si_1Ag_2$ and $Zr_{52.5}Cu_{17.9}Ni_{14.6}Al_{10}Ti_5$. The advantage of bulk metallic glass is its ability to reduce stiffness while maintaining a high strength.[10] Additional degradable metals such as magnesium, zinc, and iron-based materials have also been discussed for their use in bone-regeneration applications in the "Degradable Materials" section.

3D-Printing Technologies for Metals

Powder Bed Fusion

PBF has been the primary technology adopted for 3D printing of medical devices. PBF of metallic materials can be further divided into subcategories of technologies based on the high energy source used to achieve fusion of the powder material. The two most common are electron beam melting and laser PBF. While both technologies have been used to produce metallic medical implants and there are advantages and disadvantages to each depending on the end part and its application, laser PBF has seen wider adoption. This wider adoption can be attributed to its ability to achieve smaller feature sizes and control complex geometry, which are advantageous for the fabrication of complex porous lattices to allow for osseointegration.

While PBF has unlocked an unprecedented opportunity to produce medical devices, there are some processing-related challenges that must be considered. First, the sensitivity of reactive metals to oxidation at high temperatures must be managed. In PBF, this is overcome by use of inert gases and/or a vacuum in the build chamber to reduce the risk of oxidation. Typically, oxygen levels are well below 100 ppm throughout the duration of the build. Further, the metallic material produced from PBF usually has a microstructure that differs from that of the wrought metal. Due to the layer-wise process, anisotropy in the grain structure is often observed, as well as a non-equilibrium phase. For example, titanium alloy is a biphasic material and the as-printed microstructure is a non-equilibrium alpha resulting from rapid heating and cooling during the PBF process. To homogenize the material microstructure, reduce residual thermal stresses, and improve the material properties, PBF parts typically require postprocessing thermal treatments. These include standard stress relieving, high-temperature annealing, as well as hot isostatic pressing (HIP) processes. Lastly, the as-printed surface of parts resulting from PBF can have roughness (R_a) ranging from 5 to 50 μm due to the adherence of partially fused powder particles. While in some osseointegration applications this topography may be favorable, in those at risk of high wear, the surface of implants must be treated through chemical or physical methods.

Others

While PBF technologies have dominated the AM of implants to date, other technologies are poised to offer advantages for the production of metallic implants. Directed energy deposition (DED) has been investigated for printing of multimaterial components due to its ability to switch between feedstock more easily, which allows the local deposit of different materials or the introduction of material gradients.[11,12] One such example would be a hip stem with a porous titanium alloy stem and a CoCrMo head for articulation.

Similarly, material extrusion and binder jetting (BJ) of metallic parts have been demonstrated in both research and commercial settings.[13] However, the material selection and geometric complexity are currently limited in these processes. Further, both technologies require a postprinting workflow that includes debinding and sintering steps. One major hurdle for these technologies in implantable medical devices will be complete removal of the binder material to ensure no contamination occurs in the body.

Polymers

Introduction

A polymer is a macromolecule composed of smaller repeating units known as monomers. A polymer is formed when monomers are linked together by a primary bond that is typically covalent in nature. Colloquially, a subset of synthetic polymers is better known as plastics. Polymers are of significant interest in medical technology owing to their unique characteristics and large range of properties. For example, the mechanical properties of polymers can range from being akin to gel, rubber, or hard plastic. Many common polymers also possess good processability, making them amenable to 3D printing. These qualities have led to a vast number of commercial products and scientific research that utilize 3D-printed polymers for medical applications. In orthopedics, commercial applications of 3D-printed polymers have ranged from simple surgical guides and instruments to a bioresorbable bone graft cage implant. The types of 3D-printed polymers available for orthopedic implants are limited due to stringent biocompatibility requirements but a much larger range of polymers is available for nonimplant applications (e.g., surgical guides, surgery planning aids, orthoses).

The properties of a polymer are largely determined by its chemistry, structure, and morphology. By varying these aspects, polymers can be tuned to achieve specific objectives and improve the performance of a device. The chemistry of a polymer is the combination of atoms contained in a polymer chain and the manner in which they are bonded to one another. The structure or configuration of a polymer refers to the way the atoms in a polymer are arranged, which could vary in a polymer with the same chemistry, such as in linear versus branched polymers. The morphology of a polymer is the arrangement of polymer chains in relation to all other polymer chains and any ordering associated with it, and the morphology is strongly related to its processing history. In addition to these three factors, the property of a polymer can also be altered by using additives to achieve specific goals. For example, plasticizers are commonly added as an additive to promote plasticity and reduce the brittleness of a polymer.

Nondegradable Polymers Used in Orthopedics 3D Printing

From the perspective of orthopedic applications, there are some 3D-printable polymers that are frequently in use in both scientific research and commercial products. These polymers are described and their applications in the context of orthopedics are presented in the following section. All the polymers shown here are discussed in the context of their use as a nondegradable material, which is defined as a material that does not degrade appreciably within its service life.

Most polymers commonly used for 3D printing are not suitable for implant applications. The requirements for implant materials are much more stringent than nonimplants and include specifications spanning from biocompatibility and physical properties, to mechanical properties. Generally, nonimplant applications (e.g., surgical planning aids) only require two properties: safety for short-term contact and suitable mechanical properties (Fig. 3.4).

In this chapter, synthetic polymers are categorized into thermoplastics, thermosets, and photopolymers. This classification reflects the nature of their processing, which in turn strongly determines the 3D-printing methods available to them.

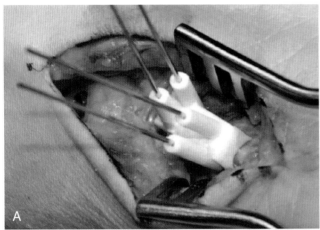

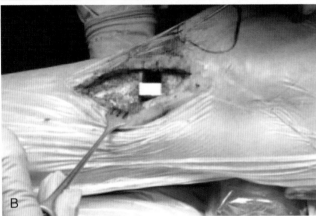

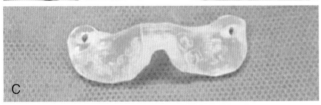

• **Fig. 3.4** Examples of 3D-printed orthopedic surgical guides in the literature. (A) Polyamide surgical guide printed via selective laser sintering and used in setting k-wires. (B) Acrylonitrile butadiene styrene wedge-shaped spacer printed via melt extrusion and used as a reference for osteotomy. (C) Stereolithography-printed part used as a marker for the entry point of a screw for surgery. (Sources: (A) Schweizer A, et al. Computer-assisted 3-dimensional reconstructions of scaphoid fractures and nonunions with and without the use of patient-specific guides: early clinical outcomes and postoperative assessments of reconstruction accuracy. *J Hand Surg Am.* 2016;41(1):59-69; (B) Pérez-Mañanes R, Burró JA, Manaute JR, Rodriguez FC, Martín JV. 3D surgical printing cutting guides for open-wedge high tibial osteotomy: do it yourself. *Knee Surg.* 2016;29(8):690-695; (C) Kaneyama S, et al. Safe and accurate midcervical pedicle screw insertion procedure with the patient-specific screw guide template system. *Spine (Phila PA)* 2015;40(6):E341-E348.)

Thermoplastics

Thermoplastics are polymers that can be melted when exposed to temperatures above their melting temperature. In thermoplastics, the polymer chains are held together by secondary bonds which form physical crosslinks such as hydrogen bonds, which are reversible. The physical crosslinks dissipate when heated past a critical temperature but reform when cooled, granting thermoplastics their reprocessable nature. Reprocessable refers to the capability of an already shaped polymer to be melted and reshaped. Because of these properties, thermoplastics lends themselves well to fused filament fabrication (FFF) and PBF 3D printing.

Nylon

Nylon is a colloquial name for a group of polymers based on aliphatic polyamides. An aliphatic polyamide is a polymer with aliphatic repeating units connected by amide bonds. There is a large variety of nylon available, the most common being PA6, PA66, PA11, and PA12. Nylon is a semicrystalline thermoplastic polymer with high toughness and strength, and is steam sterilizable. It also has a wide processing window, allowing it to be processed in a large variety of ways. Owing to this processing window, current PBF printing of polymers mainly uses nylon. In medical devices, nylon is often used in sutures and in short-term devices such as balloon catheters; nylon is rarely used long term. In orthopedics, 3D-printed nylon sees use in nonimplant applications such as surgical guides and tools due to its excellent mechanical properties and its amenability to PBF printing.

Poly(Aryl Ether Ketone) Polymers

Poly(aryl ether ketone) (PAEK) is a relatively new family of thermoplastic that is composed of a backbone of paraphenylene groups interspersed with ketone and ether groups. Prominent polymers in the PAEK family include poly(ether ether ketone) (PEEK), poly(ether ketone) (PEK), and poly(ether ketone ketone) (PEKK). Of the members of the PAEK family, PEEK is the most commonly used in commercial applications. PEEK is a polymer with a high melting temperature (allowing for steam sterilization), radiolucency, and excellent mechanical and chemical resistance properties. PEEK also has a stiffness that is closer to bone than metal, minimizing stress shielding. In medical devices, PEEK has vast applications, particularly in orthopedics.[14] It is also one of the few polymers commonly used for load-bearing orthopedic implants. PEEK has a long and established history of clinical use, exhibiting osteoconduction and biocompatibility. Some examples of PEEK implants include internal fixations for bones, spinal cages, and craniofacial implants. PEEK also has nonimplant applications as surgical instruments and its stability allows for autoclaving, enabling sterilization, and repeated use.

The most common processing method for PEEK is injection molding, which is commonly used as a benchmark for 3D-printed samples. PEEK is amenable to both extrusion and PBF 3D printing. 3D printing of PEEK is a frequent research subject because of its perceived potential for commercial applications. In past studies of PEEK FFF 3D printing, a wide variety of resulting properties have arisen because of the wide-ranging testing parameters and set up used by the authors.[15] In general, printed PEEK is highly anisotropic and has vastly inferior mechanical properties to injection-molded PEEK.[16,17] Many approaches have been proposed to mitigate the reduction in mechanical properties, such as annealing/heat treatment,[18] adjustments to the printing environment, and other print parameter optimizations[19]; however, none have yielded significant improvement on the observed anisotropy. Currently, no commercial PEEK implant is 3D printed via FFF. Studies on PBF 3D printing of PEEK have generally demonstrated mechanical properties that are superior to FFF printing.[20,21] However, although these studies did not test for anisotropy, printed PEEK is expected to be anisotropic, as has been shown in other PBF-printed materials.[22,23] Currently, to the best of the authors' knowledge, there is no commercial PBF-printed PEEK implant.

PEKK is another member of the PAEK family that is useful in orthopedic implants. Chemically it is similar to PEEK, but with one ether group and two ketone groups interspersing the paraphenylene group backbone. In orthopedics, PEKK is used in similar applications to PEEK because its properties are in many ways comparable. One of the earliest 3D-printed polymer implants cleared by the FDA is a craniofacial device (OsteoFab, Oxford Performance Materials) fabricated out of PEKK via selective laser sintering (SLS). Currently, there are also a number of FDA-cleared PEKK 3D-printed load-bearing spinal implants (SpineFab, Oxford Performance Materials; Tetrafuse, RTI Surgical) fabricated via SLS (Fig. 3.5). A key advantage for PEKK 3D printing compared to PEEK 3D printing is printed PEKK's superior properties, a direct result of its thermal behavior which is suited for PBF printing.[24]

Other Thermoplastic Polymers

Polymers that find some use in 3D printing for orthopedic research and commercial devices are discussed here:

1. *Acrylonitrile butadiene styrene (ABS):* ABS is one of the most common polymers for FFF 3D printing, especially in a home 3D printer setting. Outside of medical applications it is often used in products such as toys and enclosures for consumer electronics. In medical devices, ABS finds the most use outside of implants. In orthopedics, FFF 3D-printed ABS is used in the fabrication of surgical planning aids[25] as it is sterilizable using ethylene oxide.

2. *Polylactic acid (PLA):* PLA is another common polymer in FFF 3D printing along with ABS. It is an aliphatic polyester composed of lactic acid. It has favorable properties for processing via extrusion and molding. In medical devices, PLA is most often used in implant applications requiring bioabsorbability. In orthopedic applications without need for bioabsorbability, FFF 3D-printed PLA has been used in surgical planning aids.

3. *Ultra-high-molecular-weight polyethylene (UHMWPE):* UHMWPE is a common engineering polymer with excellent mechanical properties and good wear resistance, self-lubricating properties, and biocompatibility. In orthopedics, it is commonly used in hip, knee, and spine implants for articulating surfaces. The 3D-printing

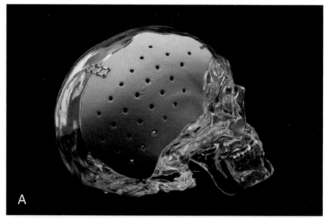

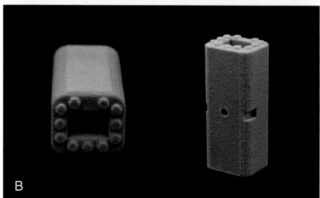

• **Fig. 3.5** Commercial 3D-printed orthopedic implants. (A) OsteoFab Patient Specific Cranial Device. (B) SpineFab VBR System. (https://oxfordpm.com/osteofab-medical-devices)

method of choice for UHMWPE is PBF. However, its high melt viscosity hinders optimal printing via PBF, resulting in inferior properties.[26-28] At its current state, 3D printing of UHMWPE appears to be unsuitable for use in common UHMWPE orthopedic implants.

4. *Polymethyl methacrylate (PMMA):* PMMA, also known as bone cement, is a ubiquitous polymer in orthopedics. PMMA is also used in other implant applications, such as in craniofacial implants (e.g., PMMA Customized Implant, Stryker). Its thermoplastic nature allows it to be printed using extrusion[29] and PBF[30] methods. PMMA can also be printed via BJ.[31] However, the printed parts possess significantly inferior mechanical properties and/or lower density compared to injection-molded samples.

5. *Polypropylene (PP):* PP is a semicrystalline polymer composed of propylene monomers and the second most produced thermoplastic in the world behind polyethylene. PP is a widely used material in FFF 3D printing. It is also one of the most used polymers in medical devices, frequently seen in sutures, packaging, noncontact devices, and implants. In orthopedics, an example of PP application is in ligament augmentation devices. SLS-printed PP shows properties close to injection-molded PP.[32]

6. Thermoplastic *polyurethane (PU)*: PU belongs to a large family of polymers that are used in a large variety of industries. PU's main characteristic is its urethane links that joins its monomers together. Polycarbonate urethane (PCU) is a member of the PU family that has garnered much attention for its potential use in orthopedics, particularly as articulating surfaces for knee implants,[33,34] and has been shown to be very amenable to FFF 3D printing, having similar properties to injection-molded samples.[35]

7. *Polysulfones (PSUs)*: PSUs are a group of high-performance polymeric materials. Similar to PAEKs, PSUs possess high hydrolytic resistance, high temperature resistance, and good mechanical properties. They are often used in reusable devices requiring sterilization such as surgical trays and sizers for implants. Commercial PSU 3D-printing filaments are available for extrusion printing, such as Ultem 9085 (Stratasys). Extrusion-printed PSUs have shown potentially similar properties to injection-molded PSUs in past studies.[36]

Thermosets

Thermosets are chemically crosslinked polymers with a highly restricted chain motion. Because of the covalent nature of the crosslinks, thermosets are not reprocessable, unlike thermoplastics and their physical crosslinks.

Silicone

Silicone, or polysiloxanes, are polymers containing a siloxane (Si-O-Si) linkage. Silicones are used in many applications owing to their very versatile properties. Medical device applications for silicones are particularly vast because of their biocompatibility and chemical stability. An example of clinical applications of silicones include contact lenses and catheters. In orthopedics, polysiloxanes are used in hand and foot joint implants. 3D printing of polysiloxanes is commonly performed via direct extrusion[37] and a base silicone material is typically mixed with substances to achieve a consistency that is suitable to be used as a printable ink.

Photopolymers

Photopolymers are polymers that are crosslinked under exposure to light of a particular wavelength and are printed using vat photopolymerization and material jetting (MJ). Most photopolymers are not reprocessable, hence they are often a subset of thermoset polymers. A photopolymerization system is typically composed of three components: a mixture of monomers and oligomers, photoinitiators, and other additives such as stabilizers and photosensitizers. Most commercial mixtures are proprietary, and their list of components are not readily searchable. The most common photopolymer systems are described here. It is important to note that, in practice, these different systems are often combined into a complex mixture to improve properties.

Currently, commercial photopolymers find most of their applications in nonimplant devices such as surgical planning aids and guides. Commercial photopolymers have a wide range of mechanical properties and are suitable for most nonimplant applications. However, to the best of the author's knowledge and at the time of writing, no commercial photopolymer has been present in an FDA-cleared human implant.

Acrylate and Methacrylate-Based Systems

(Meth)acrylate-based photopolymerization is the earliest type of system developed for vat photopolymerization (VP) and remains the most common. (Meth)acrylate-based systems polymerize via free radical photopolymerization (FRP), which is a polymerization approach where a polymer is formed by the addition of monomers into a propagating radical chain. An example resin mixture is a combination of urethane acrylate, urethane methacrylate, trimethylolpropane triacrylate, and other reactive diluents along with photoinitiators for use in continuous liquid interface production (CLIP) 3D printing.[38] (Meth)acrylate-based resins are very versatile and are used in many 3D-printing applications such as for shape-memory polymers,[39] tough polymers,[40] natural polymers,[41] and functional polymers.[42] (Meth)acrylate resins have a high rate of polymerization and exhibit long-term stability, but generally result in parts that are brittle.[43] They exhibit significant shrinkage when cured, and as a consequence they can also exhibit deformations such as curling. Some pure (meth)acrylate resins also show significant gelling even at low conversions, inducing high viscosity and limited flow of resin for optimal printing. For these reasons, meth(acrylate) resins are often combined with epoxy-based resins to improve properties.

Epoxy-Based and Vinyl Ether-Based Systems

Epoxy and vinyl ether-based systems are both facilitated via cationic photopolymerization. Cationic polymerization is chain-growth polymerization via carbocationic growing species.[44] Examples of common epoxy monomers include 3,4-epoxycyclohexane methyl 3,4-epoxycyclohexylcarboxylate (EPOX), bisphenol A diglycidyl ether (DGEBA), and 1,4-cyclohexane dimethanol divinyl ether (CDVE).[45] Epoxy-based systems and other similar ring-opening polymerization systems tend to show minimal shrinkage compared to acrylates and they are often mixed with acrylates to allow for thermal post curing and to minimize shrinkage.[46] Epoxy resins also show less inhibition by oxygen, allowing for a lower photoinitiator concentration. However, epoxy resin photopolymerization reactions tend to proceed more slowly compared to acrylate's free radical polymerization.

Thiol-ene and Thiol-yne Systems

Thiol-ene and thiol-yne systems are based on the reaction between thiols and carbon-carbon double bonds and triple bonds, respectively. These systems have a couple of advantages over (meth)acrylate systems in that they display less shrinkage and less oxygen inhibition. They also demonstrate improved biocompatibility,[47] hence the significant interest in using them for applications requiring biocompatibility and degradability.[48,49] However, these systems tend to have a poor shelf life and bad odor.[50]

3D-Printing Processes for Polymers

3D printing of polymers is available in a large variety of approaches because of the large range of available polymer properties. In this section, the most common methods of polymer 3D printing are described. Important considerations for each method are presented in the context of printing parameters, mainly from a materials perspective.

Extrusion

The main advantages of extrusion-based polymer printing are its simplicity and a large library of material that is available for use, some of which possess an established clinical use history. However, structures with overhanging sections are difficult or impossible to print via extrusion and should be minimized during device design.

Printing parameters that are important to polymer extrusion are temperatures, and print pathing and orientation. Typically, the overarching objective of adjusting these parameters are to (1) achieve good mechanical properties, and (2) print parts with good fidelity. In achieving good mechanical properties, layer bonding is the primary consideration. For good part fidelity, the extruded polymer needs to maintain its shape in a predictable way when extruded out to form layers.

Nozzle and bed temperature are considered one of the most important print parameters for melt-based extrusion. Excessively high temperature leads to polymer degradation and undesired spreading of the molten polymer, while inadequate temperature leads to low polymer flow and weak layer bonding.[51-53] In addition, temperature also has a more nuanced effect on printed polymers, such as by affecting crystallinity.[54] Print pathing and orientation are also major factors in improving print quality.[55] Print pathing includes aspects such as layer thickness, path width, raster pattern, and many others, whereas print orientation refers to the orientation at which the object is printed. Broadly speaking, parameters that maximize part density (such as smaller layer thickness) and direct mechanical loads away from layer bonding surfaces (such as via raster pattern adjustment) will improve quality.

There are a vast number of parameters that can be adjusted for extrusion printing. All these parameters are interrelated; therefore, it is important to evaluate each printed part using the exact same parameter as production parts, including the same environment, same device, and same material. In orthopedics, extrusion printing has found the most use in surgical planning models. The simplicity of extrusion systems also means it can be used on site in clinical settings. At the time of writing, to the best of the author's knowledge, no commercial orthopedic device is fabricated via extrusion printing.

Vat Photopolymerization

VP printing is a process unique to polymers. The main advantage of VP is its ability to print complex structures. VP-printed parts are also accurate, with a smooth surface finish. This has led VP parts to find use in applications that require accurate form and fitting.[46] However, photopolymers tend to be non-biocompatible for implant use. Scarce clinical usage history is a major obstacle for use as an implant by device developers. In comparison to injection-molded parts, VP parts have lower durability and strength, in addition to the anisotropy common with 3D-printing techniques.

From a processing perspective, an ideal resin mixture for VP would have low viscosity, minimize undesired light leakage, polymerize rapidly, and have no shrinkage when cured. The formulation of the resin strongly affects this. Important parameters in VP include cure depth and scan pathing. Cure depth is a commonly used VP measure that includes the effect of laser power, laser penetration, laser speed, resin cure-threshold, and laser spot size.[56] Along with cure depth, scan pathing is an important parameter that is able to minimize residual stress and shrinkage when adjusted well.[56] It is also worth noting that VP systems can use different types of radiations (e.g., ultraviolet [UV], visible light, or infrared) to initiate photopolymerization.

Research directions in VP include novel VP approaches such as two-photon microprinting. In the context of medical devices and orthopedics specifically, there is much interest in the development of novel photopolymers that are biocompatible for implant application. Some past research on this subject includes the development of biocompatible hydrogels,[57,58] biodegradable scaffolds,[59] filler-added resins,[60] and so on. In orthopedics, VP finds most often used in nonimplant applications.

Powder Bed Fusion

PBF of polymers has the distinct advantages of both being able to fabricate complex structures and having a large library of biocompatible thermoplastics. However, a limiting factor of PBF is that it requires that the polymers have a narrow set of thermal properties to print viably. The most common variety of PBF printing for polymers is SLS. For nondegradable polymers, the material that is by far the most commonly used for PBF is polyamides, making up more than 95% of the current PBF market,[61] with PA12 and PA11 being the most common varieties.

In SLS printing, the major build parameters are laser power, bed temperature, layer thickness, scan spacing, scan speed, and part raster pattern. Laser power, scan spacing, and scan speed are often bundled and expressed as the amount of energy delivered by the laser to the polymer powder. Appropriate energy delivery by laser and bed heating is important for printing serviceable parts. Powder properties are also well documented to be crucial to print quality,[61-63] which are primarily affected by powder morphology. In addition, environmental effects such as humidity and electrostatic charging should also be taken into account.[64,65] Another important consideration in polymer PBF is powder aging and reuse. The ability to reuse polymer powders from prior print runs improves the economy of PBF printing significantly. Powders that are used in a print run are subject to thermal aging[66] and often result in parts with inferior print quality,[66] but a mitigation approach that is frequently used is to mix virgin powders with aged powders to minimize the decrease in part quality. Postprinting powder removal is also important to consider.

In the context of orthopedics, polymer PBF is used in both implant and nonimplant applications, and currently it is the only printing approach that has been used for commercial orthopedic implants. For implant applications, PAEK polymers are a common choice because of their vast clinical usage history and good printed properties. Commercial PAEK devices include a suture anchor, craniofacial implants, and spinal implants. For nonimplant materials, a common choice is any nylon variety, with common applications in surgical guides. Although there is obviously much potential in the use of PBF for printing orthopedic devices, currently there are relatively few commercially available powders that are optimized for PBF, with the majority of them being nonimplant grade.

Inkjet

Inkjet (IJ) printing is considered to be the most complex yet most accurate printing method, resulting in multicolor parts with a good finish. However, the printed parts are mechanically weaker than standard injection-molded parts. Material availability is also very limited compared to other printing methods because of stringent property requirements, and commercial resins are typically proprietary and machine specific. IJ can be classified into MJ and BJ. Both use photopolymers, although BJ processes can also use other substances for binding, such as solvents. Some processing considerations of IJ are similar to VP, wherein the photopolymer needs to cure properly during the build process. A crucial difference to VP is the need to consider the jetting process. Additionally, for BJ there is also a need to take powder properties into account. Postprint powder removal is also important in medical applications. In medical devices and orthopedics specifically, IJ is most often used for planning and visualization aids.

Summary and Future Trends

A summary of some of the polymers described in this section is presented in Tables 3.1 to 3.3, for thermoplastics, thermosets, and photopolymers, respectively. Polymer data is

TABLE 3.1   Summary of 3D-Printable Thermoplastics and Their Injection-Molded Properties at Ambient Temperature

Material	Common Print Method(s)	Mechanical Properties		Applications in Orthopedics
Polyamide (nylon 66)	Extrusion, PBF	UTS Mod Failure strain	85 MPa 2.0 GPa 300%	• Surgical guide, instruments, and planning tools
PEEK	Extrusion, PBF	UTS Mod Failure strain	95 MPa 6.5 GPa 3.5%	• Craniofacial and spinal implants
PEKK	Extrusion, PBF	UTS Mod Failure strain	73 MPa 3.3 GPa 13.2%	• Craniofacial and spinal implants, interference screws
ABS	Extrusion	UTS Mod Failure strain	57 MPa 2.6 GPa 50%	• Surgical planning aid • Device enclosures
PLA	Extrusion	UTS Mod Failure strain	65 MPa 2.5 GPa 65%	• Surgical planning aid
UHMWPE	PBF	UTS Mod Failure strain	40 MPa 0.8 GPa 350%	• Articulating surfaces
PMMA	Extrusion, PBF	UTS Mod Failure strain	76 MPa 3.1 GPa 10%	• Bone cement
PP	Extrusion, PBF	UTS Mod Failure strain	30 MPa 1.7 GPa 140%	• Ligament augmentation • Orthotics
PCU	Extrusion,	UTS Mod Failure strain	50 MPa 0.08 GPa 400%	• Articulating surfaces
PSU	Extrusion	UTS Mod Failure strain	87 MPa 5.0 GPa 28%	• Surgical guide, instruments, and planning tools

ABS, Acrylonitrile butadiene styrene; *Mod*, modulus of elasticity; *PBF*, powder bed fusion; *PCU*, polycarbonate urethane; *PEEK*, poly(ether ether ketone); *PEKK*, poly(ether ketone ketone); *PLA*, polylactic acid; *PMMA*, polymethyl methacrylate; *PP*, polypropylene; *PSU*, polysulfone; *UHMWPE*, ultra-high-molecular-weight polyethylene; *UTS*, ultimate tensile strength.

TABLE 3.2	Summary of 3D-Printable Thermosets and Their Properties at Ambient Temperature			
Material	**Common Print Method(s)**	**Mechanical Properties**		**Applications in Orthopedics**
Polydim-ethylsiloxane	Extrusion, MJ	UTS	2 MPa	• Arthroplasty implants
		Mod	360 MPa	
		Failure strain	300%	

MJ, Material jetting; *Mod*, modulus of elasticity; *UTS*, ultimate tensile strength.

TABLE 3.3	Summary of 3D-Printable Photopolymers and Their Properties at Ambient Temperature			
Material	**Common Print Method(s)**	**Mechanical Properties**		**Applications in Orthopedics**
Durable (Formlabs)	VP	UTS	28 MPa	• Nonimplant applications (including surgical guide, visualization aids, instruments, etc.)
		Mod	1 GPa	
		Failure strain	55%	
Accura PEAK (3D Systems)	VP	UTS	67 MPa	
		Mod	4.5 GPa	
		Failure strain	2%	
RPU 60 (Carbon)	VP	UTS	48 MPa	
		Mod	1.6 GPa	
		Failure strain	130%	
VisiJet M3-X (3D Systems)	MJ	UTS	50 MPa	
		Mod	2.1 GPa	
		Failure strain	8.3%	
VisiJet SR200 (3D Systems)	MJ	UTS	34 MPa	
		Mod	1.7 GPa	
		Failure strain	7.3%	
VisiJet PXL	BJ	UTS	14 MPa	
		Mod	9.4 GPa	
		Failure strain	0.23%	

BJ, Binder jetting; *Mod*, modulus of elasticity; *UTS*, ultimate tensile strength; *VP*, vat photopolymerization.

available in different grades, specifications, and testing methods. The data presented in the table is meant to be used only as a broad guidance. Typical orthopedic applications of the polymer as a nondegradable are also shown. To note is that photopolymer resins used in commercial 3D printing are typically sold under trade names (e.g., VeroBlack [Stratasys], Accura [3D Systems], etc.), and their exact compositions are not publicly released. These polymers are presented under their trade names in the summary table.

In this section, common nondegradable polymers that are used in orthopedics are presented. Current 3D-printed polymeric devices are dominated by nonimplants. There are only a handful of 3D-printed implantable devices that are available commercially but some of these implants are load-bearing devices, indicating the potential for more demanding applications in the future. Although many polymers are available for 3D printing, the majority are not implantable due to (1) low biocompatibility and limited clinical use history, and/or (2) bad printability (i.e., low dimensional accuracy and inferior properties). Hence from a materials perspective, there are two research frontiers in 3D printing for orthopedics applications: the development of new biocompatible print materials and methods to improve print quality. There is also a strong push toward the combined use of bioactive substances and synthetic substances, such as in the use of bone grafts to improve osteoconductivity and the use of impregnated antibiotics to reduce infection rates.

Composites

Introduction

Composites are materials that are produced from two or more constituent phases/components. The constituent materials are typically very dissimilar in their chemical or physical properties, and when merged, they create a material with properties unlike its individual counterparts. Bone is an example of a naturally occurring composite. The matrix of bone (into which cells are embedded) is composed of collagen as the main organic component and hydroxyapatite (HA) as the main inorganic or mineral component.[67] Collagen is responsible for the relatively high tensile strength of bone, whereas HA provides bone with relatively high compressive strength. These complimentary properties arising from the combination of two (or more) different materials are the essence of the beneficial use of composites for various applications. The attractive feature of composites is this possibility to have the best of both (and multiple) worlds. For instance, adding ceramic components into polymer matrices can improve the mechanical properties of polymers as well as their bioactivity. On the other hand, adding polymers or ceramics to metal-based materials can improve their biocompatibility and reduce stiffness. Finally, adding polymer fibers or other polymer additives to ceramics typically decreases their brittleness and provides reinforcement.

Composites have found widespread use in biomedical applications due to their ability to more closely mimic the complex nature of tissues as well as provide the possibility to overcome the drawbacks of certain materials. In biomedical composites, at least one of the constituent materials should ideally be bioactive. Moreover, composites can also be fully bioresorbable if resorbable components are used for their creation. In tissue engineering applications, composites are frequently used as scaffolds; for instance, to treat defective bone tissue. Proper selection of materials can lead to favorable functions such as osteoconductivity and osteoinductivity, while the composite material can be loaded with drugs and antibiotics to improve healing and prevent infections, respectively.[68]

In orthopedic applications, composites are promising materials for bone grafts, bone fracture repair, joint prostheses, craniofacial implants, and as artificial tendons and cartilage.[68,69] The use of composites in orthopedic applications can help overcome some limitations of single-material implants, such as stress shielding, radiopacity, high strength-to-weight ratio, and limited bone integration.[69] The most frequent type of composites used for orthopedic applications are polymer matrix composites, where typically an inorganic bioactive filler is added to the polymer matrix. HA is arguably the most widely used filler for this purpose. As it is one of the main components of bone, it is used in conjunction with other materials to improve bone healing. Other popular inorganic fillers include calcium phosphate (CaP) bioceramics and bioactive glass (BAG).[68]

Additive manufacturing (AM) or 3D printing of composites for orthopedic applications is a growing and developing field, as AM allows the manufacture of patient-specific implants with customizable designs. Although there are commercially available implants based on composites that are cleared for use in the human body, they have been manufactured using conventional processing techniques.

On the other hand, AM of composite implants may not only be useful to fabricate structures specific to a certain anatomy, but also to create surface finishes and porosities for easier osteointegration.[70] This opens up new opportunities in the development of 3D-printed composite implants, which is a flourishing research field. Composites can be 3D printed using the same techniques that are used for their individual counterparts, and an overview of these techniques and examples of 3D-printed composites used for orthopedic applications are provided here.

3D Printing Technologies for Composites

3D printing of composites for orthopedic applications is a quickly growing field due to the possibility of fine tuning the properties of the material and overcoming some drawbacks of monophasic implants, such as lack of bioactivity. The same 3D-printing technologies that are applied for the printing of composite individual counterparts can be adapted to print composite materials, and these techniques were explained in more detail in the previous sections on metals and polymers. The most frequently used techniques to print composites, specifically polymer-based composites, include material extrusion and VP. Careful optimization of parameters is needed during the printing of composites in order to achieve the required porosity and mechanical strength.[69]

Material Extrusion

Extrusion-based 3D-printing methods, such as fused deposition modeling (FDM), are simple and versatile, not requiring sophisticated instrumentation. FDM is one of the most frequent techniques for printing composites for orthopedic applications, and polymer matrix composites with different fillers are typically printed using this technique. FDM was previously described in more detail. Briefly, a polymer-based filament is extruded through a heated nozzle and deposited onto a stage. The filament is molten during deposition and is solidified afterward due to cooling when in contact with the stage. 3D structures are fabricated in a layer-by-layer manner by moving the nozzle and depositing the molten filament on top of each fabricated layer according to the sliced model.

In FDM, thermoplastic polymers are used for extrusion. The most frequently used polymer for printing with this technique, aimed at biomedical applications, is PLA and its different forms (poly-L-lactide [PLLA], poly-D-lactide [PDLA], etc.).[71] Other polymers include polycaprolactone (PCL), poly(lactide-co-glycolide) (PLGA), and PEEK. These are also used as matrices for composites printed via FDM. Filler particles, typically bioceramics, are mixed with the polymer granules and extruded into a filament. One complication specific to composites, compared to printing monophasic materials, is the need to create a composite filament with a consistent diameter and well-dispersed components in order to avoid their agglomeration.[69] In the case of polymer matrix composites with ceramics, agglomeration of ceramic particles within the polymer is a challenge that must be overcome to reduce its effect on the final printed part. Another challenge is the difference in physico-chemical characteristics between the polymer and ceramic phases, which may lead to lack of interaction and adhesion at the interface between the particles and the polymer matrix.

Vat Photopolymerization

VP techniques mainly encompass stereolithography (SLA) and digital light processing (DLP), depending on the light source used (laser beam in SLA and digital light projector in DLP).[71] These methods were previously explained in more detail. In brief, a computer-driven building stage is controlled according to the model slicing results, and a pattern is illuminated on the surface of a resin (via laser beam or digital light projector). A layer of resin is thus cured in a specific area of the surface and a section of the part is formed. The stage is either lowered or elevated and the solidified layer is covered with another layer of liquid resin. This process is repeated and the part is created in a layer-by-layer fashion. UV light is typically used to cure the resin. The resin therefore needs to consist of a photosensitive material and is typically a mixture of polymer precursors (monomers), crosslinkers, and photoinitiators.

In terms of composites, VP can be used to create polymer matrix composites reinforced with different kinds of fillers, most frequently bioceramics. Fillers can be added directly to the resin and mixed. One of the challenges arising from this method is the aggregation of particles within the resin, which needs to be overcome in order to obtain a homogeneously mixed material with isotropic mechanical properties. Another challenge associated with the method in general is the requirement for relatively low viscosity of the resin for it to remain printable. This is further complicated when particles are added. Therefore, the filler amount has to be carefully tuned.

Powder Bed Fusion

PBF encompasses several printing techniques which were previously described in more detail, wherein SLS is the method frequently used to print composites for orthopedic applications. This technique uses an infrared laser as the energy source and the printable materials are in powder form. Briefly, the powder is leveled using a flattening stick and the laser beam selectively sinters the powder according to the layer information in the model. After each layer solidifies, the powder bed is lowered and fresh powder is distributed across the surface using a roller, and the next layer is sintered until the part is complete. All excess powder is removed at the end.

One of the challenges of this technique when applied to composites is the generation of a fine powder, where the powder particles have a specific size range in order to achieve evenly sized layers.[69] Finer powders also lead to better surface finish of the parts. For polymers in particular, preprocessing of materials may be necessary in order to, for instance, remove moisture from the powder, which may affect the final

mechanical properties of the construct. SLS has been used to print polymer matrix composites with bioceramics such as HA-reinforced poly ethylene composites, as well as HA combined with PCL, PLA, and polyvinyl acetate (PVA).[69,71]

Binder Jetting

Binder jetting (BJ) is an AM technique that uses a somewhat similar approach to PBF, wherein binder droplets (instead of a laser as in PBF) are selectively deposited in the form of a jet onto a powder layer that is spread over a build platform using a roller.[72] The binder droplets act as an adhesive that binds the particles together to form a solid layer. Once a layer is completed the build platform is lowered, and fresh powder is distributed over the printed layer. Finally, when the part is printed, excess powder is removed. BJ is frequently used for 3D printing of bioceramics and can be adapted for polymer-ceramic composites, especially if the polymer is not sintered away after printing.

Bioprinting

In 3D bioprinting, tissue engineering scaffolds are produced via precise 3D deposition and patterning of biomaterials, living cells, and bioactive components, typically in a hydrogel matrix. Hydrogels are 3D networks of crosslinked hydrophilic polymer chains that swell in aqueous environments. They are frequently used in bioengineering and biomedical applications as carriers for cells and other biomaterials due to their highly hydrated environment and mechanical properties similar to those of soft tissues. Techniques used to print hydrogels along with other materials in bioprinting include extrusion printing, IJ printing, SLA, and laser-assisted bioprinting.[73]

In terms of biomedical applications, bioprinting is mostly focused on soft tissues, as the mechanical properties of hydrogels are typically within that range. Bioprinting is used in regenerative medicine applications and for tissue engineering. Wound closure and wound care are also a major focus for the use of bioprinting technologies. Vascularization of new tissues and their biological linkage are the main challenges in the field, as well as addressing the mechanical robustness of the constructs in order to print more complex structures. Bioprinting is a multidisciplinary field requiring collaborations between materials scientists, tissue engineers, and clinicians.[74] An ideal tissue engineering scaffold created via bioprinting aims to mimic the mechanical and biochemical properties of the targeted native tissue.[70] Therefore, the scaffold should have a suitable architecture and porosity to allow the flow of nutrients for cell growth. This is where a combination of different materials and the use of composites is an especially promising solution.[75-78] Moreover, the use of bioceramics as fillers for hydrogel-based scaffolds fabricated through bioprinting allows the achievement of osteoconductive properties and enhanced bioactivity.[79] Extrusion-based bioprinting is the easiest way to print composites, as inorganic fillers such as bioceramics can be mixed directly into the bioink to be extruded. SLA is another technique that can be used for composites, given that appropriate viscosity of the resin/bioink is maintained after the addition of fillers.

4D Printing

Stimuli-responsive materials offer an additional level of functionality to the printed constructs. The aim of 4D printing, where time is considered as the fourth dimension, is to mimic the complex and dynamic nature of living tissues. In essence, when a structure is printed, it can transform its shape when triggered by an external stimulus. It is a relatively new and increasingly popular technique to produce tissue-engineered scaffolds that may achieve better integration in vivo. Polymers are at the heart of this technique as they are the only class of materials that can offer a broad range of responsiveness to external stimuli. Shape transformations can be triggered by heat, light, or moisture, and magnetic or electric fields.[80] Shape-memory polymers are a class of stimuli-responsive materials that can be used for 4D printing. The main feature of shape-memory polymers is the possibility to program them into a temporary shape, whereas upon application of a stimulus, they would return to their original, permanent shape. These polymers are promising for biomedical and orthopedic applications where their unique properties could be used in minimally invasive surgeries and deployment.[81] 4D printing can be accomplished using different printing techniques that mainly depend on the choice of shape-changing and shape-memory materials. In terms of composite 4D printing, the main systems are again polymer matrix composites with added functional fillers. The most frequently used strategy to 4D print such composites is extrusion-based printing, where the stimuli-responsive polymer filament is produced with a dispersed filler (e.g., a bioceramic) within the filament.

3D Printing of Composites for Orthopedic Applications

An ideal orthopedic implant material needs to rapidly induce new bone formation and integrate with juxtaposed bone. It also needs to possess sufficient initial mechanical strength for load-bearing applications and should maintain its mechanical integrity until new bone formation is complete. In some applications it is also favorable if the material fully degrades afterward to avoid the need for follow-up surgeries and implant-removal procedures. In an effort to create such implant materials, different types of composites were developed. The following sections focus on 3D printing of various composite materials aimed at biomedical applications.

Polymers and Ceramics

Polymer matrix composites are the most widespread type of composites used for biomedical applications. In particular, the combination of polymers and ceramics is favorable for various orthopedic applications. Bioceramics are typically added to polymer matrices for reinforcement and bioactivity. Considerable research efforts have been devoted to the

development of composites with suitable biomechanical characteristics for implantation. Biocompatible, strong, and tough polymers such as PEEK, PEKK, PMMA, and polyethylene (PE) have been used as matrices for various types of composites.[69] One of the benefits of these polymers over metals, in addition to their high strength, is their radiolucency, which aids in the postoperative imaging of the implants via MRI, CT, and X-ray. As these polymers are bioinert, adding bioceramics imparts them with bioactive properties and stimulates enhanced bone apposition for load-bearing orthopedic applications.[82] Aside from these nondegradable matrices, an array of biodegradable composites has been explored for orthopedic applications, including bioceramic-loaded PLA, PCL, and PLGA. These composites are discussed in more detail in the "Degradable Materials" section.

The most frequently used bioceramics that are added to polymers include HA and other CaPs, as well as BAGs.[83] HA and CaPs are known to have excellent bioactivity, they are biodegradable, and their chemical compositions are similar to the mineral phase of natural bone. They are added to polymers to provide the composite material with osteoconductivity and to facilitate better osteointegration of the implant. Aside from CaPs, other phosphates such as magnesium phosphates (MgPs) can be used as polymer fillers for orthopedic applications.[84] More information on bioceramics can be found in the corresponding section in the biodegradable materials part. Titanium dioxide or TiO_2 (titania) is also frequently added to polymers to form composites suitable for orthopedic applications.[85] However, unlike CaPs, titania is not biodegradable.

PMMA is frequently used for orthopedic applications, but it has limited osseointegration and heat is released during its polymerization reaction. To address these issues, ceramics such as BAGs, silicates, HA, and other CaPs have been added to PMMA matrices, which also results in improvement of the polymer's mechanical properties.[69] HA and tricalcium phosphate integration into PMMA can significantly reduce the amount of heat generated during polymerization and facilitate cell attachment.[69]

Composites based on PEEK are also frequently explored for their potential in orthopedic applications, particularly for load-bearing situations due to the favorable mechanical properties of PEEK.[69] The most popular reinforcement for PEEK, carbon fibers, are discussed later. In terms of bioceramics, the most frequently used filler for PEEK is HA. Medical-grade HA-reinforced PEEK is commercially available through Invibio Biomaterial Solutions under the brand name PEEK-OPTIMA HA Enhanced and is focused on spinal device technologies. Full integration of HA in the PEEK matrix, instead of just coating the polymer, makes the osteoconductivity of HA available throughout the material. Amorphous magnesium phosphate (AMP) was also explored as an additive to PEEK, and bioactive and osseointegrable PEEK-based composite filaments were melt-blended with AMP particles for 3D printing of dental and orthopedic implants (Fig. 3.6).[84]

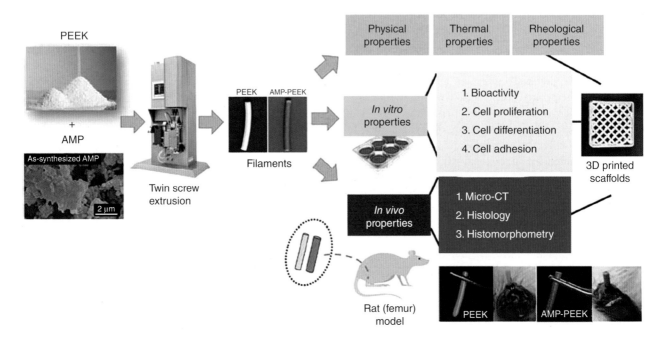

• **Fig. 3.6** Schematic illustration of the fabrication steps as well as the physical, thermal, rheological, and biological characterizations of amorphous magnesium phosphate-poly(ether ketone) composite filaments for 3D-printing applications. *AMP*, Amorphous magnesium phosphate; *PEEK*, poly(ether ether ketone). (Source: Sikder P, Ferreira JA, Fakhrabadi EA, et al. Bioactive amorphous magnesium phosphate-poly-etheretherketone composite filaments for 3D printing. *Dent Mat.* 2020;36:865-883. doi: https://doi.org/10.1016/j.dental.2020.04.008.)

Polymers and Metals

The combination of metals that are capable of load bearing and polymers that can contain bioactive species and biomaterials is a promising strategy for orthopedic applications. It is technically challenging to print both metals and polymers simultaneously, especially if hydrogels are to be used to encapsulate biomaterials. Therefore, composites of polymers and metals that are aimed at orthopedic applications typically consist of a 3D-printed porous metal framework (printed via PBF) with an infused polymer that may contain bioactive components for faster and more efficient bone healing. In this manner, the metal-based construct is imparted with bioactivity, whereas the polymer component receives mechanical reinforcement. Simultaneous printing of metals and polymers is technically challenging.

Titanium alloys have great advantages in orthopedic metal implants and have been discussed previously in the section on metals. Porous titanium alloy scaffolds and implants have been 3D printed and used for bone defect repair due to their favorable high surface areas and lower stiffness (compared to solid parts) similar to that of cortical bone. The internal porous structures also present the opportunity for filling them with bioactive components and other materials. For instance, this approach has been realized in 3D-printed porous Ti scaffolds that were filled with simvastatin/poloxamer 407 hydrogel, and the effects of bone ingrowth, osseointegration, and neovascularization were evaluated using an in vivo tibial defect rabbit model.[86] Simvastatin, when locally administered, has an excellent effect on bone formation, whereas poloxamer 407 is a thermosensitive

hydrogel with low toxicity and weak immunogenicity that is used as the carrier material for simvastatin. The composite scaffolds improved osseointegration and bone ingrowth, and were found to be promising for bone defect treatment.

In a similar approach, a hybrid polymer-metal scaffold was created via 3D printing of a Ti_6Al_4V alloy into a porous structure and the pores were subsequently filled with multifunctional polysaccharide hydrogels with incorporated bone marrow stem cells (Fig. 3.7).[87] The polysaccharide-based hydrogels were self-healable, injectable, biocompatible, and biodegradable. It was demonstrated that these composite scaffolds could depress inflammatory cytokines, restore decayed knee cartilage, and promote bone integrity capability in a rabbit rheumatoid arthritis animal model after 3 months.

Metals and Ceramics

Standard metals for orthopedic implants, such as titanium and its alloys, are durable, and nontoxic but lack bioactivity. Bioceramics, on the other hand, can strongly promote new bone formation but are susceptible to brittle failure. Thus, it may be beneficial to combine these two types of materials in a composite to gain the mechanical reliability of metals along with the bone-bonding ability of bioceramics, potentially reducing the incidence of implant failure.[88] BAG-, HA-, and CaP-based bioceramics can be used for this purpose due to their excellent bioactivity and the possibility to promote osseointegration.

Processing of metal-ceramic composites by AM approaches can lead to highly porous functional lattices, whose stiffness can be tailored to meet the mechanical properties of

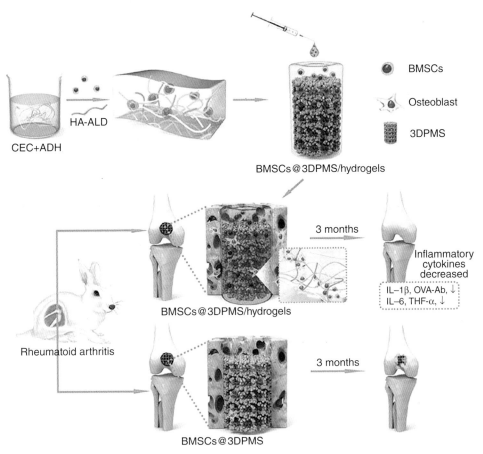

• **Fig. 3.7** Schematic illustration showing the fabrication process of hydrogels combined with 3D-printed porous metal scaffolds to deliver bone marrow stem cells for rheumatoid arthritis treatment. *3DPMS,* 3D printing porous metal scaffolds; *ADH,* adipic dihydrazide; *BMSCs,* bone marrow stem cells; *CEC,* N-carboxyethyl chitosan; *HA-ALD,* Hyaluronic acid-aldehyde. (Source: Zhao Y, Wang Z, Jiang Y, et al. Biomimetic composite scaffolds to manipulate stem cells for aiding rheumatoid arthritis management. *Adv Funct Mat.* 2019;29:1807860. doi: https://doi.org/10.1002/adfm.201807860.)

natural bone tissue. It is a technological challenge to find the AM technique that is suitable for both metal and ceramic or glass feedstocks. Laser metal deposition (LMD) can be used, as it provides the flexibility of changing the metal and ceramic or glass feedstock to print the layers alternatively. PBF, and more specifically selective laser melting (SLM), is another promising AM technique to print metal-ceramic composites. The constituent powders can be mixed beforehand in a specific composition and can then be fed into the printer. The composition of the starting phases is expected to remain unchanged upon processing, although the powders get molten under the laser beam. An alternative approach can be used based on controlled reactions that occur upon processing between the precursor powders to achieve new constituent phases.[88]

Composites With Carbon-Based Materials

PEEK is one of the more frequently used polymers for orthopedic applications. Due to its favorable mechanical properties and the possibility of use for load-bearing applications, it presents an attractive alternative to conventional metal or ceramic orthopedic implants (more information about PEEK can be found in the polymer section). To further enhance the mechanical properties of PEEK, different types of composites have been developed. In particular, carbon fiber–reinforced materials have been used for spinal and other orthopedic applications for more than two decades.[89] Carbon fiber–reinforced PEEK is a promising composite material for orthopedic applications due to its high strength and endurance, as well as stiffness range matching that of cortical bone.[90,91] It is radiolucent in all diagnostic imaging modes (MRI, CT, and X-ray), which benefits postoperative monitoring of tissues at the site of implantation. Moreover, as with other polymer-based or ceramic-based materials, it can be used where metal allergies are a risk. Carbon fiber–reinforced PEEK is the first FDA-approved composite of PEEK used for biomedical applications.[69] It has since been used for an array of commercial implants manufactured by icotec AG (Switzerland).[90] The material is known under the brand name Black-Armor and represents a clinical track record of 15 years and 20,000 implantations in spinal and fracture surgical care. However, the implants are manufactured using the company's composite flow-molding process and not 3D printed. The leading manufacturer of medical-grade PEEK, Invibio Biomaterial Solutions, offers PEEK reinforced with short carbon fibers dispersed within the polymer matrix (PEEK-OPTIMA

Reinforced), as well as continuous carbon fibers (PEEK-OPTIMA Ultra-Reinforced).

In terms of carbon fiber-reinforced PEEK 3D printing, FDM has been used to print these composite structures.[92] Tensile, bending, and compressive tests were performed to evaluate the mechanical properties of the FDM-printed composites. Compared to pure FDM-printed PEEK, the mechanical properties of carbon fiber-reinforced PEEK were significantly enhanced, making it a promising material to print implants for orthopedic applications.

Graphene oxide is another filler that can be used for polymer matrices. It is known to be an excellent antimicrobial agent that can also enhance the final mechanical properties of the composite part. For instance, graphene oxide was blended with thermoplastic PU and PLA, and the composite material was 3D printed via FDM into complex structures.[93] The addition of graphene oxide significantly enhanced the compressive and tensile modulus of the material.

Properties and Performance

Mechanical Properties

Any implanted material should exhibit excellent mechanical properties (elastic modulus, yield strength, and ultimate tensile and compressive strength) to withstand various biomechanical forces, and composites designed for orthopedic applications aim to have optimal mechanical properties in order to achieve superior biomechanical performance in vivo. Wear resistance and longevity of the implant are additional important characteristics. Composites typically consist of two phases: the matrix phase and the reinforcement phase. Reinforcing additives fill the matrix phase, which results in higher strength and stiffness of the composite material compared to the matrix material alone. Ultimately, the implant device must be capable of withstanding large torques and forces caused by compression and shear in normal loading conditions for good mechanical force transfer.[94]

Human bone has variable mechanical properties depending on its type (cortical or cancellous) or other characteristics, such as sex and age.[69] These properties need to be taken into account while designing composite 3D-printed implants. The elastic modulus of the material ideally needs to match that of bone at the site of implantation. Thankfully, the wide range of materials and their combinations that can be used for biomedical composites facilitates fine-tuning of their final mechanical properties. For example, simply altering the amount of filler in the matrix material will achieve tailorable strength, stiffness, and strain at failure of the composite under different loading scenarios. Aside from composition, the interaction between the individual phases in the composite is also important to consider as it will influence the final mechanical properties of the material.

In terms of materials, different classes can be combined into a composite material and 3D printed. Polymers, ceramics, and metals can all serve as either matrices or fillers. For orthopedic applications, polymer-ceramic composites are the most frequent system. Bioceramics not only add bioactivity

to polymer-based materials but also provide reinforcement, increasing the final strength and modulus of the material. At the same time, this helps to overcome the main challenge of ceramics, which is their brittle nature. Composites with metals and their alloys allow the addition of bioactivity to the metallic materials.

The design of the implant, which is based on the location and anatomical geometry of the defect, will also dictate the final mechanical properties of the construct. Adding more porosity to the structure decreases the strength of the material, but at the same time promotes cell infiltration and proliferation. 3D printing aids in the making of any complex shapes, while solid and porous sections can be combined in one implant for providing optimal strength and performance.[74] However, different printing techniques can result in different mechanical properties of the final construct. For instance, FDM-printed structures may have weaker mechanical properties in the Z direction due to insufficient layer fusion.

Chemical Properties

The chemical properties of orthopedic composite materials need to be considered along with their mechanical properties. Typically, this involves finding a suitable synthetic strategy for the creation of the composite. In terms of polymers, this includes synthesis of the polymer and its cross-linking strategies, which can be either chemical or physical. The interaction between the different material phases in a composite is critical for the successful processing of the material via 3D printing as well as the final mechanical properties of the construct. Relatively high adhesion and chemical interaction between the phases is favorable as this will create a more homogeneous structure with isotropic mechanical properties. It can also help to improve fracture resistance. Corrosion resistance is another chemical property that is essential for successful orthopedic implants and aging resistance is a requirement for polymer-based implant materials. For some applications, degradation resistance is also needed from polymers. On the other hand, if degradable materials are being designed, the degradation reactions need to be considered in order to avoid toxic degradation products in vivo.

Biological Properties

The implants used for orthopedic applications need to be biocompatible to be successfully implanted and maintained in vivo. Bioactivity is also preferable in order to facilitate a more efficient bone healing and remodeling process. Bioceramics are excellent candidates as fillers to add the required bioactivity to otherwise bioinert materials such as many polymers and metals. Osteoconductivity and improved osseointegration are other important characteristics of orthopedic implants, which can be added by adding bioceramic fillers such as CaPs and HA. For specific applications, biodegradability of the implants may be preferred to avoid subsequent implant-removal surgeries. In this case, biodegradable polymers along with bioceramics are typically used. Material selection then focuses on materials that have nontoxic degradation products. Infections that may occur after implantation can be avoided by using antibiotics added to the implant materials, either as coatings or fillers.

Summary and Future Trends

With the increasing use of orthopedic implants worldwide, and especially 3D-printed implants, there is great interest in developing novel materials and technologies to further improve the clinical performance of the devices. The use of composites for orthopedic applications is a growing and developing field due to the ability to tune the properties of the material and overcome limitations associated with monophasic implants. The ideal composite biomaterial should be biocompatible, durable, easily processable, and cost effective, and have sufficiently good mechanical properties. 3D printing opens up new opportunities for many of these criteria, such as cost-effectiveness, high-throughput production, and customizability. Promising results have already been obtained for 3D-printed orthopedic implants consisting of one material, where customizable implant shapes lead to a better fit and thus better postoperative outcomes. Nevertheless, limited integration with native bone is often a challenge. Implant-bone integration is critical for successful transfer of load from the implant to bone to avoid weakening of the adjacent bone and implant exposure as a result. Therefore, considerable efforts have been focused on the use of composite materials for orthopedic implants as the use of composites can enhance implant-bone integration by imparting the implant with bioactivity. As such, the main focus has been placed on polymer-based materials with ceramic fillers. For composites in general, it has been shown that adjusting the composition of multiple phases in the composite material can lead to optimal balance in terms of the final chemical-biological-mechanical properties of the implant.

Even though there are commercially available composite orthopedic implants, they are still manufactured using conventional techniques and not 3D printed. Promising research results have been obtained for 3D-printed composite implants, but they still require rigorous testing and FDA approval to be applied in surgical practice. Selecting materials for composites that have already been cleared by the FDA and used for orthopedic applications may be an option for faster translation to the clinic. The long-term effects of implanted 3D-printed composite materials should be the focus of future work to understand the critical tolerances and requirements for these implants in the clinical setting. Processability of the composite materials via 3D-printing techniques is another field where improvement is critical for the success of printed implants.

Degradable Materials

Introduction

The last couple of decades have seen a significant rise in the use of biodegradable materials in medical implants. Biodegradability in the context of medical implants is the quality of being able to disintegrate over time during implantation in the body. Bioabsorbable is a more specific term that refers to a biodegradable material whose degradation product has the capability to pass through, be metabolized, or assimilated by cells/tissues.[95] Biodegradable materials are available in many forms such as polymers, metals, and composites. The major considerations of using biodegradable materials include its degradation rate, mode, and product, in addition to all the standard considerations of using a regular stable material (biocompatibility, etc.). The degradation rate of a material needs to be suitable for the intended application of a device and should be considered in the context of required properties (e.g., mechanical property, etc.).

The use of biodegradables in an implant obviates the need for a secondary device-removal surgery, and when compared to permanent implants it reduces the chance of complications. Biodegradables are currently used for providing temporary mechanical support, delivery of bioactive substances, and tissue engineering scaffolds. Examples of commercial biodegradable implants includes suture threads, cardiovascular stents, and meshes. Biodegradable polymers are also extensively used in orthopedics, common examples being in fixation devices, interference screws, and suture anchors.

Metals

Magnesium (Mg)-, iron (Fe)-, and zinc (Zn)-based materials have been proposed as biodegradable metallics for use in implants. The primary advantage of degradable metals is the combination of initial strength while allowing for healing, with long-term bone regeneration resulting in no foreign material remaining in the body over time. Challenges associated with fine-tuning degradation rates as opposed to the associated reduction in mechanical properties require further research. For example, the rate of degradation of Mg-based materials is faster than Fe-based materials, where Zn-based materials lie somewhere in between. Thus, depending on the requirements for the application, different materials or a hybrid strategy may be appropriate.[96,97] PBF as well as extrusion 3D printing have been described in scientific literature for the fabrication of porous degradable metallic scaffolds.[13,97]

Polymers

The biodegradable device market is currently dominated by polymers. A major advantage of biodegradable polymers over other types of materials is their long and established clinical usage history. In this section, synthetic polymers that are important in orthopedics are discussed, with emphasis on aspects related to 3D printing. Polymers can be classified according to their degradation mode—hydrolytically and enzymatically degradable. The degradation of hydrolytically degradable polymers is driven by contact with water, while enzymatically degradable polymer degradation is driven by contact with enzymes. The majority of commercial biodegradable polymers today are hydrolytically degradable. In the degradation process, the bulk polymer is first hydrated, then the initially long polymer chains are broken into smaller chains, and eventually eroded from the bulk via mechanical stimuli. Typically, molecular weight loss is observed in the earliest phase of the degradation, followed by mechanical property loss, and finally mass loss. In choosing a degradable polymer, beyond the type of polymer itself, it is important to consider characteristics that are affected by processing, such as molecular weight and crystallinity.

Poly(α-ester)s

The poly(α-ester)s family of polymers are by far the most popular polymers in commercial biodegradable implants and the most widely studied. Common poly(α-ester)s are as follows:

1. *Poly(glycolide) or poly(glycolic acid) (PGA):* PGA is a thermoplastic simple linear aliphatic polyester. Its degradation products are natural metabolites, making it attractive for implant use. PGA was the first biodegradable used as a suture and has a long clinical history. PGA has been shown to be 3D printable via extrusion.[98] Although studies on PBF-printed PGA is scarce, it has been shown in a past study to be printable when mixed with PEEK.[99]

2. *Poly(lactides) or poly(lactic acid) (PLA):* PLA is one of the most ubiquitous thermoplastic polymers in both biodegradable implants and in 3D printing. However, to the best of the authors' knowledge, no 3D-printed PLA device is currently commercially available. PLA is commercially available in its two stereoisomers, PDLA and PLLA. PLLA and PDLA degrade over a relatively long timeframe of up to 2 years. In addition to PDLA and PLLA, polymerization of racemic (D,L)-lactide results in poly(D,L-lactide) (PDLLA). Due to lower crystallinity, PDLLA degrades at a much faster rate. PLA is highly amenable to 3D printing via extrusion. Extrusion-printed

parts show good mechanical properties but possess anisotropy that is characteristic of 3D printing.[100]

3. *Poly(lactide-co-glycolide) (PLGA):* PLGA is a copolymer of PLA and PGA. PLGA has a much lower degradation time than its constituents. Depending on the copolymerization ratio, PLGA can degrade very quickly, with a lifetime as low as a couple months. PLGA can be 3D printed via PBF[101] and extrusion.[102] An example of a commercial orthopedic application of PLGA is the Lactosorb Fixation System (Biomet).

4. *Polycaprolactone (PCL):* PCL is a thermoplastic semicrystalline polymer with a relatively long degradation time. The majority of commercial 3D-printed biodegradable implants are currently fabricated out of PCL. Although PCL is amenable to both extrusion and PBF printing, the majority of current FDA-cleared commercial devices are fabricated via PBF. One of the earliest in-human devices is a pediatric PCL tracheal splint. In orthopedics, 3D-printed PCL has been used in a personalized bone graft cage (TruMatch, J&J), craniofacial repair meshes (Osteomesh, Osteopore), and a cranial bone filler (TRS).

5. *Polydioxanone (PDO):* PDO is a thermoplastic with excellent mechanical properties and biocompatibility. It is considered the material of choice for fracture fixation[103] and is used in devices that are considered standard practice in surgeries[104] (e.g., Orthosorb, J&J). Dioxanone filaments used for extrusion 3D printing are widely available commercially.

In addition to these polymers, many variations exist that involve blends and copolymers containing minor components of other polymers, the properties of which are presented in Table 3.4. It is important to note that, ultimately, degradation time will strongly depend on the specifics of the device, including factors such as processing, device dimensions, and the location at which it is implanted. The degradation time presented here is intended to be used as rough guidance.

TABLE 3.4 Properties of Common Biodegradable Poly(α-ester)s[124-125]

Material	Print Method(s)	Mechanical Properties	Degradation Time (Months)	Applications in Orthopedics
PLA	Extrusion, PBF	UTS = 65.4 MPa; Mod = 2.54 GPa; FS = 10%	>24	• Fracture fixation, pins and screws, suture anchors, nails
PGA	Extrusion, PBF	UTS = 330 MPa; Mod = 7.0 GPa; FS = 20%	6–12	• Fracture fixation, pins and screws, nails, drug delivery
PLGA 85/15	Extrusion, PBF	UTS = 65 MPa; Mod = 4 GPa; FS = 10%	5–6	• Interference screws, suture anchors, drug delivery
PCL	Extrusion, PBF	UTS = 25 MPa; Mod = 0.4 GPa; FS = 500%	24–36	• Bone graft cage, craniofacial implants
PDO	Extrusion	UTS = 490 MPa; Mod = 2.1 GPa; FS = 35%	>3	• Fracture fixations

Mod, Modulus of elasticity; *PBF,* powder bed fusion; *PCL,* polycaprolactone; *PDO,* polydioxanone; *PGA,* poly(glycolide) or poly(glycolic acid); *PLA,* polylactic acid; *PLGA,* poly(lactide-co-glycolide); *UTS,* ultimate tensile strength.

Other Biodegradable Synthetic Polymers

Poly(trimethylene carbonate) (TMC) is a degradable polymer that is often used for copolymerization with poly(α-ester)s. An example is a copolymer of glycolide and TMC used in biodegradable fixation devices (e.g., Suretac, Acufex Inc.). The copolymerization process results in a polymer that is more flexible and degrades at a faster rate.[11] In addition to TMC, there are many biodegradable polymers that have seen some research interest, such as poly(hydroxyalkanoates) (PHA), poly(amino acids), polyfumarates, PUs, and polyphospazenes.

Hydrogels

Recent research in tissue engineering, has focused on using cells, signaling factors, and the scaffold material itself to better restore tissue and organ structure and function.[82,105] The types of materials, cells, and growth factors very depending on the target tissue/organ, but several requirements need to be fulfilled for the final scaffold, such as biocompatibility, mechanical support, porosity, and bioresorbability.[82] Hydrogels are crosslinked 3D hydrophilic polymer networks that swell in aqueous environments, creating a favorable hydrated environment for the encapsulation of cells and other biological materials. Hydrogels are frequently used in biomedical applications and especially in tissue engineering due to their ability to mimic the native cell environment and match the mechanical properties of soft tissues. Many synthetic hydrogels are being developed and their biomechanical properties can be adjusted by altering their material chemistries and compositions, as well as processing steps.[82] However, synthetic hydrogels are typically less biocompatible and their degradation products may be toxic. Therefore, growing focus is on the use of naturally derived polymers for hydrogels. These biopolymers are primarily based on extracellular constituents such as collagen, hyaluronic acid, fibrin, or other biologically derived components such as alginate and gelatin.[82,106] These polymers are inherently biocompatible, have limited toxicity, and most are biodegradable. However, their weak mechanical properties are a frequent challenge that can be solved, for instance, by reinforcing them with bioceramics.

Bioprinting is the AM field that is focused on hydrogel 3D printing along with living cells and other biological materials. Using this technique, cells and biomaterials are dispensed together with micrometer precision in order to form tissue-like constructs.[105] Bioprinting is gaining a lot of attention in tissue engineering applications, as it enables the fabrication of engineered tissue constructs at ambient conditions. The most common techniques used in bioprinting are extrusion printing, IJ printing, SLA, and laser-assisted bioprinting.[73] In terms of orthopedic applications, the use of hydrogel bioprinting is problematic due to their weak mechanical properties and thus lack of ability to bear adequate loads. Moreover, the low stiffness of hydrogels and hydrogel-based printed constructs could inhibit osteogenic differentiation.[105]

Bioceramics

Bioceramics are mostly used in orthopedic applications as an alternative to metals. Their compressive properties typically match those of bone and they are frequently biocompatible and bioactive, which makes them advantageous over metals. However, they are brittle and their mechanical properties are overall lower compared to native bone, which limits their use as load-bearing implant materials. Nevertheless, they have found widespread use in orthopedic applications as coating and reinforcing components, as well as bone grafts and bone cements/adhesives.[75,82,94]

HA and other CaP ceramics have been used for biomedical applications for decades due to their excellent biocompatibility, bioactivity, osteoconductivity, and mechanical strength.[82] They have been studied for use in craniofacial bone repair due to their bioactivity and as well as chemical compositions similar to the mineral phase of natural bone.[69] These bioceramics are resorbable through a cell-mediated procedure involving osteoclast activity. Tricalcium phosphates (such as a-TCP and b-TCP) have a Ca/P ratio that is close to natural bone tissue. HA and CaPs are biocompatible and biodegradable, and their degradation time depends on the composition and can be tuned to allow time for deposition of new bone.[69] However, the main drawback of CaP bioceramics is their brittle nature and low mechanical strength, which limits their application in bone repair. Injectable CaPs in the form of bone cements are used as bone substitute materials to improve their ceramic handling ability and to better fill defects in complex geometric shapes,[82] and they can provide necessary mechanical soft tissue support after hardening.[75]

Calcium sulfates are another type of bioceramic material used for orthopedic applications due to their biocompatibility, rapid resorption rate, and unique ability to stimulate osteogenesis.[82] Calcium sulfate can be combined with HA to improve its resorption rate and create faster resorbing materials. When used for bone grafts, the faster resorbing calcium sulfate will leave space for the bone tissue to grow into, while the osteoconductive HA material will guide the bone cells to grow in and onto the bone graft material.[82] MgPs have recently been explored as an alternative to CaPs. The rationale behind this is the sufficient solubility of MgP phases under in vivo conditions and the fact that Mg^{2+} is a potent inhibitor of HA crystal growth, thereby suppressing unwanted crystallization in vivo.[107]

3D printing of bioceramic-based orthopedic implants is a challenging but promising field.[108,109] The main challenge is the brittle nature of bioceramic materials. Nevertheless, bioceramics in the form of powders can be 3D printed using different techniques and used, for instance, as bone graft materials or scaffolds (Fig. 3.8).[82,110] Such patient-specific 3D-printed structures can be beneficial for the reconstruction of complex bone defects. Porous ceramic scaffolds can be produced by printing a mold with wax and subsequently infiltrating it with the ceramic slurry, and then burning out the negative matrix material. Scaffolds can also be prepared through spray-drying

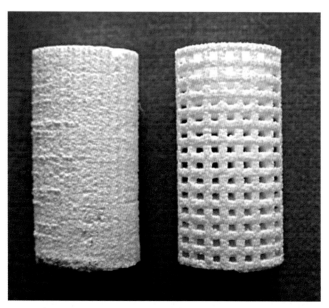

• **Fig. 3.8** 3D-printed tricalcium phosphate scaffolds with a dense *(left)* and porous *(right)* structure. (Source: Wieding J, Fritsche A, Heinl P, et al. Biomechanical behavior of bone scaffolds made of additive manufactured tricalciumphosphate and titanium alloy under different loading conditions. *J Appl Biomater Funct Mater.* 2013;11:159-166. doi:10.5301/jabfm.2013.10832.)

granules of the ceramic material which contain polymeric additives as a binder.[82] BJ is frequently used to print ceramic parts.[111] In this case, polymers are typically used as binders and the final printed constructs are then sintered at high temperatures to remove the polymer.[112] Extrusion-based printing is also common for ceramic materials. In this approach, a printing ink is created, similar to bioinks in bioprinting, where the ceramic particles are dispersed in water to form a viscous slurry, which is then extruded through a nozzle in a layer-by-layer fashion.[112] Sintering is then performed to achieve the final ceramic part. High loading of particles is needed to minimize cracks and distortion created during sintering. VP approaches such as DLP can increase shape complexity which is a challenge for ceramic FDM.[113] Using this approach, a slurry is prepared containing a photosensitive resin and ceramic powder, and is printed via DLP.[114] After printing, the green body is subjected to heat treatment involving two steps: debinding and sintering.

Bioactive Glasses

Bioactive glasses (BAGs) are another type of bioceramic frequently used either as fillers or on their own for orthopedic applications. The main components of BAGs are Na_2O, CaO, SiO_2, and P_2O_5, which are known to support osteoblast cells.[69] BAGs can also bond with the host soft tissue without the formation of fibrous tissue. BAGs are attractive scaffold materials due to their ability to stimulate angiogenesis in the presence of vascular endothelial growth factor (VEGF).[75] Similarly to bioceramics, despite their bioactivity and compressive modulus similar to that of bone, their

brittle nature makes them inappropriate for load-bearing applications. Another drawback of BAGs is their limited processability, as it is not possible to reshape them during surgery to improve the implant fit.[69] BAGs can be prepared in a range of forms, from soluble to nonresorbable, by tuning their composition. Sr- and Zn-doped BAGs have recently emerged as materials of particular interest, as these ions were shown to control bone formation. Sr can enhance osteoblastic proliferation and decrease osteoclastic turnover, whereas Zn can provide enhanced antibacterial efficacy and is linked to improved bone quality.[82] BAGs can be 3D printed using the same approaches as for bioceramics. The most common techniques include material (slurry) extrusion, SLA, and BJ.[112]

Composites

Creating bioresorbable and biodegradable orthopedic implants is a field of growing focus due to their ability to better integrate with biological tissues as well as eliminate implant-removal operations.[82] Customizing biodegradable materials through the use of composites is a promising strategy to create implants with specific biological and mechanical properties. Bioresorbable and biodegradable composites allow tuning of the final material absorption and degradation times, respectively, leading to more efficient healing in vivo. Herein, polymer matrix composites are the focus, wherein typically the matrix polymer is combined with bioactive and resorbable bioceramics. Biodegradable and resorbable polymers used as the matrix for such composites include PLA, PCL, PGA, and their copolymers (e.g., PLGA, PLCL).[115,116] Poly(ester urea)s (PEUs) are another class of polymers where degradation and mechanical behavior can be adjusted based on their chemical composition.[117] Bioceramics such as HA and other CaPs are currently one of the preferred materials for bone reconstruction. Bone graft substitutes in the form of 3D-printed scaffolds are frequently made of PCL, PLGA, and b-TCP or HA.[70] By controlling the filler content within the composite, it is possible to customize the material properties and thus the final implant properties as well.[82] Using composite fillers to modify material properties also allows challenges in the use of bioabsorbables for orthopedic applications to be addressed, such as adverse tissue reactions and degradation byproducts and time.[82]

The same 3D-printing techniques used for nondegradable composites are also used for the degradable composites. One of the most frequent techniques is FDM, where bioceramic particles are dispersed in biodegradable polymer filaments (such as PLA, PLGA, PCL, etc.).[118,119] For instance, HA and silk particles were incorporated into PLA and the composite filaments were 3D printed via FDM into bone clips,[120] and the feasibility of the printed bone clips as internal fixation devices was evaluated using an in vivo animal model. Nano-HA was recently blended with PEU and printed into porous biodegradable and bioactive scaffolds via FDM. It was shown that 3D-printed HA-containing PEU composites promoted bone regeneration and thus have the potential to be used in

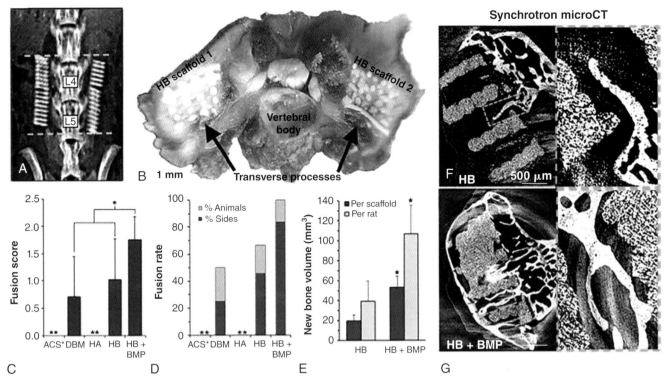

• **Fig. 3.9** Evaluation of hyperelastic bone 3D-printed scaffolds in vivo for rat spinal fusion. (Source: Jakus AE, Rutz AL, Jordan SW, et al. Hyperelastic "bone": a highly versatile, growth factor-free, osteoregenerative, scalable, and surgically friendly biomaterial. *Sci Transl Med.* 2016;8:358ra127. doi:10.1126/scitranslmed.aaf7704.)

orthopedic applications.[117] In another strategy, nano-HA was grafted onto poly(D-lactic acid) (PDLA) via in situ ring-opening polymerization of D-lactide, followed by blending with PLLA, which yielded a biocomposite with improved mechanical properties.[121] The material was processed into a filament and used for 3D printing via FDM.

Extrusion-based printing in the form of printing liquid inks was recently used to print a composite called hyperelastic bone (Fig. 3.9). It is composed of 90 wt% HA and 10 wt% PCL or PLGA, and it can be rapidly 3D printed at room temperature.[122] This material may offer promising bone-reconstruction capabilities. Extrusion-based printing of liquid inks was also used to print HA and demineralized bone matrix (DBM) particles in a PLGA matrix as potential bone graft substitutes.[116]

References

1. Ricles LM, Coburn JC, Di Prima M, Oh SS. Regulating 3D-printed medical products. *Sci Transl Med.* 2018;10:eaan6521. doi:10.1126/scitranslmed.aan6521.
2. Kelly CN, Miller AT, Hollister SJ, Guldberg RE, Gall K. Design and structure–function characterization of 3D printed synthetic porous biomaterials for tissue engineering. *Adv Healthc Mater.* 2018;7:1701095.
3. Al-Ketan O, Rowshan R, Abu Al-Rub RK. Topology-mechanical property relationship of 3D printed strut, skeletal, and sheet based periodic metallic cellular materials. *Addit Manuf.* 2018;19:167-183. doi:10.1016/j.addma.2017.12.006.
4. Speirs M, Van Hooreweder B, Van Humbeeck J, Kruth JP. Fatigue behaviour of NiTi shape memory alloy scaffolds produced by SLM, a unit cell design comparison. *J Mech Behav Biomed Mater.* 2017;70:53-59. doi:10.1016/j.jmbbm.2017.01.016.
5. Dadbakhsh S, Speirs M, Kruth JP, Schrooten J, Luyten J, Van Humbeeck J. Effect of SLM parameters on transformation temperatures of shape memory nickel titanium parts. *Adv Eng Mater.* 2014;16:1140-1146. doi:10.1002/adem.201300558.
6. Habijan T, Haberland C, Meier H, et al. The biocompatibility of dense and porous nickel-titanium produced by selective laser melting. *Mater Sci Eng C Mater Biol Appl.* 2013;33:419-426. doi:10.1016/j.msec.2012.09.008.
7. Polozov I, Sufiiarov V, Popovich A, Masaylo D, Grigoriev A. Synthesis of Ti-5Al, Ti-6Al-7Nb, and Ti-22Al-25Nb alloys from elemental powders using powder-bed fusion additive manufacturing. *J Alloys Compd.* 2018;763:436-445. doi:10.1016/j.jallcom.2018.05.325.
8. Kreitcberg A, Brailovski V, Prokoshkin S. New biocompatible near-beta Ti-Zr-Nb alloy processed by laser powder bed fusion: process optimization. *J Mater Process Technol.* 2018;252:821-829. doi:10.1016/j.jmatprotec.2017.10.052.
9. Arjunan A, Robinson J, Al Ani E, Heaselgrave W, Baroutaji A, Wang C. Mechanical performance of additively manufactured pure silver antibacterial bone scaffolds. *J Mech Behav Biomed Mater.* 2020;112:104090. doi:10.1016/j.jmbbm.2020.104090.
10. Lowther M, Loutha S, Davey A, et al. Clinical, industrial, and research perspectives on powder bed fusion additively manufactured metal implants. *Addit Manuf.* 2019;28:565-584. doi:10.1016/j.addma.2019.05.033.

11. Bandyopadhyay A, Shivaram A, Isik M, Avila JD, Dernell WS, Bose S. Additively manufactured calcium phosphate reinforced CoCrMo alloy: bio-tribological and biocompatibility evaluation for load-bearing implants. *Addit Manuf.* 2019;28:312-324. doi:10.1016/j.addma.2019.04.020.

12. Krishna BV, Bose S, Bandyopadhyay A. Low stiffness porous Ti structures for load-bearing implants. *Acta Biomater.* 2007;3:997-1006. doi:10.1016/j.actbio.2007.03.008.

13. Putra NE, Leeflanga MA, Minneboo M, et al. Extrusion-based 3D printed biodegradable porous iron. *Acta Biomater.* 2021;121:741-756. doi:10.1016/j.actbio.2020.11.022.

14. Kurtz SM, Devine JN. PEEK biomaterials in trauma, orthopedic, and spinal implants. *Biomaterials.* 2007;28:4845-4869. doi:10.1016/j.biomaterials.2007.07.013.

15. Zanjanijam AR, Major I, Lyons JG, Lafont U, Devine DM. Fused filament fabrication of PEEK: a review of process-structure-property relationships. *Polymers.* 2020;12:1665. doi:10.3390/polym12081665.

16. Arif MF, Kumar S, Varadarajan KM, Cantwell WJ. Performance of biocompatible PEEK processed by fused deposition additive manufacturing. *Mater Des.* 2018;146:249-259. doi:10.1016/j.matdes.2018.03.015.

17. Wang Y, Müller WD, Rumjahn A, Schwitalla A. Parameters influencing the outcome of additive manufacturing of tiny medical devices based on PEEK. *Materials.* 2020;13:466. doi:10.3390/ma13020466.

18. Basgul C, Yu T, MacDonald DW, Siskey R, Marcolongo M, Kurtz SM. Does annealing improve the interlayer adhesion and structural integrity of FFF 3D printed PEEK lumbar spinal cages? *J Mech Behav Biomed Mater.* 2020;102:103455. doi:10.1016/j.jmbbm.2019.103455.

19. Li Y, Lou Y. Tensile and bending strength improvements in PEEK parts using fused deposition modelling 3D printing considering multi-factor coupling. *Polymers.* 2020;12:2497. doi:10.3390/polym12112497.

20. Berretta S, Evans KE, Ghita O. Processability of PEEK, a new polymer for High Temperature Laser Sintering (HT-LS). *Eur Polym J.* 2015;68:243-266. doi:10.1016/j.eurpolymj.2015.04.003.

21. Benedetti L, Brulé B, Decraemer N, Richard R, Evans KE, Ghita O. A route to improving elongation of high-temperature laser sintered PEKK. *Addit Manuf.* 2020;36:101540. doi:10.1016/j.addma.2020.101540.

22. Ghita O, James E, Davies R, et al. High temperature laser sintering (HT-LS): an investigation into mechanical properties and shrinkage characteristics of poly (ether ketone) (PEK) structures. *Mater Des.* 2014;61:124-132. doi:10.1016/j.matdes.2014.04.035.

23. Stichel T, Frick T, Laumer T, et al. A round robin study for selective laser sintering of polyamide 12: microstructural origin of the mechanical properties. *Opt Laser Technol.* 2017;89:31-40. doi:10.1016/j.optlastec.2016.09.042.

24. Benedetti L. *Fundamental Understanding of Poly(Ether Ketone Ketone) for High Temperature Laser Sintering.* United Kingdom UK: University of Exeter; 2020.

25. Beliën H, Biesmans H, Steenwerckx A, Bijnens E, Dierickx C. Prebending of osteosynthesis plate using 3D printed models to treat symptomatic os acromiale and acromial fracture. *J Exp Orthop.* 2017;4:1-10.

26. Song C, Huang A, Yang Y, Xiao Z, Yu JK. Effect of energy input on the UHMWPE fabricating process by selective laser sintering. *Rapid Prototyp J.* 2017;23:1069-1078. doi:10.1108/RPJ-09-2015-0119.

27. Zhu X, Yang Q. Sintering the feasibility improvement and mechanical property of UHMWPE via selective laser sintering.

28. Spiegelberg S, Kozak A, Braithwaite G. *UHMWPE Biomaterials Handbook.* In: Kurtz SM, ed. *UHMWPE Biomaterials Handbook. Ultra High Molecular Weight Polyethylene in Total Joint Replacement and Medical Devices.* Norwich, NY: William Andrew Publishing; 2015:531-552. 3rd ed.

29. Kotz F, Mader M, Dellen N, et al. Fused deposition modeling of microfluidic chips in polymethylmethacrylate. *Micromachines.* 2020;11:873. doi:10.3390/mi11090873.

30. Velu R, Singamneni S. Evaluation of the influences of process parameters while selective laser sintering PMMA powders. *Proc Inst Mech Eng C J Mech Eng Sci.* 2015;229:603-613. doi:10.1177/0954406214538012.

31. Polzin C, Spath S, Seitz H. Characterization and evaluation of a PMMA-based 3D printing process. *Rapid Prototyp J.* 2013;19(1):37-43.

32. Zhu W, Yan C, Shi Y, et al. Investigation into mechanical and microstructural properties of polypropylene manufactured by selective laser sintering in comparison with injection molding counterparts. *Mater Des.* 2015;82:37-45. doi:10.1016/j.matdes.2015.05.043.

33. Elsner JJ, Mezape Y, Hakshur K, et al. Wear rate evaluation of a novel polycarbonate-urethane cushion form bearing for artificial hip joints. *Acta Biomaterialia.* 2010;6:4698-4707. doi:10.1016/j.actbio.2010.07.011.

34. Araujo Borges R, Choudhury D, Zou M. 3D printed PCU/UHMWPE polymeric blend for artificial knee meniscus. *Tribol Int.* 2018;122:1-7. doi:10.1016/j.triboint.2018.01.065.

35. Miller AT, Safranski DL, Smith KE, Sycks DG, Guldberg RE, Gall K. Fatigue of injection molded and 3D printed polycarbonate urethane in solution. *Polymer.* 2017;108:121-134. doi:10.1016/j.polymer.2016.11.055.

36. Zaldivar RJ, Witkin DB, McLouth T, Patel DN, Schmitt K, Nokes JP. Influence of processing and orientation print effects on the mechanical and thermal behavior of 3D-Printed ULTEM® 9085 Material. *Addit Manuf.* 2017;13:71-80. doi:10.1016/j.addma.2016.11.007.

37. Schaffner M, Faber JA, Pianegonda L, Rühs PA, Coulter F, Studart AR. 3D printing of robotic soft actuators with programmable bioinspired architectures. *Nat Commun.* 2018;9:878. doi:10.1038/s41467-018-03216-w.

38. Tumbleston JR, Shirvanyants D, Ermoshkin N, et al. Continuous liquid interface production of 3D objects. *Science.* 2015;347:1349-1352. doi:10.1126/science.aaa2397.

39. Zarek M, Layani M, Cooperstein I, Sachyani E, Cohn D, Magdassi S. 3D Printing of shape memory polymers for flexible electronic devices. *Adv Mater (Deerfield Beach, Fla.).* 2016;28:4449-4454. doi:10.1002/adma.201503132.

40. Patel DK, Sakhaei AH, Layani M, Zhang B, Ge Q, Magdassi S. Highly stretchable and UV curable elastomers for digital light processing based 3D printing. *Adv Mater.* 2017;29:1606000. doi:10.1002/adma.201606000.

41. Zhou Y, Liang K, Zhao S, et al. Photopolymerized maleilated chitosan/methacrylated silk fibroin micro/nanocomposite hydrogels as potential scaffolds for cartilage tissue engineering. *Int J Biol Macromol.* 2018;108:383-390. doi:10.1016/j.ijbiomac.2017.12.032.

42. Gou M, Qu X, Zhu W, et al. Bio-inspired detoxification using 3D-printed hydrogel nanocomposites. *Nat Commun.* 2014;5:3774. doi:10.1038/ncomms4774.

43. Clark Ligon-Auer S, Schwentenwein M, Gorsche C, Stampfl J, Liska R. Toughening of photo-curable polymer networks: a review. *Polymer Chem.* 2016;7:257-286. doi:10.1039/C5PY01631B.

Plast Rubber Compos. 2020;49:116-126. doi:10.1080/14658011.2020.1718321.

44. Sawamoto M, Ouchi M. Encyclopedia of Polymeric Nanomaterials. In Kobayashi S, Müllen K, eds. *Encyclopedia of Polymeric Nanomaterials.* Berlin Heidelberg: Springer; 2015:320-324.

45. Bagheri A, Jin J. Photopolymerization in 3D printing. *ACS Appl Polym Mater.* 2019;1:593-611.

46. Gibson I, Rosen D, Stucker B. *Additive Manufacturing Technologies: 3D Printing, Rapid Prototyping, and Direct Digital Manufacturing.* New York: Springer; 2014.

47. Machado TO, Sayer C, Araujo PHH. Thiol-ene polymerisation: a promising technique to obtain novel biomaterials. *Eur Polym J.* 2017;86:200-215. doi:10.1016/j.eurpolymj.2016.02.025.

48. Qin XH, Gruber P, Markovic M, et al. Enzymatic synthesis of hyaluronic acid vinyl esters for two-photon microfabrication of biocompatible and biodegradable hydrogel constructs. *Polym Chem.* 2014;5:6523-6533. doi:10.1039/C4PY00792A.

49. Bertlein S, Brown G, Lim KS, et al. Thiol-ene clickable gelatin: a platform bioink for multiple 3D biofabrication technologies. *Adv Mater (Deerfield Beach, Fla.).* 2017;29(44). doi:10.1002/adma.201703404.

50. Hoyle CE, Lee TY, Roper T. Thiol–enes: chemistry of the past with promise for the future. *J Polym Sci Part A: Polym Chem.* 2004;42:5301-5338. doi:10.1002/pola.20366.

51. Turner BN, Strong R, Gold SA. A review of melt extrusion additive manufacturing processes: I. Process design and modeling. *Rapid Prototyp J.* 2014;20:192-204. doi:10.1108/RPJ-01-2013-0012.

52. Sun Q, Rizvi GM, Bellehumeur CT, Gu P. Effect of processing conditions on the bonding quality of FDM polymer filaments. *Rapid Prototyp J.* 2008;14:72-80. doi:10.1108/13552540810862028.

53. Bachtiar EO, Erol O, Millrod M, et al. 3D printing and characterization of a soft and biostable elastomer with high flexibility and strength for biomedical applications. *J Mech Behav Biomed Mater.* 2020;104:103649. doi:10.1016/j.jmbbm.2020.103649.

54. Yang C, Tian X, Li D, Cao Y, Zhao F, Shi C. Influence of thermal processing conditions in 3D printing on the crystallinity and mechanical properties of PEEK material. *J Mater Process Technol.* 2017;248:1-7. doi:10.1016/j.jmatprotec.2017.04.027.

55. Popescu D, Zapciu A, Amza C, Baciu F, Marinescu R. FDM process parameters influence over the mechanical properties of polymer specimens: a review. *Polym Test.* 2018;69:157-166. doi:10.1016/j.polymertesting.2018.05.020.

56. Jacobs PF. *Rapid Prototyping & Manufacturing: Fundamentals of Stereolithography.* New York: Society of Manufacturing Engineers, McGraw-Hill; 1992.

57. Dhariwala B, Hunt E, Boland T. Rapid prototyping of tissue-engineering constructs, using photopolymerizable hydrogels and stereolithography. *Tissue Eng.* 2004;10:1316-1322. doi:10.1089/ten.2004.10.1316.

58. Seck TM, Melchels FPW, Feijen J, Grijpma DW. Designed biodegradable hydrogel structures prepared by stereolithography using poly(ethylene glycol)/poly(d,l-lactide)-based resins. *J Control Release.* 2010;148:34-41. doi:10.1016/j.jconrel.2010.07.111.

59. Cooke MN, Fisher JP, Dean D, Rimnac C, Mikos AG. Use of stereolithography to manufacture critical-sized 3D biodegradable scaffolds for bone ingrowth. *J Biomed Mater Res Part B Appl Biomater.* 2003;64B:65-69. doi:10.1002/jbm.b.10485.

60. Kim JY, Lee JW, Lee SJ, Park EK, Kim SY, Cho DW. Development of a bone scaffold using HA nanopowder and micro-stereolithography technology. *Microelectron Eng.* 2007;84:1762-1765. doi:10.1016/j.mee.2007.01.204.

61. Goodridge RD, Tuck CJ, Hague RJM. Laser sintering of polyamides and other polymers. *Prog Mater Sci.* 2012;57:229-267. doi:10.1016/j.pmatsci.2011.04.001.

62. Shi Y, Li Z, Sun H, Huang S, Zeng F. Effect of the properties of the polymer materials on the quality of selective laser sintering parts. *Proc Inst Mech Eng Part L: J Mater Des Appl.* 2004;218: 247-252. doi:10.1177/146442070421800308.

63. Goodridge RD, Dalgarno KW, Wood DJ. Indirect selective laser sintering of an apatite-mullite glass-ceramic for potential use in bone replacement applications. *Proc Inst Mech Eng, Part H J Eng Med.* 2006;220:57-68. doi:10.1243/095441105X69051.

64. Craik DJ, Miller BF. The flow properties of powders under humid conditions. *J Pharm Pharmacol.* 1958;10:136T-144T. https://doi.org/10.1111/j.2042-7158.1958.tb10392.x.

65. Jallo LJ, Dave RN. Explaining electrostatic charging and flow of surface-modified acetaminophen powders as a function of relative humidity through surface energetics. *J Pharm Sci.* 2015;104: 2225-2232. doi:10.1002/jps.24479.

66. Dotchev K, Yusoff W. Recycling of polyamide 12 based powders in the laser sintering process. *Rapid Prototyp J.* 2009;15:192-203. doi:10.1108/13552540910960299.

67. Kumar P, Irudhayam J Naviin. A Review on Importance and Recent Applications of Polymer Composites in Orthopaedics. Int J Eng Res Dev. 2012;5:2278-2800.

68. Saad M, Akhtar S, Srivastava S. Composite polymer in orthopedic implants: a review. *Mater Today Proc.* 2018;5:20224-20231. https://doi.org/10.1016/j.matpr.2018.06.393.

69. Jindal S, Manzoor F, Haslam N, Mancuso E. 3D printed composite materials for craniofacial implants: current concepts, challenges and future directions. *Int J Adv Manuf Technol.* 2021;112:635-653. doi:10.1007/s00170-020-06397-1.

70. Auricchio F, Marconi S. 3D printing: clinical applications in orthopaedics and traumatology. *EFORT Open Rev.* 2017;1: 121-127. doi:10.1302/2058-5241.1.000012.

71. Chen X, Chen G, Wang G, Zhu P, Gao C. Recent progress on 3D-printed polylactic acid and its applications in bone repair. *Adv Eng Mater.* 2020;22:1901065. https://doi.org/10.1002/adem.201901065.

72. Shirazi SFS, Gharehkhani S, Mehrali M, et al. A review of powder-based additive manufacturing for tissue engineering: selective laser sintering and inkjet 3D printing. *Sci Technol Adv Mater.* 2015;16:033502.

73. Bedell ML, Navara AM, Du Y, Zhang S, Mikos AG. Polymeric systems for bioprinting. *Chem Rev.* 2020;120:10744-10792. doi:10.1021/acs.chemrev.9b00834.

74. Lal H, Patralekh MK. 3D printing and its applications in orthopaedic trauma: a technological marvel. *J Clin Orthop Trauma.* 2018;9:260-268. doi:10.1016/j.jcot.2018.07.022.

75. Fahmy MD, Jazayeri HE, Razavi M, Masri R, Tayebi L. Three-dimensional bioprinting materials with potential application in preprosthetic surgery. *J Prosthodont.* 2016;25:310-318. https://doi.org/10.1111/jopr.12431.

76. Afewerki S, Magalhães LSSM, Silva ADR, et al. Bioprinting a synthetic smectic clay for orthopedic applications. *Adv Healthc Mater.* 2019;8:1900158. https://doi.org/10.1002/adhm.201900158.

77. Wang Y, Gao M, Wang D, Sun L, Webster TJ. Nanoscale 3D bioprinting for osseous tissue manufacturing. *Int J Nanomedicine.* 2020;15:215-226. doi:10.2147/IJN.S172916.

78. Curti F, Stancu IC, Voicu G, et al. Development of 3D bioactive scaffolds through 3D printing using wollastonite-gelatin inks. *Polymers (Basel).* 2020;12:2420. doi:10.3390/polym12102420.

79. Chen S, Shi Y, Zhang X, Ma J. Evaluation of BMP-2 and VEGF loaded 3D printed hydroxyapatite composite scaffolds with enhanced osteogenic capacity in vitro and in vivo. *Mater Sci Eng C*

Mater Biol Appl. 2020;112:110893. https://doi.org/10.1016/j. msec.2020.110893.

80. Lui YS, Sow WT, Tan LP, Wu Y, Lai Y, Li H. 4D printing and stimuli-responsive materials in biomedical aspects. *Acta Biomater.* 2019;92:19-36. doi:10.1016/j.actbio.2019.05.005.

81. Kirillova A, Ionov L. Shape-changing polymers for biomedical applications. *J Mater Chem B.* 2019;7:1597-1624. doi:10.1039/ C8TB02579G.

82. Ong K, Yun M, White J. New biomaterials for orthopedic implants. *Orthop Res Rev.* 2015;205:107-130. doi:10.2147/orr. S63437.

83. Bruyas A, Lou F, Stahl AM, et al. Systematic characterization of 3D-printed PCL/β-TCP scaffolds for biomedical devices and bone tissue engineering: influence of composition and porosity. *J Mater Res.* 2018;33:1948-1959. doi:10.1557/jmr.2018.112.

84. Sikder P, Ferreira JA, Fakhrabadi EA, et al. Bioactive amorphous magnesium phosphate-polyetheretherketone composite filaments for 3D printing. *Dent Mater.* 2020;36:865-883. https:// doi.org/10.1016/j.dental.2020.04.008.

85. Liu H, Webster TJ. Enhanced biological and mechanical properties of well-dispersed nanophase ceramics in polymer composites: from 2D to 3D printed structures. *Mater Sci Eng C.* 2011;31: 77-89. doi:10.1016/j.msec.2010.07.013.

86. Liu H, Li W, Liu C, et al. Incorporating simvastatin/poloxamer 407 hydrogel into 3D-printed porous Ti(6)Al(4)V scaffolds for the promotion of angiogenesis, osseointegration and bone ingrowth. *Biofabrication.* 2016;8:045012. doi:10.1088/1758-5090/8/4/045012.

87. Zhao Y, Wang Z, Jiang Y, et al. Biomimetic composite scaffolds to manipulate stem cells for aiding rheumatoid arthritis management. *Adv Funct Mater.* 2019;29:1807860. https://doi. org/10.1002/adfm.201807860.

88. Mani N, Sola A, Trinchi A, Fox K. Is there a future for additive manufactured titanium bioglass composites in biomedical application? A perspective. *Biointerphases.* 2020;15:068501. doi:10.1116/ 6.0000557.

89. Hak DJ, Mauffrey C, Seligson D, Lindeque B. Use of carbon-fiber-reinforced composite implants in orthopedic surgery. *Orthopedics.* 2014;37:825-830. doi:10.3928/01477447-20141124-05.

90. Ringel F, Ryang YM, Kirschke JS, et al. Radiolucent carbon fiber-reinforced pedicle screws for treatment of spinal tumors: advantages for radiation planning and follow-up imaging. *World Neurosurg.* 2017;105:294-301. doi:10.1016/j.wneu.2017.04.091.

91. Chan KW, Liao CZ, Wong HM, Kwok Yeung KW, Tjong SC. Preparation of polyetheretherketone composites with nanohydroxyapatite rods and carbon nanofibers having high strength, good biocompatibility and excellent thermal stability. *RSC Adv.* 2016;6:19417-19429. doi:10.1039/C5RA22134J.

92. Han X, Yang, D, Yang C, et al. Carbon fiber reinforced PEEK composites based on 3D-printing technology for orthopedic and dental applications. *J Clin Med.* 2019;8:240. doi:10.3390/ jcm8020240.

93. González-Henríquez CM, Sarabia-Vallejos MA, Rodríguez Hernandez J. Antimicrobial polymers for additive manufacturing. *Int J Mol Sci.* 2019;20:1210.

94. Shekhawat D, Singh A, Banerjee MK, Singh T, Patnaik A. Bioceramic composites for orthopaedic applications: a comprehensive review of mechanical, biological, and microstructural properties. *Ceram Int.* 2021;47:3013-3030. https://doi.org/10.1016/j.ceramint.2020.09.214.

95. ASTM F2502-05: *Standard Specification and Test Methods for Bioabsorbable Plates and Screws for Internal Fixation Implants.* Book of Standards. West Conshohocken, PA: ASTM International; 2016. 13. https://www.astm.org/f2502-05.html.

96. Li Y, Jahr H, Lietaert K, et al. Additively manufactured biodegradable porous iron. *Acta Biomater.* 2018;77:380-393. doi:10.1016/j.actbio.2018.07.011.

97. Qin Y, Wen P, Guo H, et al. Additive manufacturing of biodegradable metals: current research status and future perspectives. *Acta Biomater.* 2019;98:3-22. doi:10.1016/j.actbio.2019.04.046.

98. Jaker VL, Orrock JE, Graley CS. Polyglycolic acid support material for additive manufacturing systems. United States Patent: US9714318B2. 2017. https://patents.google.com/ patent/US9714318

99. Shuai C, Wu P, Zhong Y, et al. Polyetheretherketone/poly (glycolic acid) blend scaffolds with biodegradable properties. *J Biomater Sci Polym Ed.* 2016;27:1434-1446. doi:10.1080/0920 5063.2016.1210420.

100. Simpson RL, Wiria FE, Amis AA, et al. Development of a 95/5 poly(L-lactide-co-glycolide)/hydroxylapatite and β-tricalcium phosphate scaffold as bone replacement material via selective laser sintering. *J Biomed Mater Res Part B Appl Biomater.* 2008;84B: 17-25. https://doi.org/10.1002/jbm.b.30839.

101. Guo T, Holzberg TR, Lim CG, et al. 3D printing PLGA: a quantitative examination of the effects of polymer composition and printing parameters on print resolution. *Biofabrication.* 2017;9:024101. doi:10.1088/1758-5090/aa6370.

102. Tan L, Yu X, Wan P, Yang K. Biodegradable materials for bone repairs: a review. *J Mater Sci Technol.* 2013;29:503-513. doi:10.1016/ j.jmst.2013.03.002.

103. Martins JA, Lach AA, Morris HL, Carr AJ, Mouthuy PA. Polydioxanone implants: a systematic review on safety and performance in patients. *J Biomater Appl.* 2020;34:902-916. doi:10.1177/0885328219888841.

104. Middleton JC, Tipton AJ. Synthetic biodegradable polymers as orthopedic devices. *Biomaterials.* 2000;21:2335-2346. doi:10.1016/ S0142-9612(00)00101-0.

105. Roseti L, Parisi V, Petretta M, et al. Scaffolds for bone tissue engineering: state of the art and new perspectives. *Mat Sci Eng C.* 2017;78:1246-1262. https://doi.org/10.1016/j. msec.2017.05.017.

106. Li L, Shi J, Shen S, et al. In situ repair of bone and cartilage defects using 3D scanning and 3D printing. *Sci Rep.* 2017;7: 9416. doi:10.1038/s41598-017-10060-3.

107. Nabiyouni M, Brückner T, Zhou H, Gbureck U, Bhaduri SB. Magnesium-based bioceramics in orthopedic applications. *Acta Biomaterialia.* 2018;66:23-43. https://doi.org/10.1016/ j.actbio.2017.11.033.

108. Chang CH, Lin CY, Liu FH, et al. 3D printing bioceramic porous scaffolds with good mechanical property and cell affinity. *PLoS ONE.* 2015;10:e0143713. doi:10.1371/journal.pone.0143713.

109. Trombetta RP, Ninomiya MJ, El-Atawneh IM, et al. Calcium phosphate spacers for the local delivery of sitafloxacin and rifampin to treat orthopedic infections: efficacy and proof of concept in a mouse model of single-stage revision of device-associated osteomyelitis. *Pharmaceutics.* 2019;11:94. doi:10.3390/pharmaceutics11020094.

110. Wieding J, Fritsche A, Heinl P, et al. Biomechanical behavior of bone scaffolds made of additive manufactured tricalciumphosphate and titanium alloy under different loading conditions. *J Appl Biomater Funct Mater.* 2013;11:159-166. doi:10.5301/jabfm.2013.10832.

111. Wang YE, Li XP, Li CC, Yang MM, Wei QH. Binder droplet impact mechanism on a hydroxyapatite microsphere surface in 3D printing of bone scaffolds. *J Mater Sci.* 2015;50:5014-5023. doi:10.1007/s10853-015-9050-9.

112. Zafar MJ, Zhu D, Zhang Z. 3D printing of bioceramics for bone tissue engineering. *Materials.* 2019;12:3361.

113. Zhang J, Huang D, Liua S, et al. Zirconia toughened hydroxy-apatite biocomposite formed by a DLP 3D printing process for potential bone tissue engineering. *Mater Sci Eng C.* 2019; 105:110054. https://doi.org/10.1016/j.msec.2019.110054.

114. Guo J, Zeng Y, Li P, Chen J. Fine lattice structural titanium dioxide ceramic produced by DLP 3D printing. *Ceram Int.* 2019;45:23007-23012. https://doi.org/10.1016/j.ceramint.2019.07.346.

115. Backes EH, Pires LDN, Beatrice CAG, Costa LC, Passador FR, Pessan LA. Fabrication of biocompatible composites of poly(lactic acid)/hydroxyapatite envisioning medical applications. *Polym Eng Sci.* 2020;60:636-644. https://doi.org/10.1002/pen.25322.

116. Hallman M. Driscoll A, Lubbe R, et al. Influence of geometry and architecture on the in vivo success of 3D-printed scaffolds for spinal fusion. *Tissue Eng Part A.* 2021;27:26-36. doi:10.1089/ten.TEA.2020.0004.

117. Yu J, Xu Y, Li S, Seifert GV, Becker ML. Three-dimensional printing of nano hydroxyapatite/poly(ester urea) composite scaffolds with enhanced bioactivity. *Biomacromolecules.* 2017;18:4171-4183. doi:10.1021/acs.biomac.7b01222.

118. Ranjan N, Singh R, Ahuja IPS, et al. On 3D printed scaffolds for orthopedic tissue engineering applications. *SN Appl Sci.* 2020;2:192. doi:10.1007/s42452-020-1936-8.

119. Pitjamit S, Nakkiew W, Thongkorn K, Thanakulwattana W, Thunsiri K. Finite element analysis of traditional and new fixation techniques of the 3D-printed composite interlocking nail in canine femoral shaft fractures. *Appl Sci.* 2020;10:3424.

120. Yeon YK, Park HS, Lee JM, et al. New concept of 3D printed bone clip (polylactic acid/hydroxyapatite/silk composite) for internal fixation of bone fractures. *J Biomater Sci Polym Ed.* 2018;29:894-906. doi:10.1080/09205063.2017.1384199.

121. Gupta A, Prasad A, Mulchandani N, et al. Multifunctional nanohydroxyapatite-promoted toughened high-molecular-weight stereocomplex poly(lactic acid)-based bionanocomposite for both 3D-printed orthopedic implants and high-temperature engineering applications. *ACS Omega.* 2017;2:4039-4052. doi:10.1021/acsomega.7b00915.

122. Jakus AE, Rutz AL, Jordan SW, et al. Hyperelastic "bone": a highly versatile, growth factor-free, osteoregenerative, scalable, and surgically friendly biomaterial. *Sci Transl Med.* 2016;8:358ra127-358ra127. doi:10.1126/scitranslmed.aaf7704.

123. Mark JE. *Polymer Data Handbook.* New York: Oxford University Press; 1999.

124. Ginjupalli K, Averineni RK, Shavi GV, et al. Biodegradable composite scaffolds of poly(lactic-co-glycolic acid) 85:15 and nano-hydroxyapatite with acidic microclimate controlling additive. *Polym Compos.* 2017;38:1175-1182. https://doi.org/10.1002/pc.23681.

125. Fukushima K. Poly(trimethylene carbonate)-based polymers engineered for biodegradable functional biomaterials. *Biomater Sci.* 2016;4:9-24. doi:10.1039/C5BM00123D.

SECTION 2

Surgical Techniques

4

Isolated Total Talus Replacement

PETER D. HIGHLANDER, PAUL R. LEATHAM, RYAN J. LERCH

Definition

- Excision and replacement of the talus with a patient-specific 3D-printed metallic implant in patients without adjacent joint disease.

Indications

- Avascular necrosis (AVN) of the talus without significant arthritic changes (Fig. 4.1).
- Complex talus trauma (Fig. 4.2).
- Large osteochondral lesions with cystic formation which have failed traditional surgical procedures (Fig. 4.3).
- Malignancy requiring excision of the talus.

Anatomy

- Greater than 60% of the talus is covered with articular cartilage, which limits the surface area for vascular infiltration.[1]
- Extraosseous circulation loops all arise from branches of the posterior tibial, anterior tibial, and peroneal arteries. Vasculature within the sinus tarsi and tarsal canal in addition to deltoid branches all play vital roles for talar blood supply.
- The talus has no muscular or tendinous attachments and therefore relies on periarticular ligaments and joint morphology for stability.
- The talar dome is wider anteriorly than posteriorly, and thus mechanically more stable when the foot is dorsiflexed.

Pathogenesis

- Shah et al.[2] classified AVN etiology into six categories (Table 4.1).
- Risk factors for AVN have been identified; however, the precise pathogenesis has yet to be understood.
- It is probable that AVN occurs due to a combination of risk factors and conditions. Modifiable risk factors include excessive alcohol consumption, nicotine use, poor diet, and obesity.

- The majority of talar AVN cases occur following neck or body fracture:
  - Up to 75% of talar AVN is attributed to trauma.[3]
  - The incidence of AVN increases with coexisting adjacent joint dislocation and initial fracture displacement.[4]
  - Timing to surgical repair does not appear to influence the risk of AVN.
  - The absence of subchondral lucency, referred to as the Hawkins sign, on radiographs 6 to 8 weeks postinjury is concerning for AVN development.
- Multiple atraumatic etiologies exist but are less common for talar AVN. The most common cause of atraumatic AVN is associated with glucocorticoid use.[5]
- An underlying characteristic of AVN is insufficient and/or altered blood supply to the talus, leading to bone cell death.[1]
- Treatment may be more successful in early stages of AVN; however, early-stage AVN is more difficult to diagnose and can be asymptomatic.[5]
- Talar collapse occurs as the avascular process progresses due to the altered structural integrity of the bone.

Patient History and Physical Exam Findings

- History of trauma which required surgical intervention is common.
- Atraumatic history may include prolonged high-dose corticosteroids, alcoholism, prior irradiation treatments, and thrombophilia.
- Initially osteonecrosis is asymptomatic and will typically progress to collapse if untreated.
- Symptoms and presentation vary and may be vague until late-stage AVN, which presents with significant pain, dysfunction, and possibly deformity.
- Patients complain of a deep pain to the talar aspect of the ankle, which is exacerbated with weight bearing and range of motion (ROM).
- Decreased ROM compared to contralateral foot is common if AVN is unilateral.
- Rigid deformity may be present in late-stage talar AVN with collapse (Fig. 4.4).

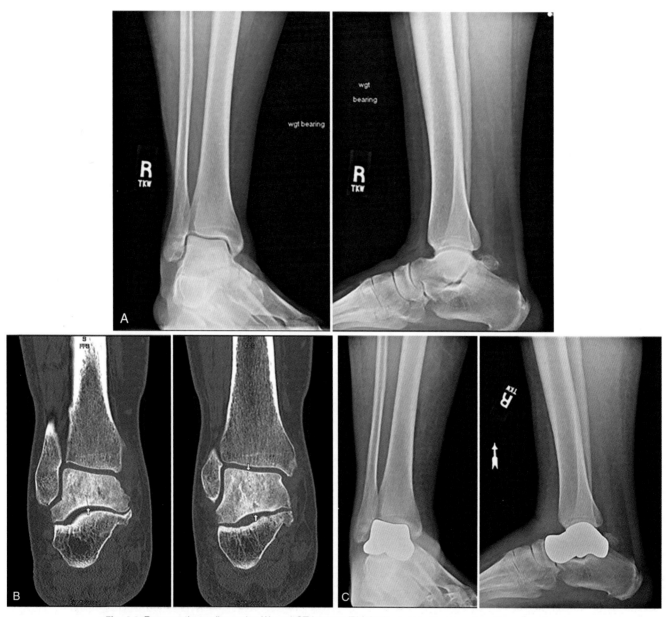

• **Fig. 4.1** Preoperative radiographs (A) and CT images (B) of talar avascular necrosis with early collapse in a 53-year-old female with history of long-term corticosteroid use for lupus. The patient failed to respond to nonoperative treatment for nearly 2 years and then underwent total talus replacement. At 1-year post-operative follow-up the patient demonstrated a significant improved in pain and function (C).

Imaging and Other Diagnostic Testing

- In the initial stage of AVN, plain radiographs are often unremarkable. If a high index of suspicion exists for talar AVN then it is critical to obtain an MRI, which is the most sensitive and specific test during the early stages (Fig. 4.5).
- In the absence of hardware, MRI can demonstrate the extent of AVN.
- An absence of the Hawkins sign 6 to 8 weeks posttrauma on plain radiographs is concerning for talar AVN.
- As the disease progresses, radiographs may demonstrate talar sclerosis, and in advanced stages may show signs of talar collapse (Fig. 4.6).
- In a posttraumatic setting, radiographs may reveal malunion or nonunion.

- Additional radiographic views, including Canale and Kelly views, can be beneficial for identifying altered talar morphology.[6]
- Contralateral radiographs are useful to compare morphology.
- CT scans are useful for determining the quality of bone and adjacent articular involvement, which aids in procedure selection and planning.

Nonoperative Management

- Non–weight bearing.
- Extracorporeal shock wave therapy.
- Noninvasive bone stimulation.
- Patellar tendon bracing or another custom rigid brace.

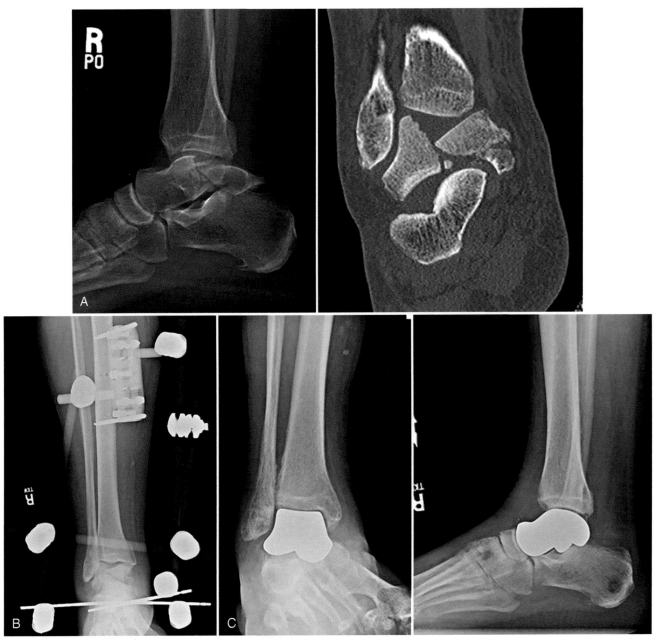

• **Fig. 4.2** Initial radiographs and CT scan of a 69-year-old male after a 10-foot fall from a ladder resulting in a comminuted talar body fracture (A). Due to the high rate of avascular necrosis and longer recovery associated with open reduction with internal fixation (ORIF) surgery, the patient decided to undergo total talus replacement (TTR). The injury was reduced and placed into a spanning external fixator (B). While the soft tissues recovered, a patient-specific 3D-printed total talus implant was designed and manufactured. Roughly 2 weeks after the injury, the patient underwent TTR. Functionally the patient remains at a preinjury activity level without a brace or assistive device at 2-year follow-up (C).

Traditional Surgical Management

- Traditional surgical options include both joint sparing and joint sacrificing
- Core decompression (CD):
  - CD may be used in AVN without collapse or adjacent articular involvement.
  - CD may slow AVN progression.
- Vascularized bone grafting:
  - Involves the introduction of new vascularized bone to the pathologic area of concern.

- Similar to CD, does not restore talar morphology and is therefore limited to early-stage AVN.
- Technically demanding.
- Arthrodesis: tibiotalar fusion, subtalar fusion, or tibiota-localcaneal arthrodesis[1]:
  - Successful fusion can be reliable for pain reduction; however, it will result in altered mechanical function and an increased demand on adjacent joints.
  - Excision of necrotic bone is essential which, if extensive, may result in a large osseous deficit. Fusion with extensive AVN may be associated with higher rates of nonunion.

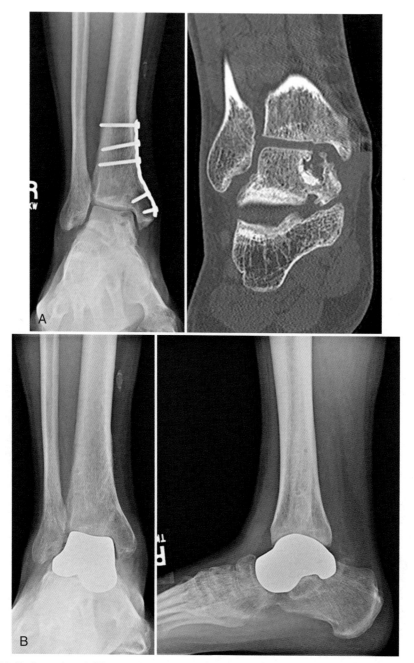

• **Fig. 4.3** Radiograph and CT scan of a 24-year-old male who failed to improve following multiple procedures for a large osteochondral defect of the medial talus (A). Due to worsening pain and function preventing the patient's ability to work, the patient elected to undergo total talus replacement (TTR). At 2 years follow-up, the patient has shown significant improvement compared to preoperative pain and function scores (B). He returned to work 4 months following TTR and remained very satisfied with his outcome.

3D-Printed Implant Design Specifications and Considerations

- 3D-printed total talus implants for global talar pathology allow restoration of normal talar morphology.
- A contralateral CT scan is used to replicate normal talar morphology. Reconstruction of the talus may be dependent on a contralateral CT scan, particularly if talar collapse is present on the affected side, therefore the contralateral talus must be free of significant pathology to be reliable.

- Total talus material selection: cobalt chromium alloy (CoCr) versus titanium alloy (Ti):
  - CoCr is currently the material of choice for 3D-printed implants that articulate with adjacent native cartilage or polyethylene joint-replacement components.
  - Achieving <50 nm of surface finish is standard for articulating implants, which can be reliably obtained for CoCr by postprint processing and polishing. The same specification can be achieved for Ti implants; however, this is not maintained over time.

TABLE 4.1	Avascular Necrosis Etiologies as Categorized
Category	**Etiology**
Direct cellular toxicity	Chemotherapy Radiotherapy Thermal injury Smoking
Extraosseous arterial	Fracture Dislocation Iatrogenic/postsurgical Congenital arterial abnormalities
Extraosseous venous	Venous abnormalities Venous stasis
Intraosseous extravascular compression	Hemorrhage Elevated bone marrow pressure Fatty infiltration of bone marrow (prolonged high-dose corticosteroid use) Cellular hypertrophy and marrow infiltration (Gaucher's disease) Bone marrow edema Displaced fractures
Intraosseous intravascular occlusion	Coagulation disorders (i.e., thrombophilia, hypofibrinolysis) Sickle cell crises
Multifactorial	A combination of two or more etiologies

Shah KN, Racine J, Jones LC, Aaron RK. Pathophysiology and risk factors for osteonecrosis. *Curr Rev Musculoskelet Med*. 2015;8(3):201-209.

- Compared to CoCr, the composition of Ti renders a higher coefficient of friction, thus it is extraordinarily difficult to obtain a surface smoothness in Ti implants that is appropriate for articulation using postprint processing and polishing.

- Other material characteristics that yield CoCr as the material of choice is its hardness, which reduces implant wear and corrosion.
- Ti alloys used for articulating implants require surface treatment to improve hardness and reduce friction. Coatings such as titanium nitride (TiN) have been shown to improve biocompatibility and wear characteristics compared to Ti alloy without surface treatment. However, multiple reports raise concern for delamination of the TiN coating leading to accelerated wear and fretting.[7-9] Additionally, TiN coatings have been associated with reduced axial fatigue strength compared to Ti alloy implants without surface coating.[10]
- The conflicting results for TiN surface treatments may be dependent on the coating process. Multiple coating processes exist, but no standard process exists. Until the surface treatment and coating application for Ti implants is optimized and standardized, the authors recommend CoCr implants for total talus replacement (TTR) in patients without allergy.[11]
- 3D printing allows implants to be customized based on patient pathology and surgeon preference. Common specifications that should be considered include:
  - Surface roughness on nonarticular aspects may be incorporated into the implant to promote soft tissue in-growth particularly for anterior talofibular (ATFL) and deltoid ligament attachment sites.
  - Eyelets may be placed at the periphery of the surface roughness. Sutures can then be passed through the implant, allowing ligaments to be reapproximated to their attachment sites (Fig. 4.7).
  - Sizing options typically range from ± 5% to 10% from nominal. In the authors' experience, nominal

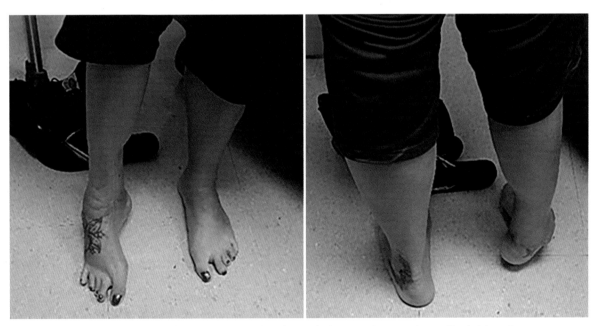

• **Fig. 4.4** Clinical presentation of a patient with advanced talar avascular necrosis, resulting in talar collapse and rigid equinocavovarus deformity.

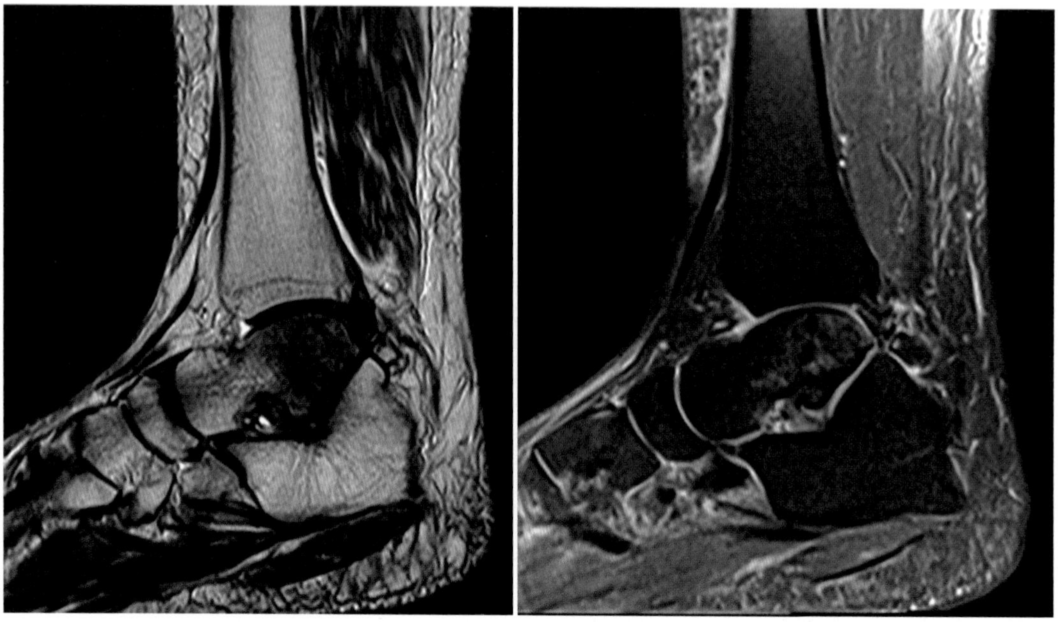

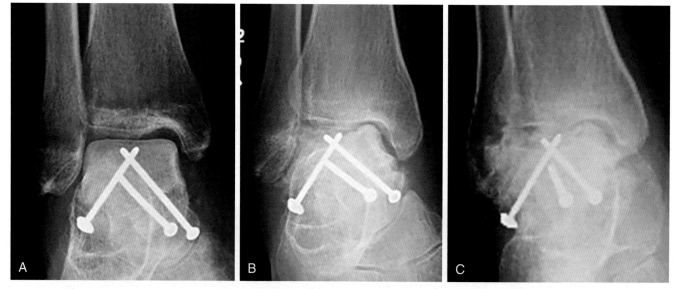

• **Fig. 4.5** Characteristic findings of early-stage talar avascular necrosis on T1- and T2-weighted MRI images in a 51-year-old female with a history of prolonged corticosteroid use.

• **Fig. 4.6** Anteroposterior ankle radiographs of a patient who sustained a talar neck fracture. Over the course of 5 years avascular necrosis progressed from sclerotic changes with preservation of normal talus morphology (A), subchondral to collapse without changes to the distal tibia (B), and finally to collapse with cartilage destruction and osteophyte formation of the distal tibia (C).

sized implants are most commonly used for isolated TTR (Fig. 4.8).
- Chapters 6 and 8 cover additional specifications if TTR is being combined with adjacent joint fusion or replacement.
- Customizable instrumentation specifications commonly used may include:
  - Polymer trials doped with barium sulfate are radiopaque, which allows clear fluoroscopic evaluation for position and fit.
  - Cut guides may be considered to improve the efficiency of talar excision, which is the rate-limiting step of the procedure.

- Impactors printed from photopolymers aid in final implant insertion while not damaging the implant.

Surgical Management With 3D-Printed Devices

- The surgeon's preference is general anesthesia with preoperative regional nerve block.
- The surgical approach is best achieved using the supine position with a hip bump.

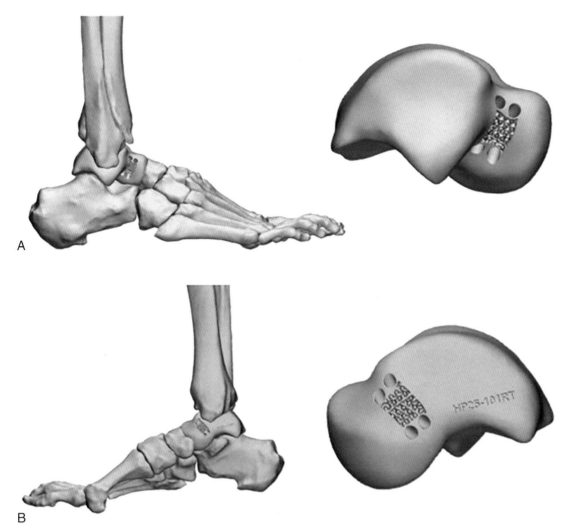

• **Fig. 4.7** Common implant specifications to consider for isolated total talus replacement include surface roughness on nonarticular aspects of the implant and eyelets for potential anterior talofibular (A) and/or deltoid ligament (B) reapproximation. (Computer-aided design images from Restor3d, Inc, Durham, NC.)

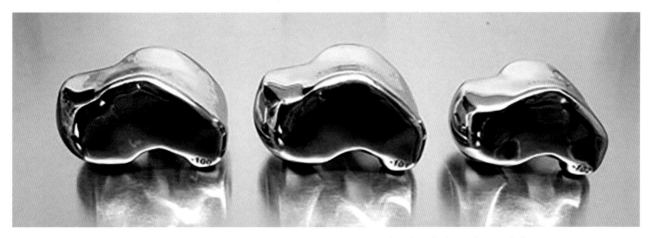

• **Fig. 4.8** Nominal sized implants are most commonly used for isolated total talus replacement; however, it is currently standard to have three different sizes available.

- Incision should be standard anterior ankle incision, utilizing the interval between the tibialis anterior tendon and the extensor hallucis longus tendon.
- Removal of the pathologic talus (Fig. 4.9):
  - The authors prefer to perform talectomy with 3D-printed cut guides due to enhanced efficiency and accuracy.
  - All visible soft tissue attachments to the talar head, neck, and body are sharply and meticulously released.
  - In a stepwise fashion, two oblique osteotomies are performed using the guide as shown in Figs. 4.9 to 4.11. It is recommended that the osteotomies are performed under fluoroscopy to prevent damage to the calcaneal facets.
  - The talar head and neck are removed via pulling traction on the talar neck with a towel clamp and/ or guidewires used during the second osteotomy (see Fig. 4.11B). An elevator or scalpel can be used to carefully release soft tissue attached to the inferior surface of the talar neck.

- A vertical osteotomy can be performed through the talar body segments to aid in removal. The anterior talar body segment is then pulled under traction while soft tissue attachments are simultaneously released. This process is then repeated for the posterior talar body (see Fig. 4.8C).
- Any bony fragments are removed and the talar space is irrigated with 3 L of normal saline.
- Implant trials are used to assess ideal fit:
  - The trial is most easily inserted by pulling via manual traction and inversion on the heel while holding the foot in maximum plantar flexion. Once the implant clears, the navicular the trial should easily pop into place.
  - With the selected trial in place, ROM and intrinsic stability is assessed. It is helpful to use radio-opaque trials for radiographic assessment. The ideal implant should place physiologic tension on the adjacent soft tissues while the ankle and subtalar joint are in a neutral position.
  - Close inspection is required to select the appropriately sized implant. If an implant is selected that is too small, this may create additional motion of the

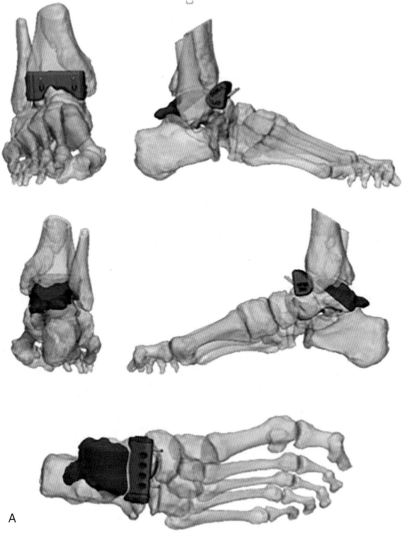

A

• **Fig. 4.9** Removal of the native talus through an anterior incision may be performed with 3D-printed custom-cut guides. Computer-aided design (CAD) images are created during the preoperative planning stage to aid in determining the trajectory of the osteotomy, as shown in *red* (A).

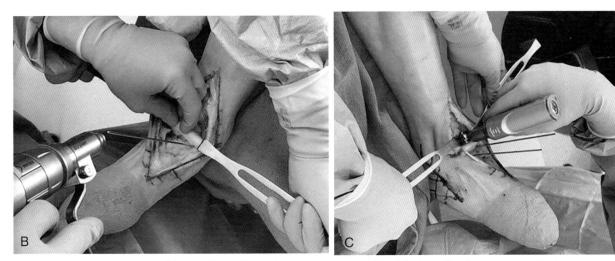

• **Fig. 4.9, cont'd** Step 1: The guide is placed on the talar neck and fixated with 2.0-mm wires on the inferior medial and lateral holes (B). An osteotomy is made through the talar dome and posterior portion of the talar body using the dorsal flat surface of the guide as a shelf for the blade (C). It is recommended to perform the osteotomy under fluoroscopy to prevent damage to the calcaneal facets. (See Fig. 4.10 for Step 2 and Fig. 4.11 for Step 3.) (CAD images from Restor3d, Inc, Durham, NC.)

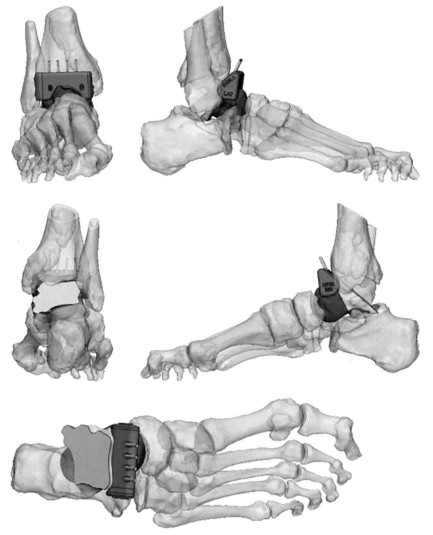

• **Fig. 4.10** Step 2: Place two 2.0-mm wires through the center superior holes and remove the two previously placed wires. Place another two 2.0-mm wires in the superior medial and lateral holes, creating four parallel wires as shown. (See Fig. 4.9 for Step 1 and Fig. 4.11 for Step 3.) (Computer-aided design images from Restor3d, Inc, Durham, NC.)

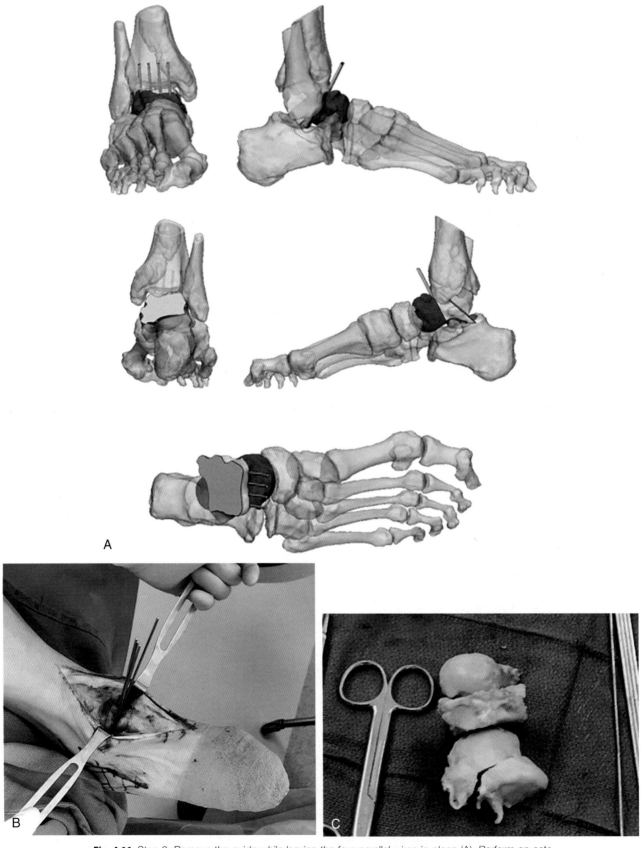

• **Fig. 4.11** Step 3: Remove the guide while leaving the four parallel wires in place (A). Perform an osteotomy along the dorsal surface of the wires. After both osteotomies have been performed, the wires may aid in removing the head and neck (B). After the talar head and neck are removed, a vertical osteotomy with an osteotome can aid in removal of the anterior and posterior talar body segments (C). (See Fig. 4.9 for Step 1 and Fig. 4.10 for Step 2.)

implant that could contribute to failure. On the other hand, if an implant is too large, then increased force is placed on the native adjacent cartilage, leading to accelerated wear. An overstuffed implant will limit the ROM and does not replicate the balanced physiologic tension of adjacent soft tissues.

- Final implantation:
  - The trial is removed and the surgical site is irrigated, taking time to ensure all osseous debris and impinging soft tissue is excised.
  - The final talar implant is inserted in a similar manner to the trial; however, this can be slightly more difficult. Impaction or instrument distraction is rarely required. Avoid any contact with metal instrumentation, which can scratch and damage the implant.
  - ROM and stability are assessed again prior to final irrigation and standard closure.
- Common adjunctive procedures are certainly variable based on the patient's presentation; however, gastrocnemius recession aids in increased ROM but can also facilitate inserting the implant.

Postoperative Protocol

- Initially the patient is placed into a well-padded posterior splint and transitioned to a fiberglass cast at the first postoperative appointment. The total time non–weight bearing is typically 3 weeks or until the incision has healed.
- Transition to a controlled ankle motion (CAM) boot once the incision is healed. At this time, the patient is to begin active ROM exercise and may weight bear as tolerated.
- Transition to a functional ankle brace with athletic shoes occurs at 6 weeks.
- Nonimpact exercise and physical therapy may begin as early as 6 weeks postoperatively. Light-impact exercise may typically begin at 12 weeks.
- X-rays should be obtained at every postoperative visit, with exception of the first postoperative visit.
- CT scans may be periodically assessed for adjacent joint changes.

Results

- In 2020 Kadakia et al. demonstrated in a retrospective review over 3 years including 27 patients with a follow-up of 22.2 months that visual analog scale (VAS) and Foot and Ankle Outcome (FAO) scores improved significantly postoperatively. FAO scores improved in terms of pain, symptoms, quality of life, and activities of daily living.[12]
- In 2021, Abramson et al. reported on a case series of eight patients who showed a mean American Orthopedic Foot and Ankle Score (AOFAS) of 79.25 and a Short Form-36 (SF-36) score of 83.25 at 23 months' follow-up. They reported no revisional surgeries. Gait analysis demonstrated a mildly abnormal gait in seven patients and moderately abnormal gait in one patient. At final follow-up, one patient had asymptomatic tibial wear on radiographs.[13]

- Huang et al. published a case report in 2021 describing a 31-year-old male diagnosed with osteoblastic osteosarcoma of the talus treated with a custom 3D-printed TTR made from titanium. This prosthesis contained tunnels for ligamentous attachment. The patient reported 93% restoration of the Musculoskeletal Tumor Society Functional Score and 93 points on the Toronto Extremity Salvage Score. At final follow-up the patient had no recurrence of osteosarcoma.[14]
- Papagelopoulos et al. demonstrated fairly successful case study results using a 3D custom talus replacement for Ewing's sarcoma of the talus with a 3.5-year follow-up in a 30-year-old female patient.[15]
- Ruatti et al. published a case report of a total talus prosthesis replacement following a talar extrusion in 2017. This prosthesis was placed into the ankle at 6 months from the initial injury, but after 2-year follow-up the patient had improved their AOFAS score from 11 to 77 and their SF-36 score from 17 to 82. This study showed that talus extrusion can successfully be treated with 3D custom replacement.[16]
- In 2021 Mu et al. published a case series on nine patients with talar necrosis and collapse who required 3D custom replacement. They demonstrated improvements in Meary's angle and talar height, improved AOFAS scores from 26.33 to 79.67, and a decreased VAS score from 6.33 to 0.83 at a mean follow-up of 23.17 months. This study had no adjacent joint degenerative arthritis, prosthetic dislocation, or other complications. Pain relief, activities of daily living, and return to physical activities were good to excellent in this study.[17]

PEARLS AND PITFALLS	
Indications and contraindications	• Avascular necrosis of talus • Selected patients with complex talar fracture • Contraindicated in cases of active infection • Use prudence in patients with a history of deep infection
Implant design	• CoCr • Use contralateral CT and CAD images to determine nominal implant size in all planes • Eyelets can be incorporated for ligament reattachment and/or augmentation
Surgical technique	• Standard anterior ankle incision • Ensure all talar bone is removed • Drill direct fixation for screws and pegs through trial implants • The ideal implant size yields physiologic tension within the adjacent soft tissues, provides inherent stability, and allows for range of motion at all corresponding articulations

CAD, Computer-aided design; *CoCr*, cobalt chromium.

References

1. Gross CE, Sershon RA, Frank JM, Easley ME, Holmes GB Jr. Treatment of osteonecrosis of the talus. *JBJS Rev.* 2016;4(7):e2.

2. Shah KN, Racine J, Jones LC, Aaron RK. Pathophysiology and risk factors for osteonecrosis. *Curr Rev Musculoskelet Med.* 2015; 8(3):201-209.

3. Adelaar RS, Madrian JR. Avascular necrosis of the talus. *Orthop Clin North Am.* 2004;35(3):383-395, xi.

4. Clare MP, Maloney PJ. Prevention of avascular necrosis with fractures of the talar neck. *Foot Ankle Clin.* 2019;24(1):47-56.

5. Weinstein RS. Glucocorticoid-induced osteonecrosis. *Endocrine.* 2012;41(2):183-190.

6. Canale ST, Kelly FB Jr. Fractures of the neck of the talus. Long-term evaluation of seventy-one cases. *J Bone Joint Surg Am.* 1978; 60(2):143-156.

7. Komotori J, Lee BJ, Dong H, Dearnley PA. Corrosion response of surface engineered titanium alloys damaged by prior abrasion. *Wear.* 2001;250(1-12):1239-1249.

8. Williams S, Tipper JL, Ingham E, Stone MH, Fisher J. In vitro analysis of the wear, wear debris and biological activity of surface-engineered coatings for use in metal-on-metal total hip replacements. *Proc Inst Mech Eng H.* 2003;217(3):155-163.

9. Galvin A, Brockett C, Williams S, et al. Comparison of wear of ultra-high molecular weight polyethylene acetabular cups against surface-engineered femoral heads. *Proc Inst Mech Eng H.* 2008; 222(7):1073-1080.

10. Costa MYP, Venditti MLR, Cioffi MOH, Voorwald HJC, Guimaraes VA, Ruas R. Fatigue behavior of PVD coated Ti-6Al-4V alloy. *Int J Fatigue.* 2011;33:759-765.

11. van Hove RP, Sierevelt IN, van Royen BJ, Nolte PA. Titanium-nitride coating of orthopaedic implants: a review of the literature. *Biomed Res Int.* 2015;2015:485975.

12. Kadakia RJ, Akoh CC, Chen J, Sharma A, Parekh SG. 3D printed total talus replacement for avascular necrosis of the talus. *Foot Ankle Int.* 2020;41(12):1529-1536.

13. Abramson M, Hilton T, Hosking K, Campbell N, Dey R, McCollum G. Total talar replacements short-medium term case series, South Africa 2019. *J Foot Ankle Surg.* 2021;60(1): 182-186. doi:10.1053/j.jfas.2020.08.015.

14. Huang J, Xie F, Tan X, Xing W, Zheng Y, Zeng C. Treatment of osteosarcoma of the talus with a 3D-printed talar prosthesis. *J Foot Ankle Surg.* 2021;60(1):194-198. doi:10.1053/j.jfas.2020.01.012.

15. Papagelopoulos PJ, Sarlikiotis T, Vottis CT, Agrogiannis G, Kontogeorgakos VA, Savvidou OD. Total talectomy and reconstruction using a 3-dimensional printed talus prosthesis for Ewing's sarcoma: a 3.5-year follow-up. *Orthopedics.* 2019;42(4): e405-e409. doi:10.3928/01477447-20190523-05.

16. Ruatti S, Corbet C, Boudissa M, et al. Total talar prosthesis replacement after talar extrusion. *J Foot Ankle Surg.* 2017;56(4):905-909. doi:10.1053/j.jfas.2017.04.005.

17. Mu MD, Yang QD, Chen W, et al. Three dimension printing talar prostheses for total replacement in talar necrosis and collapse. *Int Orthop.* 2021;45(9):2313-2321.

5

Total Talus Replacement With a Titanium Nitride-Coated 3D-Printed Titanium Implant

NAJI S. MADI, SELENE G. PAREKH

Definition

- Total talus replacement (TTR) is a surgical procedure which involves the removal of a pathologic talus and replacement with a patient-specific 3D-printed titanium (Ti) prosthesis coated with titanium nitride (TiN).
- DICOM data from a CT scan is used with specialized software to determine the size and dimensions of a TTR prosthesis.
- CT scans of bilateral ankles are preferable and recommended; however, data only from a CT scan of the ipsilateral (pathologic) talus may be used if there is no collapse, deformity, or bony deficit.

Indications and Contraindications

- Diffuse talus avascular necrosis (AVN) is a primary indication for TTR; however, other causes of bony deficit within the talus may be an indication for TTR, such as high-level trauma or malignancy.
- Isolated TTR may be considered in patients with talar pathology but without pathology of the adjacent joints.
- TTR may be combined with a total ankle replacement in the setting of talar pathology with secondary changes to the distal tibia.
- Contraindications for TTR include active infection, neuropathy, gross deformity in the sagittal or coronal planes, and AVN of the calcaneus, distal tibia, or navicular bones.[1]

Anatomy

- The talus (*Taxillus*, referring to the ankle bone of a horse) is the second largest bone in the hindfoot with an irregular saddle-shaped architecture. It is composed of a head that forms the talonavicular joint with the navicular

bone anteriorly and the anterior talocalcaneal joint inferiorly; a neck that connects the head and the body. The latter has three processes (medial, lateral, posterior), two facets (middle and posterior), two tubercles, and one talar dome (Figs. 5.1 to 5.3).[2]
- The middle facet articulates with the sustentaculum tali. The posterior facet forms with the calcaneus the posterior talocalcaneal joint.
- The talar dome or trochlea located superiorly forms the tibiotalar joint with the tibia and fibula.
- The talus is covered by more than 60% of articular cartilage.
- There are no muscle attachments, but the talus does possess multiple ligament attachments, including the deltoid complex and spring ligaments medially, and the anterior talofibular and posterior talofibular ligaments laterally.
- The modified Boyan Classification is used to describe the variable morphology of the subtalar joint facets based on the number of facets present and the distance between those facets.
- The tenuous blood supply is provided by three arterial sources (Fig. 5.4):
  - The posterior tibial artery breaks into the tarsal canal artery that supplies most of the talar body except the medial third, which is supplied by the deltoid branch of the tarsal canal artery.
  - The anterior tibial artery (becoming the dorsalis pedis artery) gives off the lateral tarsal artery, which anastomoses with the peroneal artery to form the tarsal sinus artery.
  - The tarsal sinus and tarsal canal arteries anastomose in the sinus tarsi.
  - The medial branches of the dorsalis pedis artery supply the superomedial talar neck.
  - The inferior talar neck branches of the tarsal sinus artery or tarsal canal artery supply the inferolateral talar neck.

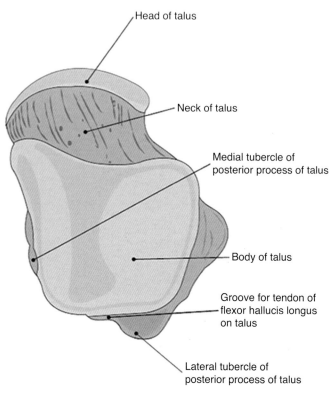

• **Fig. 5.1** Superior view of the talus showing the body of the talus, the talar neck, and head.

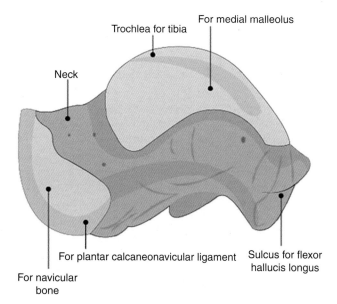

• **Fig. 5.2** Medial view of the talus showing the medial side of the talar head and the articular surface with the medial malleolus.

Pathogenesis

- The tenuous vascularity combined with a lack of periosteal blood supply increases the risk of talar AVN.
- AVN may be secondary to fractures and trauma, prolonged steroid use, alcoholism, or vasopressors.
- The extent of necrosis along with the severity of bone compromise dictates treatment management.

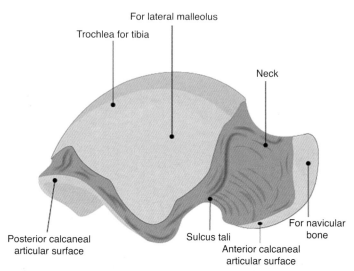

• **Fig. 5.3** Lateral view of the talus showing the lateral side of the talar head, the talar neck, the articular surface with the lateral malleolus, and the posterior facet.

- Extensive AVN has a higher risk of talar dome collapse, which can lead to degenerative changes in the ankle and subtalar joints.[2]

Patient History and Physical Exam Findings

- The clinical presentation of AVN may be quite variable.[3]
- A high level of suspicion is the key to establish an early diagnosis in nontraumatic cases.
- Deep, aching, or sharp ankle pain is a common initial complaint.
- Locking and catching might be felt with more advanced disease.
- A thorough history must be undertaken to look for systemic diseases, substance abuse, or corticosteroid use.
- The physical exam may be unremarkable in the early stages. Effusion and talar tenderness may be present in later stages.
- Limited ankle and subtalar range of motion with malalignment is seen in severe cases.
- In posttraumatic cases, several signs and symptoms may be noted, including ankle and hindfoot pain, effusion, limited range of motion, and crepitus.

Imaging

- Plain radiographs:
  - Multiple weight-bearing views of the ankle to assess for talar sclerosis, collapse, fragmentation, malunion, or nonunion. Early AVN is commonly missed on plain radiographs.
  - Specific views,[4] such as the Canale view, could be obtained to assess talar neck varus malunion.
  - Hawkin's sign might be present at 6 to 8 weeks on an anteroposterior ankle view. It is a sign of subchondral bone resorption in the setting of revascularization.[5]

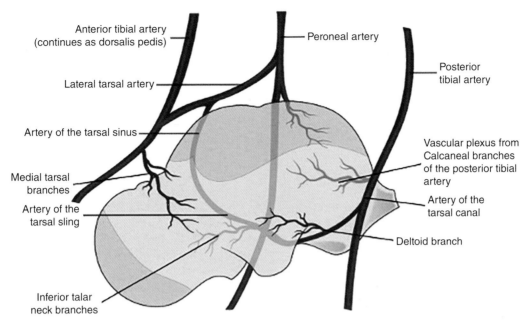

• **Fig. 5.4** Medial view of the talus showing the posterior tibial artery giving off the artery of tarsal canal, which supplies the talar body and branches into the deltoid artery. The anterior tibial artery becomes the dorsalis pedis artery, which gives off the lateral tarsal artery that anastomoses with the perforating branch of the peroneal artery to form the artery of tarsal sinus. The tarsal canal and tarsal sinus arteries anastomose in the sinus tarsi.

• CT scan:
  • This is routinely obtained to assess the extent of the necrosis, the quality of the talar bone, and articular changes.
  • Weight-bearing CT scans provide a better assessment of the ankle/hindfoot alignment and arthritic changes.
  • A contralateral talus CT scan is to be requested for a 3D-printed, custom-made TTR, especially in the setting of talar collapse or anatomic abnormalities of the talus.
• MRI:
  • MRI is the most sensitive modality to assess bone edema, loss of cartilage, quality, and viability of the talar bone.[6]
  • Gadolinium contrast might be considered to differentiate bone edema from an early stage of osteonecrosis.

Nonoperative Management

• Etiology, severity of pathology, and patient comorbidities may guide decision making for nonoperative (conservative) versus operative treatment. In cases of talar AVN, nonoperative treatment may include:
  • Protected weight bearing
  • Patellar tendon-bearing bracing
  • Extracorporeal shock wave therapy.[7]
• Extracorporeal shock wave therapy has been shown to be superior to physical therapy.[8]
• In cases of talar neck fracture complicated by AVN, Hawkins reported that only 12.5% had good or excellent outcomes.[6]

• Patients without talar dome collapse who were treated nonoperatively for a greater period of time (more than 6 months) were not found to have a poorer outcome when an intervention was needed.[8]
• Therapeutic strategies have been suggested to manage talar AVN, but there is no consensus with regard to the ideal treatment algorithm.[9]

Traditional Surgical Management

• Traditional surgical treatment may be divided into joint-sparing and joint-destructive procedures. Traditional joint-sparing procedures include vascularized and nonvascularized bone grafting, core decompression, intraosseous injections, and bone stimulation.
• Vascularized and nonvascularized bone grafting:
  • Different types of vascularized bone graft (VBG) have been described.
  • Nunley et al. successfully used a vascularized cuboid bone graft in 13 patients with AVN involving <60% of the talus.[9]
  • Other techniques using VBG from the medial femoral condyle graft,[10] first cuneiform,[11] and distal tibia[12] have been described with satisfactory outcomes in the treatment of talar AVN.
  • VBG is limited to talar AVN without collapse as these techniques will not alter the morphology of the talar bone.
• Core decompression (CD):
  • CD is used to reduce intraosseous pressure and promote neovascularization of the necrotic zone.

- CD is limited to treatment of early-stage, nontraumatic talar AVN without talar collapse.[13-15]
- Intraosseous stem cell and platelet-rich plasma (PRP) injection therapy[16]:
  - This treatment may be considered in early-stage talar AVN.
  - The treatment should be done under fluoroscopic guidance.
  - May be combined with CD.
- Bone stimulation:
  - Bone stimulators create an exogenous electric current across the osteonecrotic bone that would cause differentiation of the progenitor cells into osteoblasts and enhancement of bone healing.[16]
  - Internal implantation of a bone stimulator into the talus with bone grafting has been described.[17]
- Joint-destructive procedures—arthrodesis:
  - Arthrodesis may be considered as a last-line salvage treatment.
  - Arthrodesis is often used in advanced talar AVN with collapse and/or adjacent joint arthritis.
  - Arthrodesis leads to gait abnormalities and adjacent joint arthritis.
  - A variety of techniques and considerations may be considered:
    - Rarely a limited subtalar or talonavicular joint arthrodesis is indicated.
    - Blair's technique for tibiotalar arthrodesis has a reported high rate of pseudoarthrosis but modifications of this surgical technique have improved fusion rates.[18] These modifications include arthroscopic joint preparation[19] and fixation with a retrograde intramedullary nail to enhance compression and stability.[20] The use of allograft such as femoral head or metal cages to maintain limb length and alignment have shown variable fusion rates.
    - Subtalar arthrodesis following an ipsilateral ankle arthrodesis has a markedly high nonunion rate (40%).[18]

3D-Printed Implant Design Specifications and Considerations

- First-generation implants:
  - In 1997, the first stainless steel talar prosthesis was reported. The implant was designed to replace the talar body with a peg for fixation into the talar head and neck with bone cement.
  - The authors reported only five failures among their 33 patients with a 10- to 36-year follow-up.[19]
- Second-generation implants:
  - The design was similar to the first generation in replacing the talar body but did not include a peg fixation.
  - Taniguchi et al. reported satisfactory results on 12 patients with a 7-year follow-up.[20]

- Third-generation implants:
  - TTR with 3D-printed alumina ceramic prosthesis was first described by Taniguchi in 2015[21]:
    - The dimensions of the prosthesis were determined from bilateral CT scans. A 3D-printed stereolithographic model was created as a negative cast which was then filled with alumina ceramic, creating the prosthesis. The manufacturing process took 4 weeks.
    - Alumina ceramic has been shown to have less wear than stainless steel.[22]
  - The use of 3D-printed cobalt chromium molybdenum (CoCrMo) and Ti implants for TTR has been described. Manufacturing of CoCrMo and Ti implants incorporates use of electron beam melting (EBM), which uses a high vacuum setting to produce metallic materials with a high affinity to oxygen.
  - In 2019, Ti implants with TiN coating were made available.[23] The coating showed improved wear properties in Ti implants and minimized friction on adjacent joint cartilage.[24]
  - Third-generation implants can be used in isolation or combined with a total ankle prosthesis and may be considered constrained or unconstrained:
    - Constrained implants utilize additional fixation into the calcaneus or through ligamentous reconstruction.[25] In 2017, Regauer et al. described design modifications that allow attachment of ligaments to the implant, which may enhance stability.[26]
    - Unconstrained implants are press fitted into the mortise and have no supplemental attachment to adjacent bones or ligaments.

Surgical Management With 3D-Printed Devices

- Positioning: supine
- Anesthesia: general and regional
- A direct anterior approach to the ankle is utilized (Fig. 5.5):
  - A midline skin incision is made 4 cm proximal to the tibiotalar joint and extended to the level of the navicular tuberosity.
  - A sharp dissection is made down to the extensor hallucis longus (EHL) sheath, which is opened and retracted laterally.
  - Identify and protect the superficial peroneal nerve branches in the distal part of the incision and the anterior neurovascular bundle underneath the extensor tendons. The vascular branches travelling medially need to be cauterized and the neurovascular bundle mobilized, protected, and retracted laterally.
  - A large Gelpi retractor can be used.
  - Sharp dissection down to the tibiotalar joint and the capsular flap should be elevated with caution to allow for repair later.
  - All capsuloligamentous attachments of the talus need to be freed from the talonavicular joint.
  - The medial and lateral gutters are debrided.

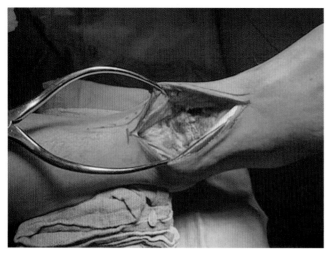

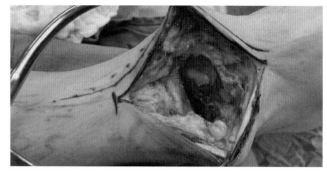

• **Fig. 5.7** Intraoperative photograph after talectomy has been completed. Care was taken not to injure the subtalar facets.

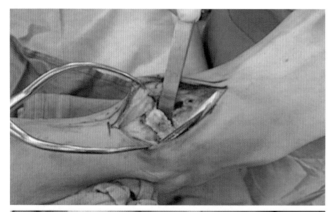

• **Fig. 5.5** Standard anterior ankle approach. The extensor retinaculum was opened on top of the extensor hallucis longus (EHL). The neurovascular bundle and EHL are retracted laterally. The joint capsule was opened longitudinally. The ankle joint is seen with advanced osteoarthritis.

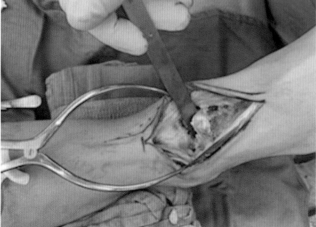

• **Fig. 5.6** Intraoperative photographs of the talus being removed in a segmental fashion.

• Talectomy:
  • The senior author (S.G.P.) recommends removing the talus in a segmental fashion (Fig. 5.6).
  • Excision of the talar neck:
    • A closing wedge osteotomy of the neck is created by first creating a horizontal osteotomy through the distal neck followed by an oblique osteotomy starting at the body-neck junction (approximately 2 cm proximal to the first osteotomy).
    • Take care to avoid injuring the subtalar joint inferiorly.
    • The neck is then removed with a rongeur.
  • Excision of the talar head:
    • A Cobb elevator is placed in the talar-navicular joint, and the head is distracted while sharply releasing soft tissue attachments from the head.
    • The head can then be easily removed.
    • Take care to avoid injury to the navicular cartilage.
  • Excision of the talar body:
    • A horizontal osteotomy is made in the residual talar body with an osteotome. The talar dome and a portion of the dorsal body is then removed. Take care to avoid injury to the tibial plafond cartilage.
    • A vertical osteotomy is used to split the remainder of the body in half. The body can then be removed while avoiding injury to the posterior calcaneal facet. The posteromedial talar body fragment is often scarred and must be carefully removed (Fig. 5.7).
  • Thorough inspection followed by irrigation are necessary to ensure that all small bony fragments are removed.
  • Special care should be made to preserve the medial and lateral ligaments and tendons around the talus.
• Insertion of the total talus prosthesis (TTP):
  • Plastic trials are available with every 3D-printed TTP.
  • One is identical size, one is a 10% smaller implant, and one is a 10% larger implant (Fig. 5.8).
  • The handle on the trials helps with insertion and reduction (Fig. 5.9).
  • The reduction maneuver is a combination of plantarflexion of the foot with traction (Fig. 5.10).
  • After reduction, stability needs to be assessed by taking the ankle in full range of motion.
  • The correct-sized implant gives an audible "thud" when reduced.
  • The final implant is then placed (Figs. 5.11 to 5.12).
  • Final fluoroscopic views are taken (Fig. 5.13).

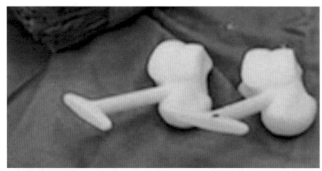

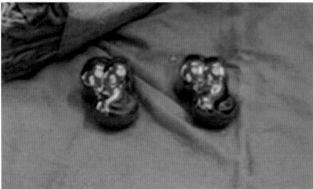

• **Fig. 5.8** The implant trials (white trials) and the final implants (gold) in different sizes.

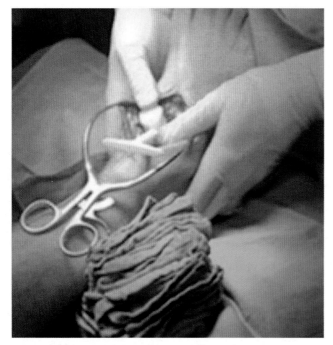

• **Fig. 5.9** Inserting the implant trial into the ankle joint.

• Closure:
  • Layered closure is achieved starting with the capsule, then the extensor retinaculum, then the subcutaneous layer, followed by the skin.
  • A bulky jones splint is applied.

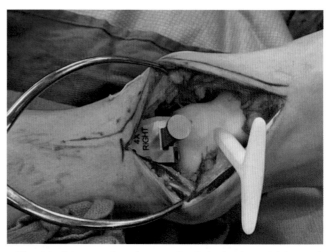

• **Fig. 5.10** Intraoperative photograph of the implant trial inserted. Adequate size and stability confirmed. Note the tibial tray component in this case of a combined total ankle and talus replacement.

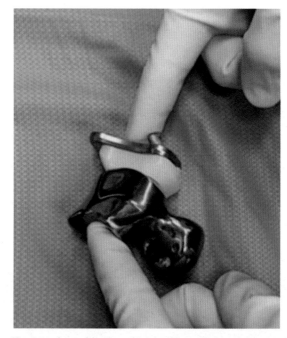

• **Fig. 5.11** A combination of total ankle and talus replacement.

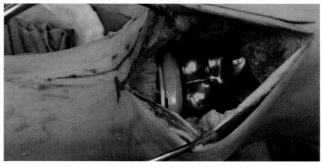

• **Fig. 5.12** The final implant is placed.

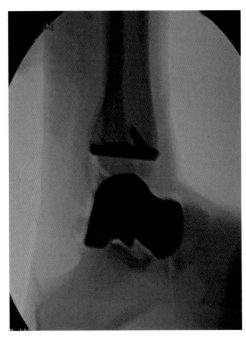

• **Fig. 5.13** Intraoperative lateral fluoroscopy view demonstrating a total ankle total talus replacement (TATTR). Note the congruent talonavicular and subtalar joints.

Postoperative Protocol

- The patient is placed in a non–weight-bearing splint for the first 3 weeks for swelling control and wound healing.
- At 3 weeks:
  - The sutures are usually removed.
  - Routine non–weight-bearing radiographs are taken.
  - The patient is placed in a removable controlled ankle motion (CAM) boot.
  - A shower is allowed without soaking the extremity.
  - The patient can begin weight bearing in the CAM boot.
  - Crutches can be discontinued as soon as the patient feels comfortable.
  - The boot is to be removed three times per day and the patient should attempt to spell out the alphabet with the big toe as a range of motion exercise.
- At 6 weeks:
  - The patient should transition to weight bearing in the CAM boot.
  - On day 1 of week 7, the patient may be out of the boot for a maximum of 2 hours; progressing to 4 hours the next day; then 6, 8, 10, and 12 hours etc.
  - The patient should begin physical therapy.
- Phase 1 (6 to 10 weeks):
  - The patient can begin range of motion (ROM) work, which comprises:
    - Active ROM, ankle circle exercises and alphabet exercises.
    - Intrinsic foot muscles stretching with towel scrunch exercises.
    - Edema control.
    - Ankle strengthening.
    - Aerobic conditioning (stationary bicycle) and proprioceptive exercises.
    - Additional seated leg press can begin later during this phase.
- Phase 2 (10 to 14 weeks):
  - The patient may begin weight-bearing proprioceptive exercises on static and dynamic surfaces.
  - Strengthening may continue to increase in intensity to include standing heel raises, squats, lunges, and step-ups.
  - At 12 weeks, assessment should be made to check that orthotics are maintaining appropriate arch alignment.
- Phase 3 (14 to 16+ weeks):
  - The patient should undergo nonimpact sports-specific training with sport cords including lunges and semicircles.
  - Discharge from therapy:
    - Normal gait without assistive device or bracing.
    - Minimal to no pain during activities of daily living.
    - Minimal swelling.
    - Adequate proprioceptive awareness.

Results/Outcomes

- The senior author's (S.G.P.) experience with 3D-printed TTR for AVN has been published. Twenty-seven patients underwent TTR with a mean follow-up of 22.2 months. Pain score and Foot and Ankle Outcome Scores (FAOSs) with regard to pain, symptoms, quality of life, and activities of daily living significantly improved postoperatively. Three complications required reoperation for superficial peroneal nerve neuroma, residual pain, and deformity in a revision surgery and revision to a combined total ankle total talus for distal tibia AVN.[27]
- Satisfactory results were seen with the alumina Ceramic 3D-printed prosthesis in 55 ankles with talus AVN followed for an average of 52.8 months. The mean scores on the Japanese Society for Surgery of the Foot ankle-hindfoot scale improved for pain, function, alignment, and total score.[28]
- The radiographic parameters after 3D-printed TTR were studied in 14 patients. The custom-made implant restored the talar height and the talar tilt in the setting of AVN and normal alignment of nonpathological joints was maintained.[28]
- Cases of 3D-printed TTR due to severe traumatic loss of the entire talus have been reported.[29,30] At 4 months follow-up of a custom anatomic stainless steel total talar prosthesis, the 25-year-old patient was able to stand and walk without gait aid and the total ankle ROM increased to 21 degrees.[31] A 14-year-old female sustained a talar extrusion but then failed reimplantation and required talectomy and antibiotic spacer due to persistent infection. Later, she underwent a custom-made total talar

prosthesis. Eleven years postoperatively she was doing well.[27] 3D-printed ceramic TTR was used to replace a comminuted talar dome fracture in six patients. With at least 1 year of follow-up, patients were doing well, with an average of 10 degrees dorsiflexion and 31 degrees of plantarflexion. Three patients returned to sports activities.[32]

- 3D-printed modular TTR was successfully used in a 43-year-old female with mesenchymal sarcoma of the talus.[33]

PEARLS AND PITFALLS

Indications and contraindications	• In diffuse talar AVN, as an isolated implant • In combination with a total ankle replacement • In complete talar destruction due to a malignancy or traumatic loss • Isolated total talus replacement is contraindicated in active infection, gross deformity, osteonecrosis of the calcaneus, distal tibia, or navicular bones
Implant design	• Titanium implants with titanium nitride are preferred by the senior author (S.G.P.) • The implant shape should be customized to the patient's anatomy • Use contralateral CT scan to generate 3D-printed talar components • The implant will be press fitted into the ankle mortise • At least 4 weeks are needed to finalize the 3D-printed design
Surgical technique	• Direct anterior approach to the ankle • Complete talectomy in a piecemeal fashion • Care should be taken not to the disrupt the surrounding joint cartilage or to leave parts of the native talus behind • Two sizes trials are available based on the preoperative templating • The ideal sized implant, based on stability, should be used
Postoperative protocol	• Compliance with postoperative instructions, including the initial phase of non-weight bearing, is essential

AVN, Avascular necrosis.

TIPS AND TRICKS

Indications	Diffuse talar avascular necrosis or talar destruction
Goal of reconstruction	Restore anatomy Pain relief Improve function Preserve motion
Imaging	Preoperative bilateral CT scan is necessary for implant planning and assessment of bone quality MRI is necessary for diagnosis
Labs/work up	Rule out infectious etiology
Design	We recommend a press-fitted titanium talar implant with titanium nitride coating
Implantation	We recommend complete removal of the talus. Bone fragments can block reduction The correct size will give an audible "thud" when reduced

References

1. Lachman JR, Parekh SG. Total talus replacement for traumatic bone loss or idiopathic avascular necrosis of the talus. *Tech Foot Ankle Surg.* 2019;18(2):87-98. doi:10.1097/BTF.0000000000000203.
2. Adelaar RS, Madrian JR. Avascular necrosis of the talus. *Orthop Clin North Am.* 2004;35(3):383-395.
3. Chiodo C, Herbst SA. Osteonecrosis of the talus. *Foot Ankle Clin.* 2004;9(4):745-755.
4. Canale ST, Kelly FB Jr. Fractures of the neck of the talus. Long-term evaluation of seventy-one cases. *J Bone Joint Surg Am.* 1978;60(2):143-156.
5. Hawkins LG. Fractures of the neck of the talus. *J Bone Joint Surg Am.* 1970;52(5):991-1002.
6. Pearce DH, Mongiardi CN, Fornasier VL, Daniels TR. Avascular necrosis of the talus: a pictorial essay. *Radiographics.* 2005;25(2):399-410.
7. Gross CE, Sershon RA, Frank JM, Easley ME, Holmes GB. Treatment of osteonecrosis of the talus. *JBJS Rev.* 2016;4(7):e2.
8. Hai L, Sun N, Zhang BQ, Wang JG, Xing GY. Effect of liquid-electric extracorporeal shock wave on treating traumatic avascular necrosis of talus. *J Clin Rehabil Tissue Eng Res.* 2010;14(17):3135-3158.
9. Nunley JA, Hamid KS. Vascularized pedicle bone-grafting from the cuboid for talar osteonecrosis: results of a novel salvage procedure. *J Bone Joint Surg Am.* 2017;99(10):848-854. doi:10.2106/JBJS.16.00841.
10. Struckmann VF, Harhaus L, Simon R, et al. Surgical revascularization—an innovative approach to the treatment of talar osteonecrosis dissecans stages II and III. *J Foot Ankle Surg.* 2017;56(1):176-181.
11. Zhang Y, Liu Y, Jiang Y. Treatment of avascular necrosis of talus with vascularized bone graft. *Zhongguo Xiu Fu Chong Jian Wai Ke Za Zhi.* 1998;12:285-287.

12. Kodama N, Takemura Y, Ueba H, Imai S, Matsusue Y. A new form of surgical treatment for patients with avascular necrosis of the talus and secondary osteoarthritis of the ankle. *Bone Joint J.* 2015;97-B:802-808.

13. Mont MA, Schon LC, Hungerford MW, Hungerford DS. Avascular necrosis of the talus treated by core decompression. *J Bone Joint Surg Br.* 1996;78(5):827-830.

14. Marulanda GA, McGrath MS, Ulrich SD, Seyler TM, Delanois RE, Mont MA. Percutaneous drilling for the treatment of atraumatic osteonecrosis of the ankle. *J Foot Ankle Surg.* 2010;49(1):20-24. doi:10.1053/j.jfas.2009.07.004.

15. Grice J, Cannon L. Percutaneous core decompression: a successful method of treatment of stage I avascular necrosis of the talus. *Foot Ankle Surg.* 2011;17(4):317-318.

16. Kesani AK, Gandhi A, Lin SS. Electrical bone stimulation devices in foot and ankle surgery: types of devices, scientific basis, and clinical indications for their use. *Foot Ankle Int.* 2006;27(2):148-156.

17. Holmes GB, Wydra F, Hellman M, Gross CE. A unique treatment for talar osteonecrosis: placement of an internal bone stimulator: a case report. *JBJS Case Connect.* 2015;5(1):e4. doi:10.2106/JBJS.CC.N.00092.

18. Zanolli DH, Nunley JA, Easley ME. Subtalar fusion rate in patients with previous ipsilateral ankle arthrodesis. *Foot Ankle Int.* 2015;36(9):1025-1028. doi:10.1177/1071100715584014.

19. Harnroongroj T, Vanadurongwan V. The talar body prosthesis. *J Bone Joint Surg Am.* 1997;79:1313-1322. doi:10.2106/00004623-199709000-00005.

20. Taniguchi A, Takakura Y, Sugimoto K, et al. The use of a ceramic talar body prosthesis in patients with aseptic necrosis of the talus. *J Bone Joint Surg Br.* 2012;94(11):1529-1533.

21. Taniguchi A, Takakura Y, Tanaka Y, et al. An alumina ceramic total talar prosthesis for osteonecrosis of the talus. *J Bone Joint Surg Am.* 2015;97(16):1348-1353. doi:10.2106/JBJS.N.01272.

22. Yoshinaga K. Replacement of femoral head using endoprosthesis (alumina ceramics vs metal)–an experimental study of canine articular cartilage. *Nihon Seikeigeka Gakkai Zasshi.* 1987;61(5):521-530.

23. Kadakia RJ, Akoh CC, Chen J, Sharma A, Parekh SG. 3D printed total talus replacement for avascular necrosis of the talus. *Foot Ankle Int.* 2020;41(12):1529-1536.

24. Van Hove RP, Sierevelt IN, Van Royen BJ, Nolte PA. Titanium-nitride coating of orthopaedic implants: a review of the literature. *Biomed Rest Int.* 2015;2015:485975.

25. West TA, Rush SM. Total talus replacement: case series and literature review. *J Foot Ankle Surg.* 2021;60(1):187-193.

26. Regauer M, Lange M, Soldan K, et al. Development of an internally braced prosthesis for total talus replacement. *World J Orthop.* 2017;8(3):221-228.

27. Gadkari KP, Anderson JG, Bohay DR, et al. An eleven-year follow-up of a custom talar prosthesis after open talar extrusion in an adolescent patient: a case report. *JBJS Case Connect.* 2013;3(4):e118. doi:10.2106/JBJS.CC.L.00331.

28. Tracey J, Arora D, Gross CE, Parekh SG. Custom 3D-printed total talar prostheses restore normal joint anatomy throughout the hindfoot. *Foot Ankle Spec.* 2019;12(1):39-48.

29. Stevens BW, Dolan CM, Anderson JG, Bukrey CD. Custom talar prosthesis after open talar extrusion in a pediatric patient. *Foot Ankle Int.* 2007;28(8):933-938. doi:10.3113/FAI.2007.0933.

30. Ruatti S, Corbet C, Boudissa M, et al. Total talar prosthesis replacement after talar extrusion. *J Foot Ankle Surg.* 2017;56(4):905-909.

31. Angthong C. Anatomic total talar prosthesis replacement surgery and ankle arthroplasty: an early case series in Thailand. *Orthop Rev (Pavia).* 2014;6(3):5486. doi:10.4081/or.2014.5486.

32. Katsui R, Takakura Y, Taniguchi A, Tanaka Y. Ceramic artificial talus as the initial treatment for comminuted talar fractures. *Foot Ankle Int.* 2020;41(1):79-83. doi:10.1177/1071100719875723.

33. Fang X, Liu H, Xiong Y, et al. Total talar replacement with a novel 3D printed modular prosthesis for tumors. *Ther Clin Risk Manag.* 2018;14:1897-1905. doi:10.2147/TCRM.S172442.

6

Primary Constrained Total Talus With Subtalar Joint Arthrodesis

PATRICK R. BURNS

Definition

- Patient-specific 3D custom-printed metallic constrained total talus replacement includes modifications to implant design and technique in order to incorporate subtalar arthrodesis.

Anatomy

- The talus, through its articulations, is the link between foot and ankle motion.
- The talus is covered by approximately 60% cartilage, with little area remaining for soft tissue attachments or penetration of blood supply.[1,2]
- The neck of the talus allows for ligament attachment such as the deltoid and the anterior talofibular, which aid in ankle stability. It also contains the interosseous talocalcaneal ligament on its undersurface for portions of subtalar joint stability. A majority of the blood supply to the talus enters through this region, making it vulnerable during injury and surgery.
- The posterior tubercles of the talus allow posterior ligaments such as the posterior talofibular and components of the deep deltoid to aid in ankle stability, as well as the posterior talocalcaneal ligament of the subtalar joint.
- Medial support of the subtalar joint comes from the corresponding talocalcaneal ligament, while the lateral talocalcaneal ligament is aided in its support by the calcaneal fibular ligament.
- The blood supply to the talus is fragile and easily compromised by trauma and surgery.[1,2]
- The main blood supply to the body of the talus is from the posterior tibial artery and its branches through the medial deltoid, in addition to its supply to the artery of the tarsal canal.[3,4]
- The dorsalis pedis artery supplies the dorsal neck and sinus taris region of the talus through the artery of the tarsal sinus.

- The perforating peroneal artery supplies blood to the posterior body as well as to the tarsal sinus plexus.
- The inferior surface of the talus contains facets for articulation with the calcaneus to form the subtalar joint.
- The subtalar joint has an oblique axis that allows for supination and pronation, working in conjunction with the ankle, talonavicular, and calcaneal cuboid joints.
- The subtalar joint axis runs anterior and superomedial from the posterolateral tubercle toward the neck of the talus and is dynamic, changing as the joint progresses through motion.
- The average axis of the subtalar joint is 16 degrees from the sagittal plane, 42 degrees from the transverse plane.[5]
- The accepted range of motion of the subtalar joint is approximately 30 to 40 degrees total, with it divided one-third eversion and two-thirds inversion from neutral.
- Subtalar joint fusion can be a useful procedure and is performed in deformity corrections, to decrease pain in arthritis, to aid in rearfoot stability, and to provide a stable platform for the talus in complicated reconstructions.
- Altered mechanics are still debated after subtalar fusion, with conflicting data. Long-term arthritic changes may not be as definite as once thought but pressure studies show loading shifts after fusion, which may have implication on the ankle joint or implant arthroplasty following fusion. The effects on adjacent joints need to be considered when incorporating subtalar joint fusion into constrained total talus replacement.[6]

Pathogenesis

- Large talar deficits that may necessitate the need to incorporate subtalar arthrodesis include:
  - Severe osteoarthritis including both the ankle and subtalar joints.
  - Avascular necrosis of the talus with concomitant subtalar arthritis or deformity.
  - Other destructive pathology with extensive cystic changes to adjacent bone, such as other arthritides, hemophilic joint pathology, and neoplastic processes.

- Failed arthrodesis with subsequent bone loss.
- Failed total ankle arthroplasty with component subsidence violating the subtalar joint.
- Trauma is the most common cause of talar avascular necrosis (AVN), occurring in approximately 75% of cases, with medication and idiopathic trauma also being described.[1,2]
- Arthritides such as rheumatoid arthritis and osteoarthritis can affect both the ankle and subtalar joints leading to cystic changes and joint destruction, which in some cases involves both the ankle and subtalar joints concurrently.
- With the increasing number of total ankle joint arthroplasties being performed annually, more complications are being reported. The development of revision techniques is essential and, for certain cases, total talar replacement is a possibility. For implants that have violated or subsided into the calcaneus and subtalar joint, incorporating subtalar arthrodesis has been a valuable tool to add fixation and provide a stable platform for the revision.
- Talar deficiency is a challenging dilemma, with surgical options including talectomy, tibiotalocalcaneal arthrodesis with or without bone grafting, tibiocalcaneal arthrodesis, or even major amputation.
- Arthrodesis of the ankle and subtalar joints has been the standard of treatment for large talar deficits and patients with concomitant ankle and subtalar pathology.
- Local bone quality and quantity can make fixation for arthrodesis around the talus challenging. Without adequate fixation, fusion is more likely to fail.
- Unreliable blood supply adds to the challenges of talar deficiency and surgery to address these deformities may disrupt blood supply, further compromising results.
- Long-term consequences of arthrodesis include the potential for limb shortening, stress on adjacent structures, and chronic pain.
- Arthrodesis can lead to increased disability, decreasing overall dorsiflexion by 63% and plantarflexion by 82%.[7]
- Fusion for large talar deficits can have high failure rates including nonunion of 16% to 52%, increased infection rates up to 21.8%, and hardware complications of 14%.
- Fusion for large talar deficits can have an overall high rate of reoperation up to 39.6%, or even conversion to major amputation of up to 16%.[8-10]

Patient History and Physical Exam Findings

- A complete history must be obtained including history of trauma, arthritis, prior surgeries, and any complications encountered.
- Patients will have localized pain to the ankle and subtalar joints. Typically there is loss of motion, but attempting to isolate the ankle from the subtalar joint can be useful.
- Any deformity of the ankle and subtalar joint is noted. Differentiating soft tissue from bone deformity, or rigid from flexible, can assist with surgical planning.

- Equinus is one of the most common associated deformities and should be addressed surgically.
- Instability of the ankle and subtalar joints should be evaluated, which may be caused by soft tissue, loose implant components, or bone loss.
- The range of motion of adjacent joints should be assessed to understand the patient's ability to compensate.
- Joint effusion or crepitation may be noted.
- Consideration of old incisions is important in preoperative planning. Scars from prior fracture care, fusion attempts, or implant surgery may influence your subsequent approach.
- Understanding the patient's activity level and discussing their expectations in particular without long-term data available for patient-specific implants is an important element of the informed decision.

Imaging and Other Diagnostic Testing

- Radiographs:
  - Standard radiographs of the foot and ankle will allow initial assessment of the problem. These images give a sense of the overall mechanics as well as basic deformity planning measurements.
  - Evaluate any angular deformities of the ankle and foot, as these may need to be addressed with additional procedures.
  - The need for refinement with osteotomies and soft tissue work is common when trying to achieve the best outcome in complicated revisions.
  - Take note of shortening or loss of height due to AVN collapse, failed total ankle replacement with component subsidence or similar.
  - Note all hardware as it may require removal for revision. Having an understanding of the current hardware can aid in its removal. Obtaining old reports or notes can benefit the planning process.
  - Understanding the bone quality and quantity is paramount. This can have a bearing on implant design if voids need to be accommodated. Bone may be entirely missing or severely compromised, requiring different configurations of implant surfaces. Violation and variations to the calcaneus, in particular for the purpose of this chapter, require the custom total talus implant to be constrained. Being fixed to the calcaneus and having the appropriate choice of implant surface will promote fusion and stability to the implant, encouraging better outcomes.
- Advanced imaging:
  - MRI may be useful in the diagnosis of AVN. This can be challenging, however, in cases of talus fracture with history of open reduction and internal fixation (ORIF). Hardware can limit the usefulness of MRI and due to interference, the true extent of bone involvement may be disguised by poor image quality.
  - MRI may be useful to evaluate the extent as well as monitor the progression of treatment in reconstructions where infection is an element of the pathology.

- CT scan is the standard of care for evaluating bone, making it useful for peritalar pathology. CT scans give more accurate information regarding bone quality in the presence of large cysts and will often reveal larger cysts or an increased number from what is seen on conventional radiographs.
- CT scan can be more useful in determining nonunion and aids in establishing bone quality with regard to loosening around implants.
- CT scan is the modality of choice for planning and manufacturing patient-specific 3D implants. It is utilized to model the abnormal anatomy and then calculate the more "normal" desired position and size implant to achieve the surgeon's goals.
- Other testing:
  - Infection work-up for any nonunion or failed total ankle arthroplasty is warranted. This includes appropriate laboratory values and inflammatory markers such as complete blood count (CBC), erythrocyte sedimentation rate (ESR), C-reactive protein (CRP), and others at the surgeon's discretion.
  - In cases of infection or concern for infection, infectious disease consultation should be coordinated.
  - If desired, joint aspiration can be performed and analyzed.
  - Likewise if there is concern, surgery may be staged so that hardware can removed and appropriate cultures taken. This should include frozen sections from the surrounding soft tissue for more complete information.[11]
  - Hardware removed should also be sent for sonication and subsequent culture.[12]
  - In cases that are staged, external fixation is considered. This allows for stability and maintenance of the correction. Stability will limit inflammation, and since the deformity has already been reduced and held by the external fixator, the definitive surgery is easier to finalize.
  - In cases of concern, vascular testing may be judicious and an appropriate vascular consultation scheduled where necessary.
  - Nutrition can be monitored with appropriate laboratories including total protein, albumin, and prealbumin.
  - Decisions can be made by the surgeon to monitor and address any smoking history. In particular, in cases of arthrodesis smoking may have a role in failure to fuse.[13]

Nonoperative Management

- Upright ankle bracing, hinged or solid.
- Custom bracing such as Arizona bracing or similar.
- Assistive devices to aid in ambulation, including a cane or walker.
- Pain-management modalities.

Traditional Surgical Management

- For large talar voids and simultaneous subtalar pathology, the standard has been arthrodesis of the ankle and subtalar joints with internal fixation.

- External fixation has been utilized but requires knowledge and comfort with this form of fixation. Depending on the construct, external fixation can add significant cost.
- In situ tibiotalocalcaneal fusion may require a bone graft, which may be from local bone if a lateral incision is utilized. The fibula can be harvested and then utilized to aid in height loss and to fill voids, but this option has limits.
- For larger deficits including talectomy, allograft bone has been described.[14]
- A large allograft utilized for arthrodesis has limitations as far as the overall size of graft that can be incorporated. In addition, the bone has to heal at two locations, increasing the possibility for one end to fail union.
- Tibiocalcaneal fusion is an alternative but leads to significant loss of length to the affected limb. This may be balanced by shoe lifts, but has a mechanical cost and may not be tolerated well.
- Distraction osteogenesis is a possibility but requires a lengthening osteotomy and a procedure more proximal. It also requires advanced knowledge of deformity correction. Generating length proximally while performing a distal arthrodesis is more challenging. Complications exist with external fixation, including pin site infection, and in the case of distraction osteogenesis, there is now potential for complications at the proximal surgical site. The distraction performed proximal must regenerate bone with appropriate quality and quantity to have a successful outcome.
- Below-knee amputation is an option but is generally reserved for severe infection or nonreconstructable cases, such as those with bone loss that cannot be overcome or failed revisions. Major amputation can lead to a slower gait, a shorter stride length, and increased energy expenditure.[15]

3D-Printed Implant Design Specifications and Considerations

- Titanium and cobalt chrome are the materials of choice for 3D-printed implants (Fig. 6.1).
- In the case of an implant surface being utilized for arthrodesis, the surface to interface with the native bone must be able to accept bone ingrowth. There have been many materials applied to implants over the years, but the exposed porous surfaces of metal seem to be the most popular and studied.
- Because most of the total talus implant requires articulation, cobalt chrome is the best option as the surfaces can be polished to meet medical standards.
- For constrained total talus applications, the talus articulates with the navicular distal and the tibia or total ankle component dorsally; however, the undersurface requires a porous exposed surface for integration with the calcaneus (Fig. 6.2).
- The porous style preferred by the author is a "gyroid" design that allows for maximum bone ingrowth to the implant. The amount and location of the porous structure is

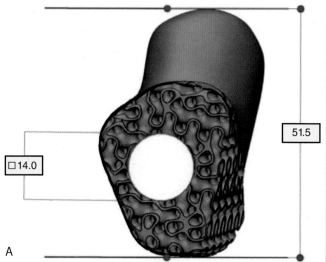

• **Fig. 6.1** Clinical image of a (A) cobalt chrome and (B) titanium total talus implant.

defined by the anatomy and aided in construction by a CT scan.

- Most constrained total talus cases have three sizes of implant for trial and subsequent placement. This allows flexibility for the surgeon and it is the surgeon's decision regarding what is to be made available. Based on CT scans, the implant can be made "nominal" or what is thought to be the actual size of the native talus. One size larger and one size smaller are typical alternatives that can be produced and made available, typically 5% smaller and 5% larger (Fig. 6.3).
- At the time of surgery there are typically three sizes of implants available and the surgeon decides on the best "fit" after trialing them intraoperatively (Fig. 6.4).
- If there is significant destruction or bone loss, the contralateral extremity can be imaged with a CT scan and the implant to be utilized is fabricated to mirror that side.
- Preoperative imaging reveals all bone defects which are then "filled" in using available data from the remaining talus or the contralateral side to generate the implant (Fig. 6.5).
- To incorporate subtalar fusion, the corresponding posterior facet of the calcaneus requires intraoperative preparation. This is done using the surgeon's preferred technique. It is the author's preference to be certain that subchondral bone of the calcaneus is exposed to allow bone ingrowth into the porous undersurface of the 3D talus implant.
- The corresponding joint surface can be prepared and then drilled or fishscaled to promote the arthrodesis discussed later in Technique 1.
- An alternative is to prepare the posterior facet with an acetabular reamer, discussed later in Technique 2. This is useful to expose increased amounts of subchondral bone and for those with larger calcaneal cysts or loss. This technique also allows for a modification to the undersurface of the total talus implant. The plantar portion of the

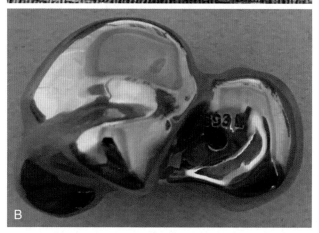

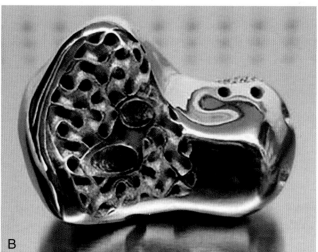

• **Fig. 6.2** Preoperative planning and (A) CAD drawing of a planned implant with a gyroid surface covering areas for projected fusion. (B) Clinical image of a custom implant undersurface with a gyroid surface for bone integration. *CAD*, Computer-aided design. (Reprinted with permission from Restor3d, Inc, Durham, NC.)

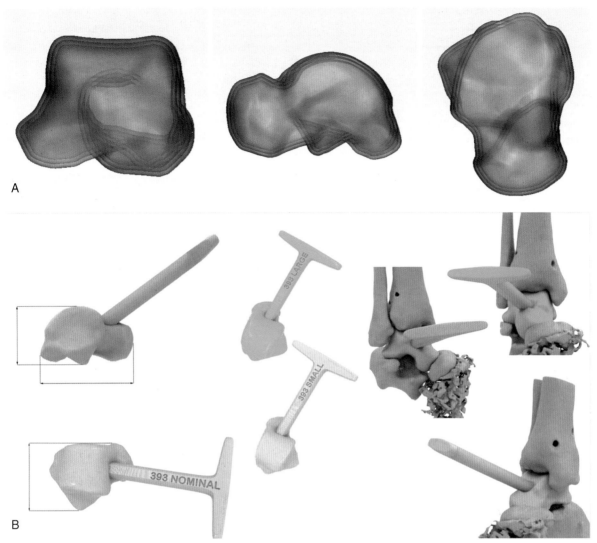

• **Fig. 6.3** Preoperative CAD planning with suggested implant sizes (A) along with proposed trials (B). *CAD,* Computer-aided design. (Reprinted with permission from Additive Orthopaedics, LLC, Little Silver, NJ).

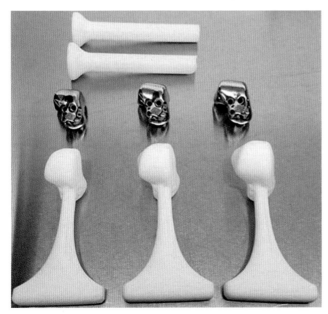

• **Fig. 6.4** Custom total talus implants with corresponding sizers.

implant can then be made convex, increasing the amount of porous undersurface having contact with the fusion surface of the calcaneus. This also allows for more surgeon adjustment, as the surface is rounded compared to a more traditional saddle-shaped talus design.

• Custom talus implants designed to incorporate subtalar fusion must also be designed to accommodate some form of fixation. The implant in this fashion is then considered "constrained" as it is fixated to the calcaneus.

• Through the design process and utilizing CT scans, holes to accommodate screw fixation can be included in the implant. The trajectory and screw size to be utilized is decided on by the surgeon and anatomy available. The author prefers two large screws (Fig. 6.6).

• Appropriate-sized holes with corresponding drill guides are provided at the time of surgery to constrain the total talus implant.

• For placement purposes, screws must originate in the implant, with screw threads ending in native bone. Threads cannot end in the custom implant.

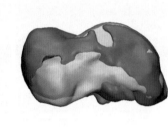
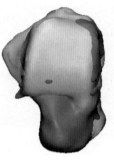

• **Fig. 6.5** Preoperative CAD showing missing or damaged areas *(blue)*, of the affected talus using the contralateral side to aid in filling in missing information. *CAD,* Computer-aided design. (Reprinted with permission from Additive Orthopaedics, LLC, Little Silver, NJ).

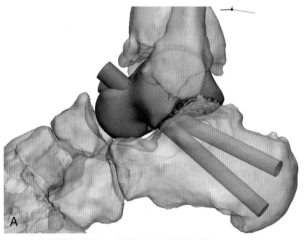

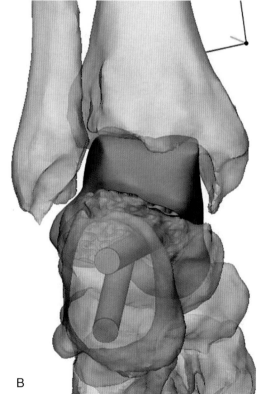

• **Fig. 6.6 (A and B)** CAD images with proposed fixation for a constrained custom 3D total talus implant. The screw size and trajectory are planned preoperatively. *CAD,* Computer-aided design. (Reprinted with permission from Restor3d, Inc, Durham, NC.)

- From the author's experience, it has not been necessary to require soft tissue attachment methods for this style of implant, although it has been described.
- Consideration of constrained versus unconstrained should be made. Incorporating the subtalar joint fusion to create a constrained implant is necessary when there is concomitant bone loss or structural concerns regarding the posterior facet and subtalar joint. A constrained total talus can then achieve multiple goals of replacing a large void and maintaining ankle and talonavicular range of motion, yet fusing a compromised subtalar joint.
- Long-term metal-on-cartilage wear as well as the need for stability have been considerations for constraining all custom total talus implants, but it is the surgeon's decision with limited data available to guide.[16] It is the author's preference to incorporate subtalar fusion only when there is concern for the structural integrity of the calcaneus.

Surgical Management With 3D-Printed Devices

- Equipment required:
  - Usual instrument set and joint distractor.
  - Appropriate saw and drill system.
  - Screw set for subtalar fixation; the author prefers large 6.5-mm cannulated screws.
  - Fluoroscopy.
  - 3D custom implant, corresponding sizers, and prefabricated drill guides for selected screws (Fig. 6.7).
- Position: supine with a bump under the ipsilateral hip to ensure the anterior ankle is in the proper position.
- Anesthesia: general and regional.
- Approach: the majority of 3D total talus implants incorporating subtalar fusion are performed from an anterior approach. This can vary depending on prior incisions but anterior is preferred, allowing the most complete access to anatomy.
- Technique 1:
  - The incision utilized most often is the standard anterior ankle approach between the tibialis anterior and extensor hallucis longus tendons (Fig. 6.8).

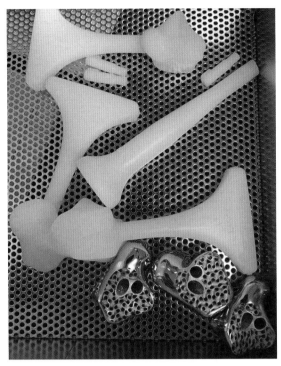

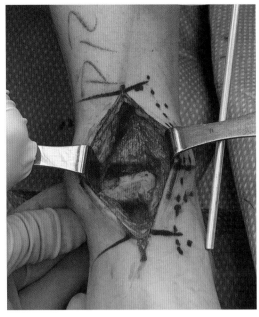

• **Fig. 6.9** Intraoperative image of the anterior incision. Note that the tendons remain in their sheath while gaining access to the talus.

• **Fig. 6.7** Intraoperative image of implants for a constrained total talus. Note the availability of multiple sizers, implants, impactor, and prefabricated drill guides for eventual screw fixation.

- If possible, tendons are kept protected in their tendon sheaths.
- The anterior ankle joint capsule is opened to reveal the anterior dome of the talus (Fig. 6.9).
- This capsule reflection is continued distal over the talonavicular joint to expose the entire dorsal surface of the talar head and neck.

- If there is obvious hardware from a previous ORIF or implant arthroplasty, some may be able to be removed. Otherwise, hardware remaining in the talus may be removed during the talus explant itself and can be disregarded.
- The talus is removed completely. This may require one or more osteotomies through the neck and body. This can be performed with a saw or osteotome. Smaller pieces may be easier to remove (Fig. 6.10).

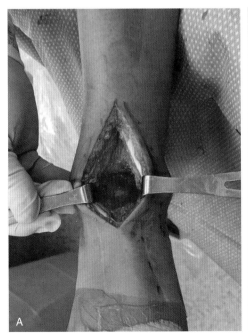

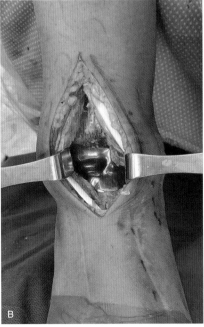

• **Fig. 6.8** (A and B) Intraoperative images of the typical anterior approach to the talus for custom total talus implant. This gives access to the talus itself as well as the subtalar joint for fusion. Note the prior healed incisions common in talar pathology.

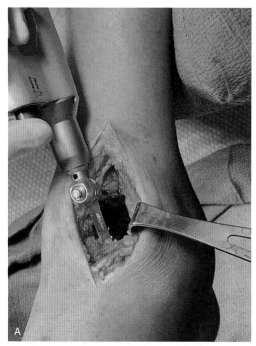

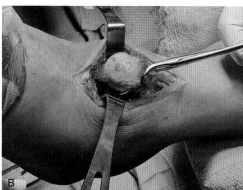

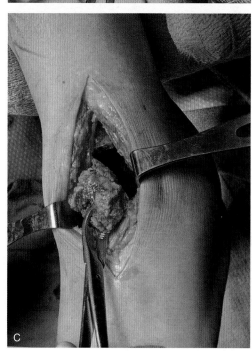

• **Fig. 6.10** (A–C) The talus is removed, often being cut into smaller pieces to facilitate removal.

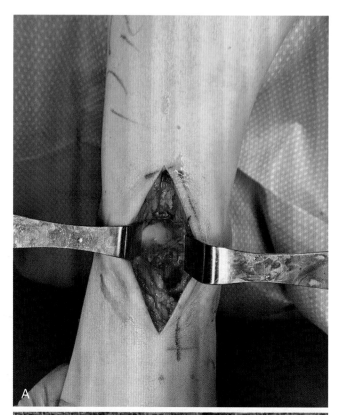

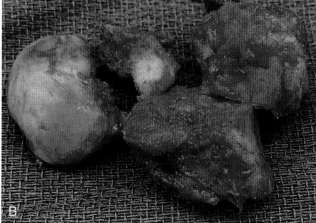

• **Fig. 6.11** Intraoperative image of a talectomy. (A) Note the posterior facet of the calcaneus is now accessible in the wound. (B) The talus was removed in pieces.

- Care is taken to remove all fragments and then an inspection is performed on the soft tissue and remaining void (Fig. 6.11).
- If this surgery is staged, cultures and pathology may be taken.
- For primary surgery, the posterior facet is identified and any remaining cartilage is removed using the surgeon's preferred method.
- The posterior facet is drilled or fishscaled to allow access to the subchondral bone, which aids bone ingrowth to the undersurface of the talus implant (Fig. 6.12).
- The foot is typically plantarflexed and inverted to permit placement of the trials.

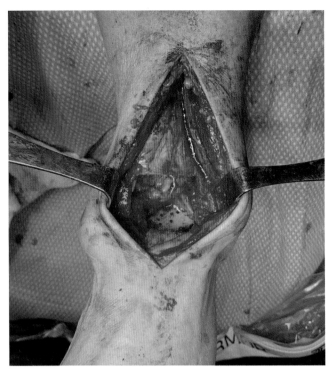

• **Fig. 6.12** Intraoperative image of the posterior facet of the calcaneus after cartilage has been removed. Note the subchondral drilling to facilitate bone fusion and ingrowth once the constrained total talus implant is placed and fixated.

- Radio-opaque sizers are then placed through the anterior incision and assessed.
- The overall fit of the implant is evaluated using both fluoroscopy and direct visualization. All contact surfaces are assessed and stability is examined throughout the range of motion (Fig. 6.13).
- If being done with a tibial component as part of ankle arthroplasty, this can be performed before placement of the custom total talus.
- Once a decision is made, the appropriate implant can be prepared. At the surgeon's preference bone graft can be applied to the plantar surface of the implant along the porous surface to aid ingrowth.
- The actual implant may be slightly more difficult to place as the undersurface is rough and designed to have a coefficient of friction (Fig. 6.14).
- With the implant placed, the custom-printed targeting guides can be placed in the appropriate prearranged holes in the neck of the talus implant. These are typically 3D-printed "sleeves" that fit into the holes within the custom implant. They are designed to match the guide pin for the predetermined screw. Once the guide pins are placed through these guides, fluoroscopy is utilized to accurately determine the screw length (Fig. 6.15).
- The targeting guide pin sleeves are removed from the implant and the screws are placed over the guide pin and tightened.
- Guide pins for the cannulated screws are removed.

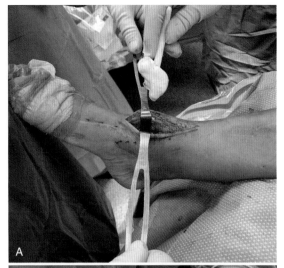

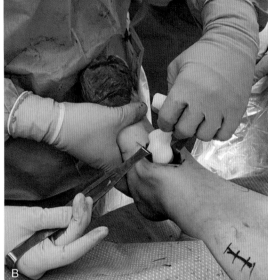

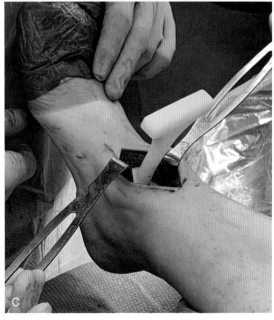

• **Fig. 6.13** Placement of trials through the anterior incision. (A) It is usually helpful to plantarflex and invert the foot for placement. (B) The trial is placed and then (C) fit and range of motion is evaluated.

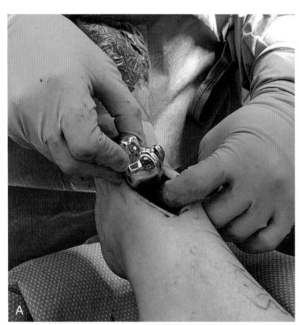
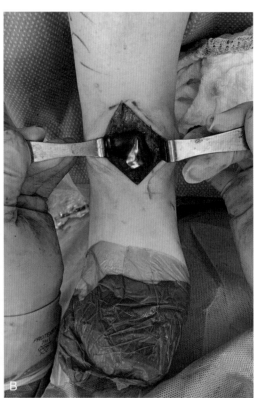

• **Fig. 6.14** (A) Placement of the final custom implant and (B) an intraoperative picture of the implant in place.

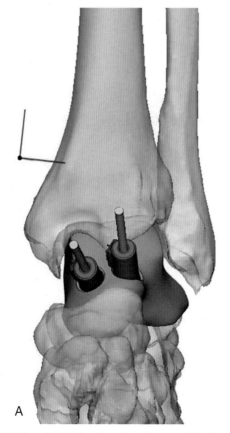

Drilling for 6.5 mm synthes screws

1. Place implant in the anatomy
2. Place k-wire guides into holes for screws
3. Shoot 2.8 mm k-wires through guides
4. Slide guides off over k-wires
5. Drill over k-wires using 5.0 mm cannulated drill

• **Fig. 6.15** (A and B) CAD schematic of proposed fixation. Note the custom-designed drill guide sleeves to be used intraoperatively. These guides are designed to accept the predetermined guide pin. The guides protect the implant and ensure appropriate screw placement into the calcaneus.

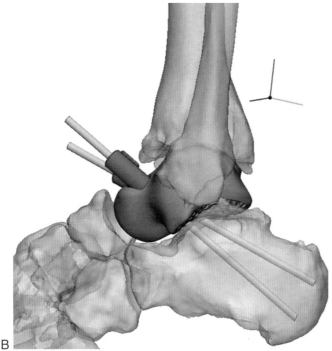

Drilling for 6.5 mm synthes screws

1. Place implant in the anatomy
2. Place k-wire guides into holes for screws
3. Shoot 2.8 mm k-wires through guides
4. Slide guides off over k-wires
5. Drill over k-wires using 5.0 mm cannulated drill

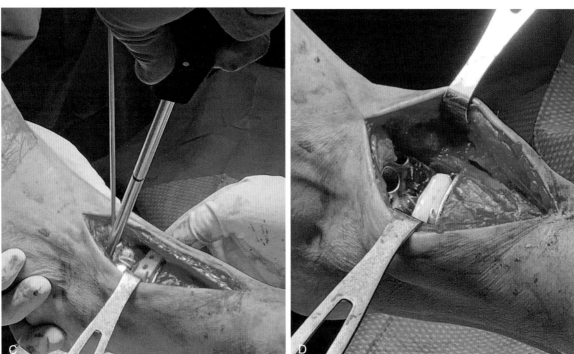

• **Fig. 6.15, cont'd** (C) Intraoperative photos of a constrained total talus implant with guide pins placed and the screw being inserted. The pins and screws follow the planned trajectory. (D) In the final image of the constrained implant, note the screw holes in the talar neck area with a recess to prevent prominence of the screw head. *CAD*, Computer-aided design. (Reprinted with permission from Restor3d, Inc, Durham, NC.)

- Fluoroscopy then confirms placement of the implant and screws.
- The construct is again tested for range of motion and stability.
- Adjunctive procedures are performed as needed.
- Layered closure and the use of a drain is then performed according to the surgeon's preference.

- Radiographs of an example of Technique 1 are provided in Figs. 6.16 to 6.19.
- Technique 2:
  - The approach and removal of the damaged talus is performed in a similar manner.
  - Once the posterior facet of the calcaneus is exposed, it is prepared utilizing an acetabular reamer. The size

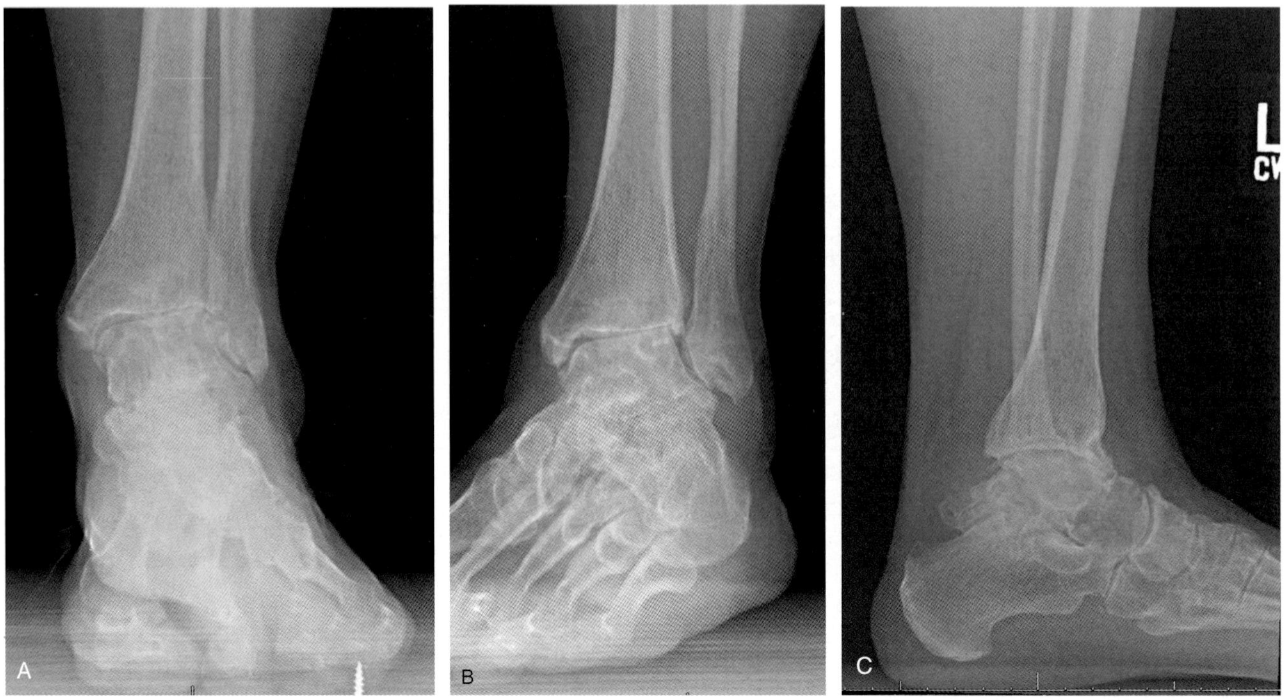

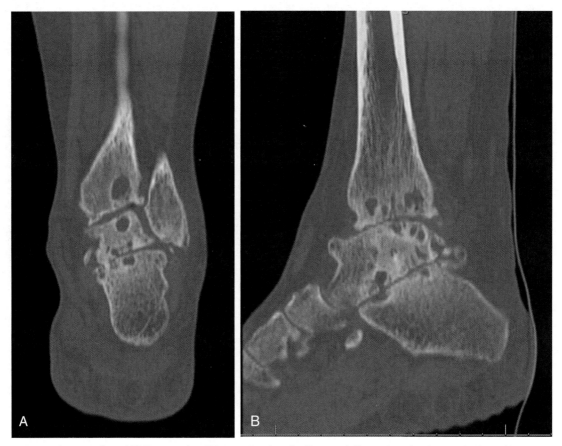

• **Fig. 6.16** (A–C) Preoperative radiographs revealing arthritic and cystic changes to both the ankle and subtalar joints. Mild valgus deformity is noted as well.

• **Fig. 6.17** (A and B) Preoperative CT scan showing significant arthritic and cystic changes in the ankle and subtalar joints.

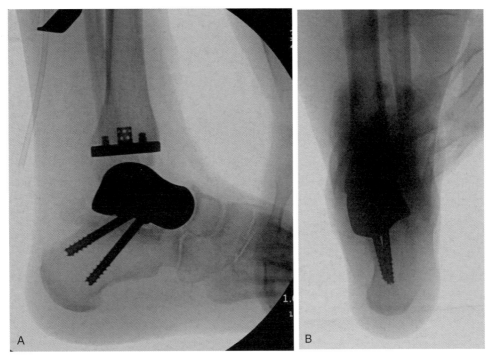

• **Fig. 6.18** (A and B) Intraoperative fluoroscopy to confirm implant and screw fixation for constrained total talus implant.

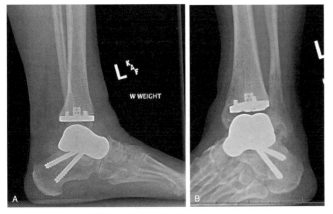

• **Fig. 6.19** (A and B) Weight-bearing images of a restrained total talus implant matched with a tibial component for combined arthrodesis of the subtalar joint and ankle arthroplasty.

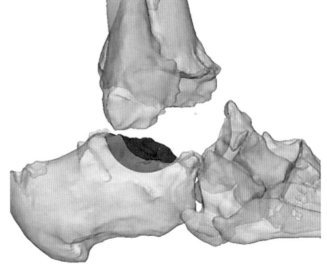

• **Fig. 6.20** CAD image with a proposed resection and size reamer, in this case a 36-mm reamer was selected. *CAD*, Computer-aided design. (Reprinted with permission from Restor3d, Inc, Durham, NC.)

of the reamer is determined preoperatively using a CT scan (Fig. 6.20).

- The reamer is placed through the anterior incision and monitored using fluoroscopy to ensure appropriate orientation and that the appropriate amount of subchondral bone is removed (Fig. 6.21).
- It is useful during reaming to frequently reevaluate the resection depth.
- Trials are placed and assessed.
- If a tibial component is necessary, it is implanted after reaming and copious irrigation is performed.
- The final talar implant is then packed with bone graft. The author prefers morselized autograft from the proximal or distal tibia. The graft is collected and separated into solid and liquid components using

the Hensler Bone Press (Hensler Surgical Technologies, Wilmington, NC). The solid graft is then easily packed into the trabecular/porous aspect of the implant.

- The talar implant is then placed. Under fluoroscopy it is aligned and the provided custom targeting guides are placed.
- Utilizing the provided guides, the talar component is then fixated or constrained to the calcaneus with predetermined screws (Fig. 6.22).

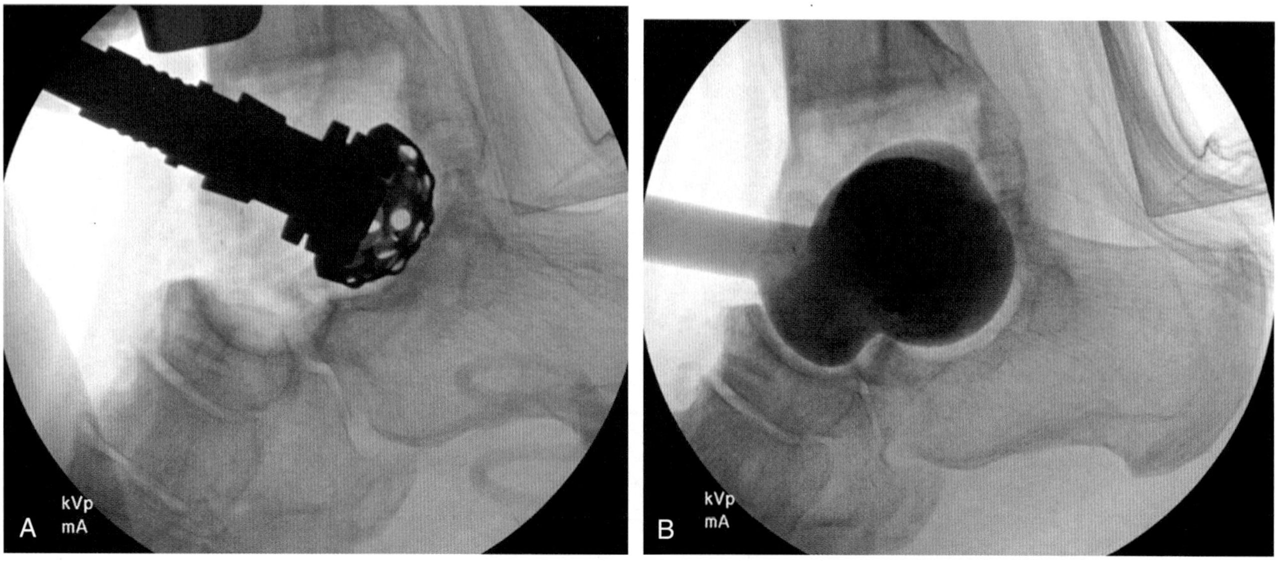

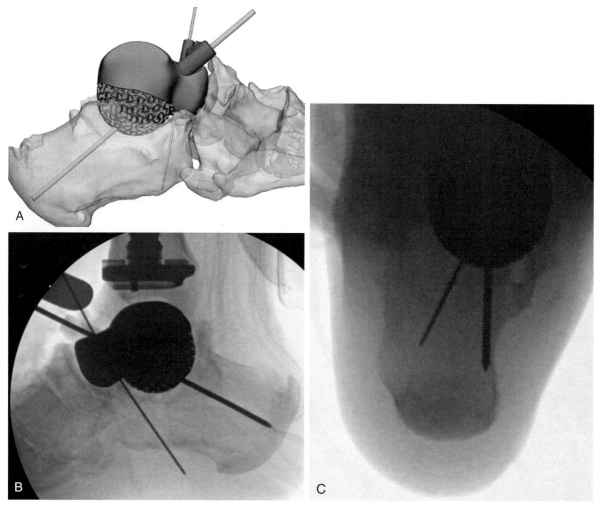

• **Fig. 6.21** Intraoperative fluoroscopy showing the (A) reamer utilized through the anterior incision used to contour the (B) calcaneus for testing of the implant trials. This technique allows the surgeon to have more flexibility with implant alignment while maximizing surface area for bone ingrowth.

• **Fig. 6.22** (A) CAD drawing of proposed screws and their trajectory. (B & C) Intraoperative fluoroscopy showing guide pins and the predetermined trajectory and placement of screws for a constrained total talus implant. *CAD*, Computer-aided design. (Reprinted with permission from Restor3d, Inc, Durham, NC.)

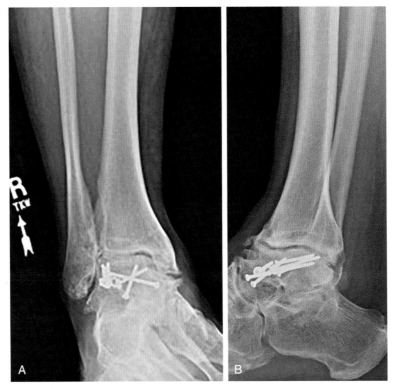

• **Fig. 6.23** (A and B) Preoperative radiographs of a posttraumatic arthritic ankle and subtalar joint after talar fracture and subsequent open reduction and internal fixation.

- The targeting guides are removed and appropriate screws placed.
- Fluoroscopy then confirms placement of the implant and screws.
- The construct is again tested for range of motion and stability.
- Adjunctive procedures are performed as needed.
- Layered closure and the use of a drain is then performed according to the surgeon's preference.
- Radiographs of an example of Technique 2 are provided in Figs. 6.23 to 6.28.

Postoperative Protocol

- Patients are placed in a non–weight-bearing compression splint.
- Many patients are kept overnight for observation to help with pain control as well as to evaluate the splint the next morning.
- Anticoagulation is initiated the next day unless there are contraindications.
- The patient is followed according to the surgeon's protocol. The author's preference is to follow-up in 1 week.
- A below-knee cast is then applied for 2 weeks, and the patient is kept non–weight bearing.
- The sutures are removed when the anterior skin is healed.
- The usual non–weight bearing period is 6 weeks due to the arthrodesis component.
- Transition to a walking boot occurs after week 6.
- Protected weight bearing is then at least 4 weeks.

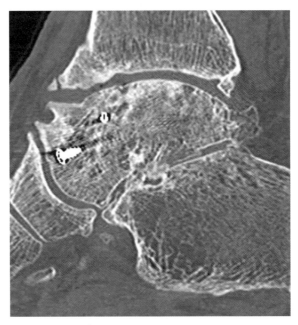

• **Fig. 6.24** CT scan revealing significant changes to both the ankle and subtalar joints.

- Radiographs are typically performed at monthly intervals or at the surgeon's discretion.
- A CT scan may be beneficial to evaluate incorporation, but it is not the author's routine practice to order advanced imaging unless there is a concern.
- The patient is transitioned to shoe gear and activity depending on tolerance, starting with low impact.
- Physical therapy as appropriate.

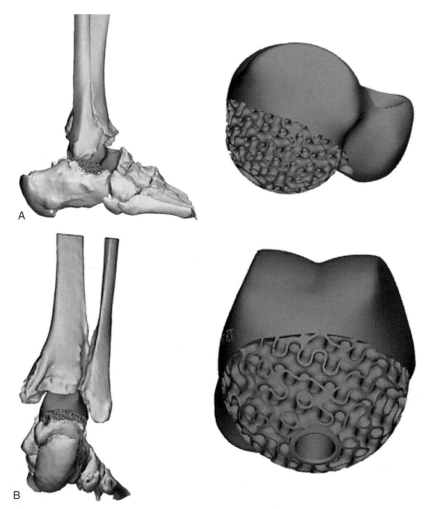

• **Fig. 6.25** Preoperative CAD images with a proposed constrained total talus design. **(A and B)** Note the concave gyroid inferior surface and the implant. This design allows more flexibility with intraoperative correction as well as an increased surface area for bone integration with the implant. *CAD*, Computer-aided design. (Reprinted with permission from Restor3d, Inc, Durham, NC.)

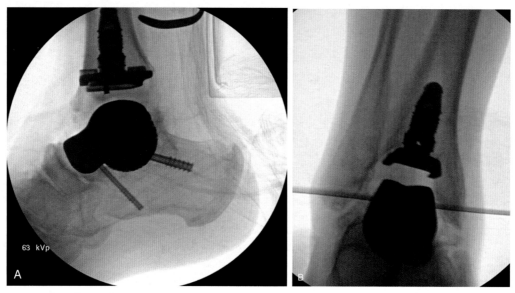

• **Fig. 6.26** (A and B) Intraoperative images after appropriate fit and placement of the implant was confirmed. Screw fixation adds stability and compression to the constrained custom implant.

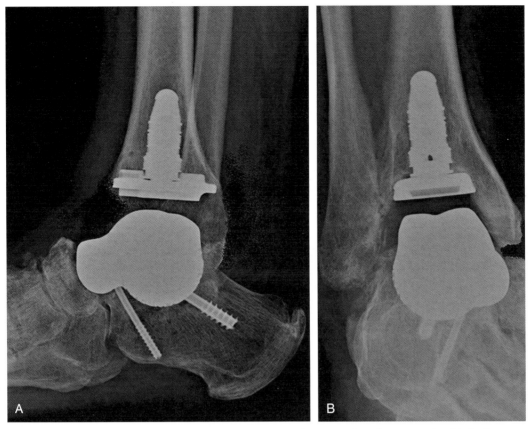

• **Fig. 6.27** (A and B) Postoperative radiographs demonstrating appropriate alignment and stable fixation.

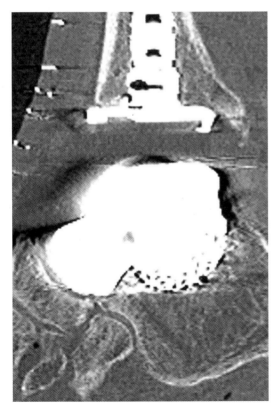

• **Fig. 6.28** Postoperative CT scans can be obtained to evaluate osseous integration. Note the increased surface area achieved by this style of constrained total talus implant.

Considerations

- Replacement of the entire talus is reserved for patients with severe deformity or bone loss affecting the ankle and subtalar joints.
- In appropriate patients a constrained total talus implant can provide an alternative to the more limiting extended fusions or even amputation.
- In the author's practice custom talar implants have been very useful, in particular for the younger patient after trauma. In past years, we have been limited to extended arthrodesis in these unfortunate younger patients after trauma. With extensive arthritis and at times collapse after AVN, custom talus replacement has become a welcome addition to the treatments available.
- With increasing numbers of total ankle arthroplasty being performed, the vulnerability of the talus has been exposed. The talus in some cases is not strong enough to support the prosthesis and in others there may have been excessive bone removal from the talar body. The author has seen several cases of component subsidence eroding through the talar body into the calcaneus. This results in a difficult salvage where constrained total talus implants would have given the option of successful revision.
- Constraining the implant to the calcaneus has advantages in patients with concomitant subtalar pathology.

The long-term sequalae of a constrained talus implant is not known but should mimic subtalar joint fusion. Longer follow-up and serial imaging should be performed.

- The surgeon must take an active role in interpreting the CT scan and subsequent computer-aided drawing (CAD) images. The more information that is discussed and shared, the better the implant design and surgical plan.

- There is limited data on outcomes, with mostly case or series reports on constrained total talus patient-specific implants.[16-19]

- In the author's experience, there have been no intraoperative issues with implantation. The custom-printed target guides have allowed for quick, accurate screw placement.

- Modifying the plantar surface of the implant as in Technique 2 has been a progression in thought process and design. This has allowed for more controlled implant placement. It has also allowed for a larger surface area to facilitate bone migration into the implant. This more closely matches other total joint surgery where larger areas of subchondral or cancellous bone have been exposed with bone cuts. Although drilling and fishscaling have been a mainstay of fusion surgery, exposing additional subchondral bone seems a reasonable progression.

References

1. Kadakia RJ, Akoh CC, Chen J, Sharma A, Parekh SG. 3D printed total talus replacement for avascular necrosis of the talus. *Foot Ankle Int.* 2020;41(12);1529-1536.

2. Gross CE, Haughom B, Chahal J, Holmes GB. Treatment for avascular necrosis of the talus. A systematic review. *Foot Ankle Spec.* 2014;7(5):387-397.

3. Mulfinger GL, Trueta J. The blood supply of the talus. *J Bone Joint Surg Br.* 1970;52(1):160-167.

4. Shnol H, LaPorta GA. 3D printed total talar replacement: a promising treatment option for advanced arthritis, avascular osteonecrosis, and osteomyelitis of the ankle. *Clin Podiatr Med Surg.* 2018; 35(4):403-422.

5. Kirby KA. Subtalar joint axis location and rotational equilibrium theory of foot function. *J Am Podiatr Med Assoc.* 2001;91(9):465-487.

6. Hutchinson ID, Baxter JR, Gilbert S, et al. How do hindfoot fusions affect biomechanics: a cadaver model. *Clin Orthop Relat Res.* 2016;474:1008-1016.

7. Chou LB, Mann RA, Yaszay B, et al. Tibiotalocalcaneal arthrodesis. *Foot Ankle Int.* 2000;21(10):804-808.

8. Pitts C, Alexander B, Washington J, et al. Factors affecting the outcomes of tibiotalocalcaneal fusion. *Bone Joint J.* 2020; 102-B(3):345-351.

9. Bussewitz B, DeVries JG, Dujela M, McAlister JE, Hyer CF, Berlet GC. Retrograde intramedullary nail with femoral head allograft for large deficit tibiotalocalcaneal arthrodesis. *Foot Ankle Int.* 2014;35(7):706-711.

10. Devries JG, Philbin TM, Hyer CF. Retrograde intramedullary nail arthrodesis for avascular necrosis of the talus. *Foot Ankle Int.* 2010;31(11):965-972.

11. Musso AD, Mohanty K, Spencer-Jones R. Role of frozen section histology in diagnosis of infection during revision arthroplasty. *Postgrad Med J.* 2003;79:590-593.

12. Evangelopoulos DS, Stathopoulos IP, Morassi GP, et al. Sonication: a valuable technique for diagnosis and treatment of periprosthetic joint infections. *Scientific World J.* 2013;2013:375140.

13. Pearson RG, Clement RG, Edwards KL, Scammell BE. Do smokers have a greater risk of delayed and non-union after fracture, osteotomy and arthrodesis? A systematic review with meta-analysis. *BMJ Open.* 2016;6:1-10.

14. Jeng CL, Campbell JT, Tang EY, Cerrato RA, Myerson MS. Tibiotalocaneal arthrodesis with bulk femoral head allograft for salvage of large defects in the ankle. *Foot Ankle Int.* 2013;34(9): 1256-1266.

15. Waters RL, Perry J, Antonelli D, Hislop H. Energy cost of walking of amputees: the influence of level of amputation. *J Bone Joint Surg Am.* 1976;58:42-46.

16. West TA, Rush AM. Total talus replacement: case series and literature review. *J Foot Ankle Surg.* 2021;60:187-193.

17. Scott DJ, Steele J, Fletcher A, Parekh SG. Early outcomes of 3D printed total talus arthroplasty. *Foot Ankle Spec.* 2020;13: 372-377.

18. Patel H, Kinmon K. Revision of failed total ankle replacement with a custom 3-dimensional printed talar component with a titanium truss cage: a case presentation. *J Foot Ankle Surg.* 2019; 58:1006-1009.

19. Ruatti S, Corbet C, Boudissa M, et al. Total talar prosthesis replacement after talar extrusion. *J Foot Ankle Surg.* 2017;56:905-909.

7

3D-Printed Custom Hemi-Talus Replacement

JAMES M. COTTOM, CHARLES A. SISOVSKY

Definition

- Resection of damaged cartilage and subchondral bone in the talus which is then replaced with a metallic, patient-specific, 3D-printed implant without the need for malleolar osteotomy.

Indication(s)

- Chronic, medium-to-large osteochondral defects (OCDs) of the talar dome which are often uncontained (i.e., involving the talar shoulder) and have mixed cystic and sclerotic subchondral bone.
- Prior failed arthroscopic OCD repair which may include debridement, microfracture, or morselized cartilage allografting.
- Prior failed open treatment of the OCD which may include structural allograft resurfacing or osteochondral transfer.

Anatomy and Pathogenesis

- 60% of the talus is covered by articular (hyaline) cartilage which contains no nervous, vascular, or lymphatic vessels.
- The exact etiology of talar OCDs has been theorized to be direct trauma, microtrauma secondary to instability or deformity, and spontaneous focal avascular necrosis (AVN).
- With time, OCDs may progress in size, develop cystic bone and sclerosis, subchondral collapse, and higher, asymmetric contact stresses.
- There is concern for the development of localized arthritis but, in general, OCDs do not progress to diffuse arthritis.
- Classically, acute lateral OCDs tend to be more shallow and anteriorly located, whereas acute medial lesions are cup-shaped, deeper, and located in the central to posterior aspects of the talar dome. In our experience, chronic lesions, especially if prior surgical intervention, are more

irregularly shaped, have a variable/nonuniform depth, and a degree of local AVN.

Patient History and Physical Exam Findings

- In the authors' experience, patients complain of anterior or "deep" aching ankle pain with or without clicking, popping, or catching of the ankle, which is worse with activity.
- If trauma is reported, which often is not, it most often involves remote or recurrent ankle sprain. Less often the patient will report a previous malleolar fracture.
- Patients may limp or complain of inability to perform athletic or recreational activities.
- Stiffness is a common symptom, especially with chronic OCDs.
- Stability testing may elicit guarding, pain, or frank laxity.
- Immobilization often improves but does not eliminate symptoms.
- Patients may report that prior corticosteroid injection provided temporary relief.

Imaging and Diagnostic Tests

- Chronic, large OCDs are often seen on X-rays depending on their size and location, but detailed description of the lesion is not clear with X-rays alone and advanced imaging is indicated.
- MRI is great for diagnosis of OCDs and assessment of common concurrent problems such as lateral collateral ligament and/or peroneal tendon pathologies. However, bone marrow edema may cause an overestimation of size and decrease the clarity of the lesion's shape and location.
- CT is the preferred imaging modality to determine size and characterize the depth and extent of subchondral bone involvement.

- In the authors' experience, obtaining both MRI and CT scans is very beneficial in preoperative planning and gives an excellent overview of the extent of talar pathology.
- Diagnostic injections can be considered and may alleviate symptoms temporarily, but, in the authors' opinion, injections should be avoided if possible due to the deleterious effect of intra-articular local anesthetics and corticosteroids on chondrocytes.

Nonoperative Management

- In the authors' experience, conservative treatment modalities may show temporary improvement but are unsuccessful in younger or more active patients with chronic talar OCDs. However, they should still be attempted.
- Rest, ice, compression and elevation (RICE) therapy.
- Activity modification.
- Bracing.
- Oral or topical nonsteroidal antiinflammatories (NSAIDs).

Traditional Surgical Management

- Bone marrow stimulation (BMS) techniques such as microfracture, subchondral drilling, and abrasion chondroplasty are often a reasonable option for smaller, contained OCDs:
  - BMS techniques encourage fibrocartilage ingrowth, which is inferior to native hyaline cartilage.
  - BMS may lead to an increase in lesion size and depth within 1 year.[1]
  - Long-term results for BMS have mixed functional results and are associated with the development of arthritis and decreased athletic activity.[2]
- BMS plus cellular allograft, acellular allograft, scaffold, and/or growth factors:
  - To encourage ingrowth of "hyaline-like" cartilage augmentation with an allograft, scaffold or growth factors may be considered; however, few are commercially available in the United States compared to Europe and other countries.
  - BMS plus graft or scaffold is a good option for small primary OCDs of the talus and may yield satisfactory results in select patients.
- Autologous chondrocyte implantation/transplantation (ACI):
  - First described by Brittberg et al. for treating deep cartilage defects in the knee.[3]
  - Arthroscopic ACI has led to the possibility of a valid option for regenerating the osteochondral layer with less morbidity than open-field surgery.[4]
  - Staged procedures have been described, which in the authors' opinion is a disadvantage to this technique as it puts the patient through an additional procedure despite there being satisfactory outcomes.[4,5]

- Subchondral cysts may be treated with subchondral drilling and retrograde bone grafting:
  - Treatment of subchondral cysts was first described in the knee and was performed in an effort to prevent patients from having to undergo a total knee arthroplasty (TKA).
  - The procedure involves percutaneous injection of a flowable nanocrystalline calcium phosphate synthetic bone graft into the cancellous trabeculae of the subchondral bone. It is hypothesized that the calcium phosphate improves the structural integrity and biomechanical strength of pathologic subchondral bone without damaging the existing bone scaffold.[6]
  - It is important to note that the subchondral bone provides support for the overlying articular cartilage and absorbs most of the mechanical force transmitted during joint loading.[7]
- Osteochondral transfer with allograft or autograft:
  - Osteochondral autograft transfer/transplantation has also been described as a method to replace damaged cartilage with either allograft or autograft.
  - Autograft transplantation, also known as knee-to-ankle mosaicplasty, has been described, but not without caution. In a study by Valderrabano et al., they concluded that there was significant donor-site morbidity at the knee joint which potentially led to incipient patellofemoral osteoarthritis.[8]
  - In addition, elevated graft placement leads to significant increases in joint contact pressure at the graft site. Recessed graft placement leads to transfer of pressure from the graft site to the opposite facet of the talus.[9]

3D-Printed Implant and Instrumentation Considerations

Materials:
- Cobalt-chromium is used owing to its low coefficient of friction, which reduces wear with adjacent bones of the foot that need to be kept intact to preserve motion in the joint (i.e., subtalar and talonavicular joints).[10]

Polished versus rough surfaces:
- Articulating aspects of the implant should be polished to lower the coefficient of friction over the adjacent cartilage.
- Rough and porous surfaces are needed where bony ingrowth is desired.

Pore size:
- The gyroid is porous and measures 6 mm $\times$ 6 mm $\times$ 6 mm, with a 0.5-mm separation of pores.

Shape:
- The shape of the implant must match that of the resected area of the talus. Naturally, the superior surface of the implant must be convex to be continuous with the remaining portion of the talus

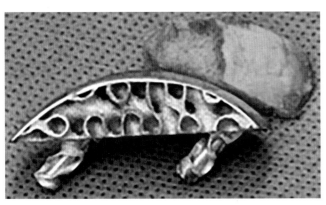

• **Fig. 7.1** Implant design correlating with the contour of a resected portion of the talus.

and to articulate appropriately with the tibia. The inferior surface of the implant is flat, with two 10 mm–long pegs for fixation into the body of the talus and associated pores to facilitate bone ingrowth (Fig. 7.1).

Sizing:
- The surgeon's preference is nominal ± 5% to 10%.

Special features:
- The pegs can be placed in any orientation depending on the patient's given anatomy.
- Options for screw fixation may be advantageous where additional/increased stability may be needed.

• Rationale for patient-specific instrumentation:
  - CT and CAD images are extremely useful to determine nominal sizing in all planes.
  - Patient-specific imaging also aids in accurately cutting an appropriately sized portion of the talus (Fig. 7.2).

Surgical Management With 3D-Printed Devices

- Special off-the-shelf instrumentation:
  - The authors recommend utilizing a Hintermann distractor to help distract the ankle joint for better exposure of the ankle joint and for easier retrieval of the resected portion of the talus.
  - A power rasp can be used to smooth the area of resected talus for easier insertion of implant and for quick adjustments to the resected surface of the talus.
  - A 4-mm osteotome can be used for mobilization of the resected portion of talus.
- Positioning and anesthesia:
  - The patient is positioned supine with a well-padded thigh tourniquet and ipsilateral thigh bump to ensure the foot and ankle are perpendicular to the operative table.
  - General anesthesia with a local block is administered for postoperative pain control.
- Approach and technique:
  - A mini anterior ankle incision is made between the interval of the tibialis anterior and extensor hallucis longus tendons.
  - The ankle capsule is reflected utilizing sharp dissection and a Cobb elevator.
  - Exposure is maintained using Gelpi and Weitlaner retractors placed deep so as not to compromise healing of the incision.
  - A Hintermann distractor is utilized to maintain exposure of the ankle joint. Usually the distractor is placed on the side of the talus that is being replaced (Fig. 7.3).

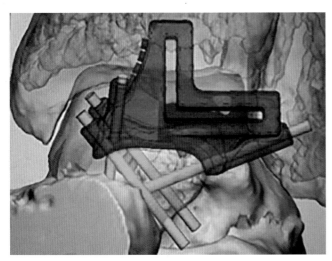

• **Fig. 7.2** Preoperative CAD image showing appropriate positioning of guide and respective talus cuts. *CAD,* Computer-aided design. (Reprinted with permission from restor3d, Inc, Durham, NC.)

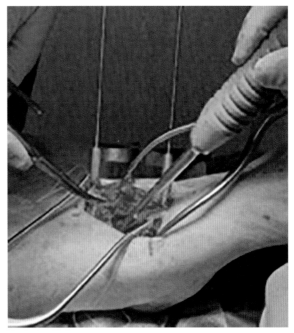

• **Fig. 7.3** A Hintermann distractor being used to maintain distraction of an ankle joint.

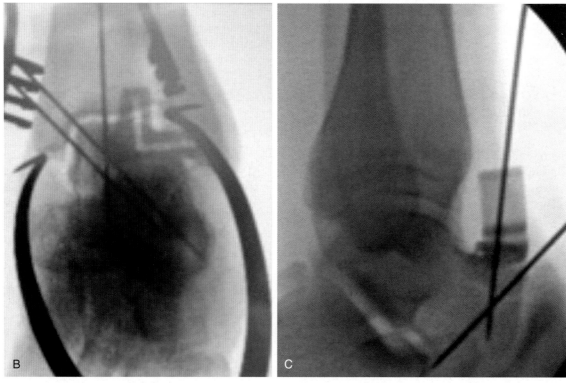

• **Fig. 7.4** (A) A cut guide pinned in place. (B and C) Anteroposterior and lateral fluoroscopic images showing the cut guide pinned in place.

- Carefully remove any osteophytes from the distal tibia and talar neck, ensuring not to remove any bony landmarks for the cut guide.
- Place appropriate-sized custom-cut guides and confirm using fluoroscopic guidance (Fig. 7.4A–C).
- Perform the cut using a reciprocating or sagittal saw, being careful not to damage the tibial plafond (Fig. 7.5A,B).
- Utilizing the Hintermann distractor, distract the ankle joint to aid in retrieving the resected talus.
- Once the cut is complete, remove the cut guide, mobilize the resected portion of talus, and remove.

- It is the senior author's recommendation to use a 4-mm straight osteotome at this step if needed to mobilize the resected portion of talus.
- Once the resected portion of talus is removed, the power rasp can be utilized to smooth any pieces that may not have been captured by the cut guide.
- Resection of pathological anatomy and/or preparation for implantation
  - Sizing and trials:
    - Once the resected portion of the talus and any remnants have been removed, sizing of the implant ensues (Fig. 7.6).

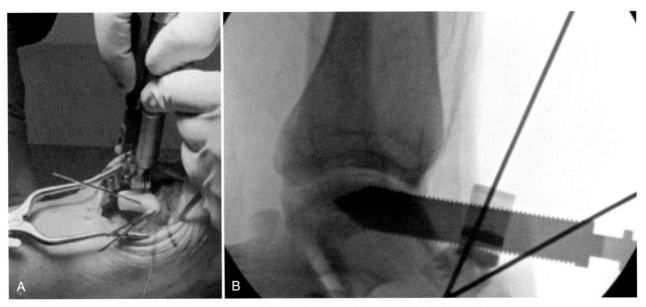

• **Fig. 7.5** (A) Utilizing a custom-cut guide to make appropriate cuts within the talus using a sagittal saw. (B) Intraoperative fluoroscopy is recommended while using the reciprocating saw for the sagittal cut in the body of the talus to ensure preservation of tibial cartilage.

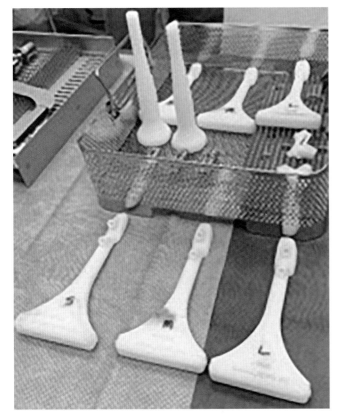

• **Fig. 7.6** Small, medium, and large implant trials, cut guides, and impactors.

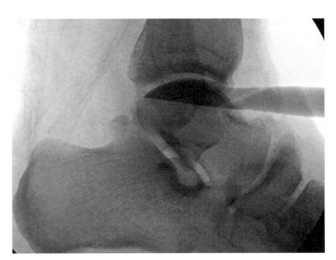

• **Fig. 7.7** Lateral fluoroscopic image showing an implant trial.

- Fluoroscopic guidance is utilized to ensure the proper size is selected (Fig. 7.7).
- Once the size is determined and confirmed using fluoroscopy, it is secured in place (Fig. 7.8A,B).
- Utilizing the appropriate reamer, peg holes are drilled through the guide (see Fig. 7.8). It is important to note that the wires may need to be trimmed to allow access for the reamer (Fig. 7.9).
- Final implantation and fixation:
  - The appropriate-sized custom hemi-talus is grafted with a mixture of bone marrow aspiration, autologous bone graft, and demineralized bone matrix, which is placed on the porous surface of the graft.
  - The pegs of the graft are then inserted into the drilled holes and impacted accordingly until the dorsal surface of the implant is adjacent/slightly below the native talar cartilage (Fig. 7.10).
  - Placement of the graft is confirmed utilizing dry arthroscopy (Fig. 7.11).
- Common adjunct procedures:
  - If there remains significant lateral ankle instability, a direct open anterior talofibular ligament (ATFL) repair is performed utilizing a pants-over-vest technique.

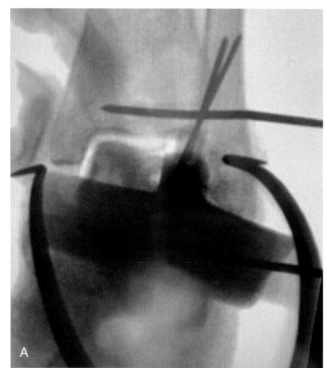

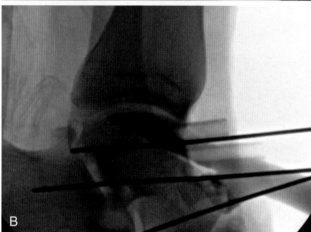

• **Fig. 7.8** (A) Anteroposterior fluoroscopic view showing an implant trial. (B) Lateral fluoroscopic view showing an implant trial secured in place.

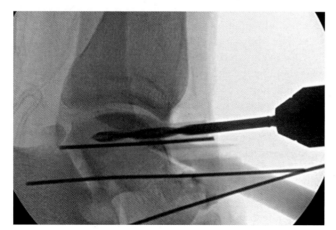

• **Fig. 7.9** The introduction of a reamer through a trial guide. Notice that the wires have been cut in order to allow access for the reamer. (With permission from Dr. Peter Highlander.)

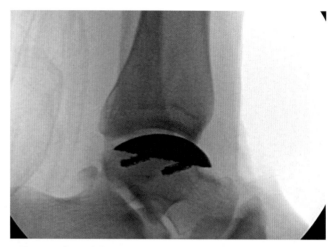

• **Fig. 7.10** Lateral fluoroscopic image showing an implant inserted with the inferior aspect of the graft flush to the resected talus. (With permission from Dr. Peter Highlander.)

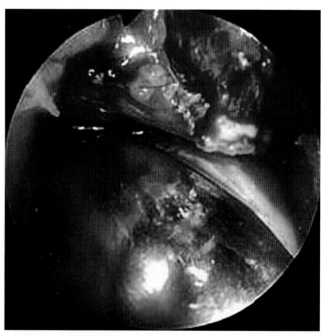

• **Fig. 7.11** Dry arthroscopic image showing anatomic alignment of the graft relative to the native talus. In this image it is important to note that the graft is flush to slightly depressed with the adjacent cartilage.

- Release of any equinus contracture.
- Appropriate osteotomies above and below the ankle joint.

Postoperative Protocol

- Strict non-weight-bearing for 1 week in a posterior splint. Radiographs are taken at the first postoperative visit.
- The patient remains non–weight-bearing in a below-knee cast for 4 weeks and then a boot non–weight-bearing with dorsiflexion and plantarflexion of the ankle allowed. The patient is followed on a biweekly basis until radiographs demonstrate osteointegration into the custom implant. This usually takes 6 to 8 weeks.

- Once deemed appropriate, weight bearing is allowed in a pneumatic controlled ankle motion (CAM) boot for a period of 1 to 2 weeks and physical therapy is also initiated. After 5 to 6 sessions, the patient can transition into an ankle brace and complete their physical therapy.
- The ankle brace is worn for daily activities for 4 to 6 months after the initial procedure.

CASE STUDY: HEMI-TALUS

A 70-year-old female presented to the office complaining of left ankle pain that has been present for over 2 years. She underwent a flatfoot reconstruction in 2016 with a gastrocnemius recession, subtalar joint fusion, and posterior tibial tendon repair with a flexor digitorum tendon transfer that healed uneventfully. Her ankle pain was treated in the past with bracing, NSAIDs, physical therapy, injections, and activity modification without relief. A CT scan of the ankle demonstrated a 2.4 cm × 2.0 cm × 1.5 cm area of AVN of her lateral talus including cortical collapse and fragmentation of the shoulder. Treatment options were discussed with the patient and she did not want to pursue a fusion or allograft bone block procedure. A custom 3D-printed hemi-talus was discussed with her in detail and she elected to proceed with that option.

Preoperative X-rays (Figs. 7.12 and 7.13)

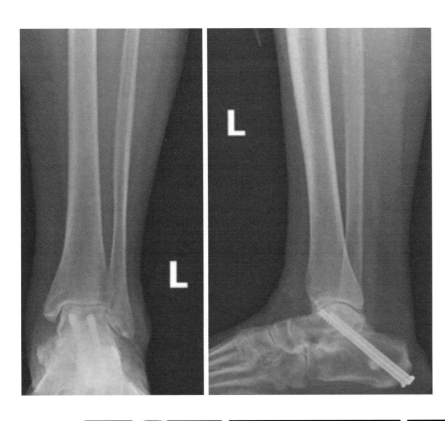

• **Fig. 7.12** Preoperative anteroposterior and lateral weight-bearing radiographs. The patient had a previous subtalar joint fusion and was complaining of long-standing pain in the lateral aspect of the ankle joint.

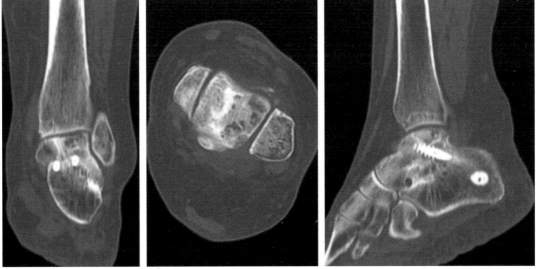

• **Fig. 7.13** CT scan demonstrating a large lateral talar lesion with cortical collapse and fragmentation. The subtalar joint is fused in the anatomic position.

Preoperative Planning (Figs. 7.14 to 7.16)

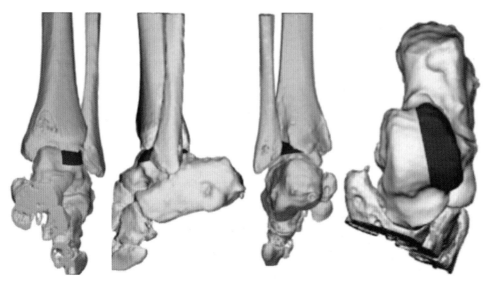

• **Fig. 7.14** Preoperative CAD images based on a CT scan demonstrating the patient's anatomy. The proposed resected area of the avascular necrosis of the talus is shown in red. *CAD*, Computer-aided design. (Reprinted with permission from restor3d, Inc, Durham, NC.)

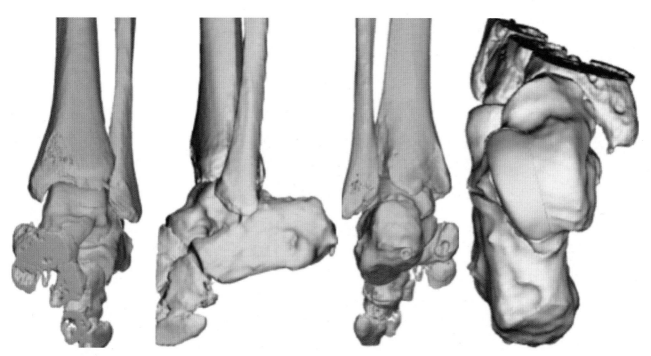

• **Fig. 7.15** Proposed hemi-talus implant. *(Left to right)* Anterior view, lateral view, posterior view, and superior view of the resected talus. A retained screw fixation from a previous subtalar joint fusion is in teal, which was removed before insertion of the hemi-talus implant. (Reprinted with permission from restor3d, Inc, Durham, NC.)

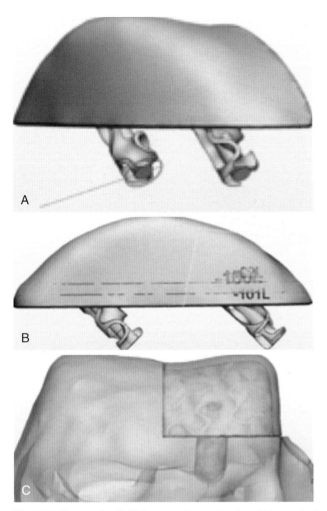

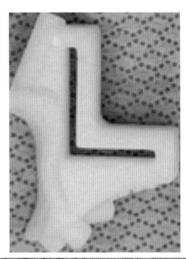

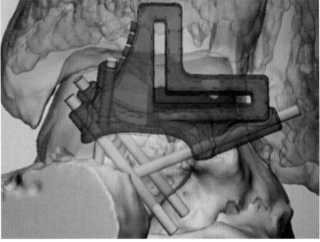

• **Fig. 7.16** Preoperative CAD images of a custom hemi-talar implant. (A, B) Note the inferior aspect of the custom implant has two 4-mm pegs to press fit into the resected talus. (C) Anterior view of the proposed implant seated in the lateral talus. CAD, Computer-aided design. (Reprinted with permission from restor3d, Inc, Durham, NC.)

• **Fig. 7.18** The cutting guide for resection of the talus was selected and pinned into position. Note on the CAD rendering the multiple options for pin stabilization of the cutting guide. *CAD,* Computer-aided design.

Intraoperative Images (Figs. 7.17 to 7.25)

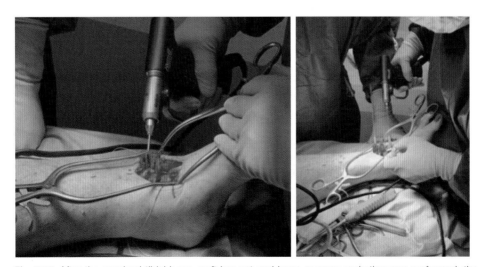

• **Fig. 7.17** After the proximal tibial bone graft harvest and bone marrow aspiration was performed, the ankle was approached with a standard anterior incision between the anterior tibial tendon and the extensor hallucis longus. A large pin distractor was utilized to obtain increased access to the lateral ankle joint. The superior pin was placed in the lateral distal tibia and the inferior pin in the lateral talar neck.

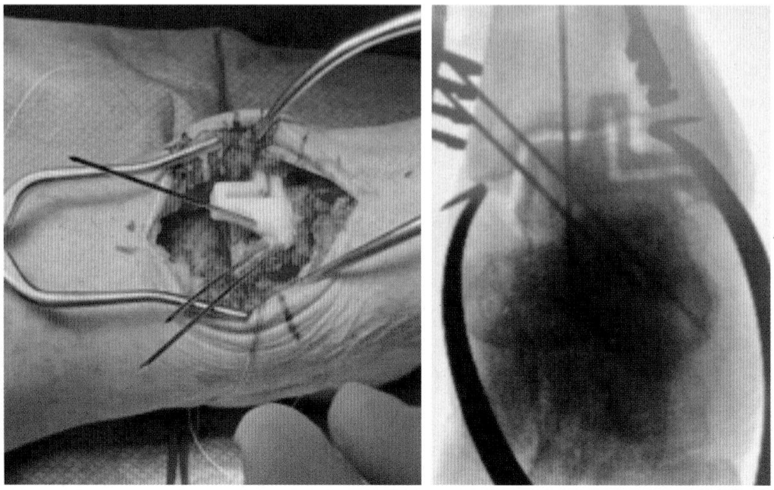

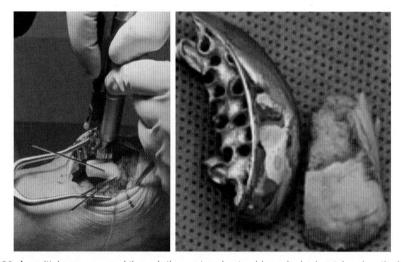

• **Fig. 7.19** The cutting guide was inserted and pinned with radiographic confirmation of placement and resection.

• **Fig. 7.20** A sagittal saw was used through the captured cut guide and a horizontal and vertical cut was made in the lateral talus *(left)*. The resected talus was removed and placed next to one of the definitive hemi-talar implants. Note the extensive loss of cartilage on the resected talus. In addition, the bone was soft and brittle, which is consistent with avascular necrosis.

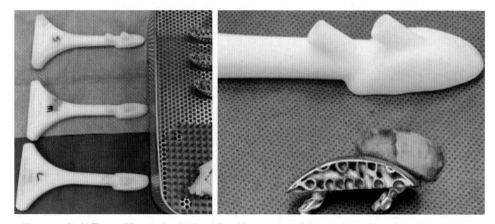

• **Fig. 7.21** *(Left)* Three different-sized talar drill guides were available to determine what size would best fit the patient. *(Right)* Note the slots on the superior aspect of the drill guide for peg drilling of the definitive hemi-talar implant.

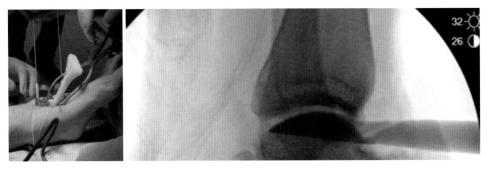

• **Fig. 7.22** The talar sizer was placed into the resected talus and confirmed with intraoperative fluoroscopy.

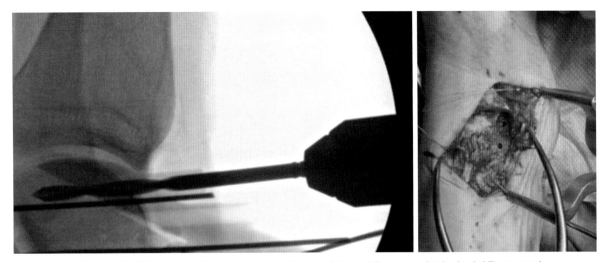

• **Fig. 7.23** *(Left)* The talar drill guide was pinned into position and the appropriately sized drill was used through the provided guide. *(Right)* Superior view of the drill holes for the definitive hemi-implant.

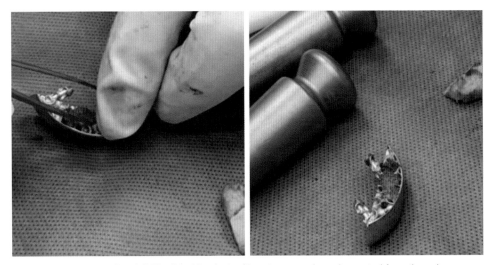

• **Fig. 7.24** Packing the definitive hemi-implant with autogenous bone harvested from the calcaneus.

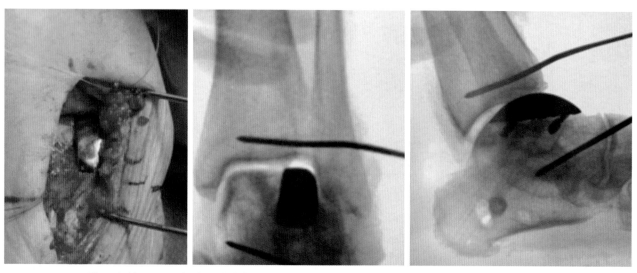

• **Fig. 7.25** Intraoperative image of the final implant in place. The superior aspect of the implant is sitting flush to slightly below the native cartilage. The anteroposterior and lateral intraoperative fluoroscopy images demonstrate the excellent position of the implant.

Postoperative X-rays (Fig. 7.26)

• Possible complications:
  • Infection.
  • Nonunion.

• Hardware failure/need for removal, which may necessitate conversion to a total talus replacement or ankle fusion.
• Raised or subsidence of the implant, which could lead to referred pain elsewhere in the ankle secondary to transfer pressure.

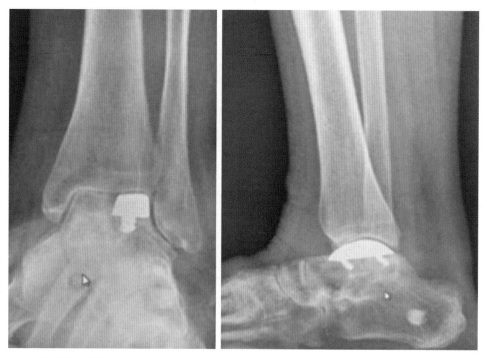

• **Fig. 7.26** Final weight-bearing films demonstrating the excellent bone ingrowth position of the implant. The patient has resumed daily activities without pain.

PEARLS AND PITFALLS

Indications and contraindications	• Avascular necrosis of the talus • Osseous deficits of the talus which has led to pain and dysfunction • Contraindicated in cases of active infection • Use prudence in patients with a history of deep infection
Implant design	• Take your time when planning these cases. Work with the company that is producing your implant and do not rush the planning. The authors carry out multiple meetings when planning these cases. Attention to detail is critical for a good outcome. • Cobalt-chromium with a polished surface • Implant shape and porosity should provide inherent stability and enhance bony ingrowth • Use CT and CAD images to determine the nominal implant size in all planes • Direct fixation will enhance stability at the bone-implant interface but may reduce the amount of bony ingrowth and biological fixation
Surgical technique	• Ensure all compromised bone is removed but do not resect bony landmarks that correlate with the cut guide • Use instrumentation that replicates the shape and size of the implant to promote optimal bone-implant contact • Utilize a Hintermann distractor to distract the ankle joint for visualization and to protect adjacent healthy cartilage • Perform dry arthroscopy to ensure appropriate positioning of the graft relative to native cartilage • Try and seat the implant just below the native talar cartilage

CAD, Computer-aided design.

References

1. Reilingh ML, van Bergen CJA, Blankevoort L, et al. Computed tomography analysis of osteochondral defects of the talus after arthroscopic debridement and microfracture. *Knee Surg Sports Traumatol Arthrosc.* 2016;24(4):1286-1292.

2. Polat G, Erşen A, Erdil ME, Kızılkurt T, Kılıçoğlu Ö, Aşık M. Long-term results of microfracture in the treatment of talus osteochondral lesions. *Knee Surg Sports Traumatol Arthrosc.* 2016;24(4):1299-1303.

3. Brittberg M, Lindahl A, Nilsson A, Ohlsson C, Isaksson O, Peterson L. Treatment of deep cartilage defects in the knee with autologous chondrocyte transplantation. *N Engl J Med.* 1994; 331(14):889-895.

4. Pagliazzi G, Vannini F, Battaglia M, Ramponi L, Buda R. Autologous chondrocyte implantation for talar osteochondral lesions: comparison between 5-year follow-up magnetic resonance imaging findings and 7-year follow-up clinical results. *J Foot Ankle Surg.* 2018;57(2):221-225.

5. Giannini S, Buda R, Ruffilli A, et al. Arthroscopic autologous chondrocyte implantation in the ankle joint. *Knee Surg Sports Traumatol Arthrosc.* 2014;22(6):1311-1319.

6. Chan JJ, Guzman JZ, Vargas L, Myerson CL, Chan J, Vulcano E. Safety and effectiveness of talus subchondroplasty and bone marrow aspirate concentrate for the treatment of osteochondral defects of the talus. *Orthopedics.* 2018;41(5):e734-e737.

7. Farr J, Cohen SB. Expanding applications of the subchondroplasty procedure for the treatment of bone marrow lesions observed on magnetic resonance imaging. *Oper Tech Sports Med.* 2013;21(2):138-143.

8. Valderrabano V, Leumann A, Rasch H, Egelhof T, Hintermann B, Pagenstert G. Knee-to-ankle mosaicplasty for the treatment of osteochondral lesions of the ankle joint. *Am J Sports Med.* 2009; 37(suppl 1):105-111.

9. Latt LD, Glisson RR, Montijo HE, Usuelli FG, Easley ME. Effect of graft height mismatch on contact pressures with osteochondral grafting of the talus. *Am J Sports Med.* 2011;39(12): 2662-2669.

10. McAlister J. A closer look at a total talar replacement and ankle arthroplasty. *Podiatr Today.* 2020;33(3). https://www.podiatrytoday.com/closer-look-total-talar-replacement-and-ankle-arthroplasty.

8

Primary Total Ankle Total Talus Replacement

JEFFREY E. McALISTER, JAMES M. COTTOM, JOSEPH R. WOLF, PETER D. HIGHLANDER

Definition

- Surgical treatment of end-stage ankle arthritis with concomitant avascular necrosis (AVN) of the talus utilizing a combination of patient-specific 3D-printed and off-the-shelf (OTS) components for joint preservation and restoration of function.
- 3D printing has evolved and now allows surgeons to partner with technology that facilitates a continuity of care to maintain ankle joint range of motion (ROM) and avoid the need for tibiotalar calcaneal joint arthrodesis.
- This chapter focuses on the niche situations that involve significant talar body loss from AVN or posttraumatic changes where plafond and arthritic changes are evident.

Anatomy

- The talus is a uniquely shaped bone that articulates with the tibial plafond, fibular malleolus, calcaneus and navicular bones.
- The talus is without tendon attachments therefore stability is provided by its articulations and ligament attachments.
- Sixty percent of the talar surface is covered by cartilage, thus minimizing available area for vascular perforators.
- The primary source of vascular influx is provided by the posterior tibial artery via perforators within the deltoid ligament and to the tarsal canal. The dorsal neck and sinus tarsi rely on vascular supply from the dorsalis pedis artery while the perforating peroneal artery serves the posterior body.

Pathogenesis

- AVN results from a temporary or permanent loss of vascular supply to a bone. Interruption in any part of the vascular supply (arteries, capillaries, sinusoids, or veins) can lead to AVN. Bones with a single terminal vascular source are known to be at higher risk for AVN.

- Within 3 hours of vascular impairment, anoxia causes osteocyte necrosis. Over time the resultant osteonecrosis can progress to subchondral fracture, loss of normal bony architecture, and collapse, leading to cartilage destruction and arthritis.[1]
- Much of the pathogenesis is not fully understood, although trauma, drug-induced, and idiopathic causes can result in vascular impairment. Trauma remains the most common cause of talar AVN. The more severe talar trauma, the more likely AVN will develop.[1]
- The physiologic response to AVN is to resorb necrotic bone by revascularization and reossification, which can be observed radiographically.

Patient History and Physical Exam Findings

- Patients will typically present with a history of isolated injury to the ankle, or a history of drug-induced ankle pain only sought out upon further investigation of the patient's past medical history, typically a high dose of steroid. Presentation will almost always be very similar to posttraumatic arthritis or secondary arthritis of the ankle.
- Patients often have failed to respond to nonsurgical treatment including but not limited to corticosteroid and/or regenerative injection therapy, rigid ankle-foot orthoses, various braces, nonsteroidal antiinflammatory drugs (NSAIDs), and physical therapy.
- Particularly in the chronic and more advanced cases, patients often have failed to respond to previous surgical intervention aimed at revascularizing the talus, such as core decompression.
- Early stages of AVN may be somewhat vague but often present as generalized ankle/hindfoot pain, which is worse with weight-bearing activity and ROM. As the disease advances, the symptoms become more apparent.
- Limited and painful ROM of the ankle and/or hindfoot.
- Antalgic gait.

- Deformity may or may not be apparent on exam depending on the presence and degree of collapse.
- Patients with AVN often have an unremarkable dermatologic and neurovascular exam.

Imaging

- Currently, no radiographic classification system exists for talar AVN, however plain radiographs reveal characteristic areas of opacity or sclerosis of the talar dome and/or body. As the disease advances and collapse occurs, AVN is more apparent and can cause secondary deformity.
- Advanced AVN will demonstrate collapse with articular degeneration of the tibiotalar and/or subtalar joints while the talonavicular joint is least commonly affected.
- Advanced imaging is indicated for diagnostic and treatment planning purposes. Prior to the advent of 3D printing, AVN was a strict contraindication for total ankle replacement (TAR).
- The authors recommend CT and MRI, which will highlight areas of osteoblastic and osteoclastic activity within the talus and surrounding bones.
- MRI is the imaging modality of choice for early diagnosis. When AVN is apparent on plain radiographs CT may be more valuable for surgical planning (Fig. 8.1).
- In addition to imaging, infection is ruled out with blood work and, if necessary, a joint aspiration or bone biopsy.

Nonoperative Management

- Immobilization and non–weight bearing.[2]
- Bracing.

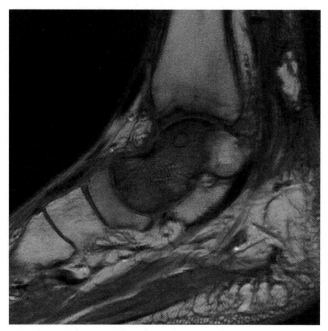

- **Fig. 8.1** Talar avascular necrosis seen on this MRI T1-weighted sequence. This patient underwent previous core decompression, which failed to alleviate symptoms and slow progression of the avascular necrosis.

- NSAIDs and other pain-management modalities.
- Shoe and activity modification.
- Over-the-counter versus custom orthotics.

Traditional Surgical Management

- Core decompression may be indicated in early-stage AVN without evidence of collapse. In these select cases, core decompression with adjunct injection of bone marrow mesenchymal stem cells (MSCs) did improve the natural history of the disease compared to core decompression alone.[3]
- AVN with collapse is not an indication for core decompression. Advanced cases with collapse have traditionally been treated with fusion with a variety of fixation options, including plates/screws, intramedullary nails, and external fixation.
- Tibiotalar calcaneal (TTC) fusion may be considered when AVN is focal. Necrotic bone must be excised with preservation of the talus to maintain limb length.
- If AVN is geographic, which requires talectomy, tibiocalcaneal (TC) fusion has traditionally been recommended. TC fusions historically have lower fusion rates, require more extensive bone grafting, and result in limb length discrepancy.
- Contaminant distraction osteogenesis may be considered to maintain limb length when TC fusion is necessary. However, this requires staged treatment, prolonged external fixation, which carries increased risk of pin site infection, and patient intolerance ("cage rage") in addition to increased cost.
- Below-knee amputation should be considered but is generally not recommended as a primary option. In the authors' practice, below knee amputation (BKA) is reserved for failed fusions, infections, and those patients not amenable to reconstruction.

3D-Printed Implant and Instrumentation Considerations

- As per previous chapters, preoperative planning involves partnering with industry to create a 3D-printed custom talus based on the contralateral and ipsilateral CT scans.
  - The 3D printing manufacturer can provide radiographic specifications to ensure the necessary data points are obtained.
  - CT scans should include the tibial tubercle, which will accurately establish alignment and location of the ankle joint axis.
- It is the surgeon's preference as to which OTS tibial and polyethylene components will be used. The talar dome will mirror the size and shape of the polyethylene component.
- Three sizes of the total talus implant are typically available and the authors prefer nominal and ±5% by volume or by implant height alone.
  - In the authors' experience nominal is most commonly used (Fig. 8.2).

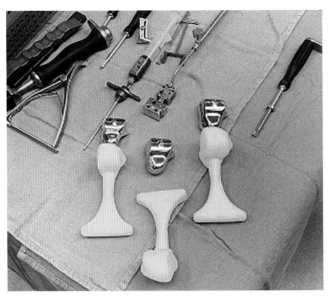

• **Fig. 8.2** Intraoperative sizing of custom talar implants is important. Typically three sizes are offered based on preoperative templating and sizing.

- Sizes may differ (based on surgeon's preference) on total volume where all aspects of the implant are larger or smaller versus only differing in talar implant height. By maintaining a constant anterior-to-posterior length, the surgeon may prevent increasing friction on the navicular bone while having some degree of freedom to restore the anatomic axis of the tibiotalar joint.
- If requested sizing differs on height alone, consider nominal ±2 mm or another absolute value based on the patient's needs and planned tibial resection.
- Additional features, such as eyelets to accommodate suture passage for ligament attachment, may be surgeon or patient specific. For nonarticular portions of the talus corresponding to attachment of the deltoid slips and anterior talofibular ligaments, the authors recommend considering focal areas of roughness and porosity to promote soft tissue ingrowth, which may help stabilize the talar implant (Fig. 8.3).

- The authors recommend a cobalt chrome (CoCr) 3D-printed talus. CoCr can be highly polished and yields a lower coefficient of friction compared to titanium. Titanium may lead to expedient polyethylene wear, which may result in aseptic loosening.
- In cases where a previous wound infection was present, these may require a staged approach to AVN of the talus with tibial plafond arthritic changes. The authors recommend a staged approach, with the first stage being resection of talar bone, bone biopsy, wound debridement, and closure with placement of an antibiotic cement spacer. An antibiotic cement spacer is placed for 6 weeks as well as intravenous antibiotics for 6 weeks. If blood work is still negative, the authors will move forward with the second stage of talus implantation (Fig. 8.4).

Surgical Management With 3D-Printed Devices

- The incisional approach for a primary total ankle arthroplasty with custom total talus involves a standard 10- to 12-cm incision overlying the anterior ankle with dissection through the superior extensor retinaculum. The interval is taken down between the tibialis anterior tendon and extensor hallucis longus. The extensor hallucis longus is maintained within its sheath. Dissection is carried down medial to the neurovascular structures, which are maintained in adipose tissue. An anterior capsulotomy is performed with resection of any hypertrophic anterior capsule. Deep retraction is utilized with a sharp self-retaining retractor on deep tissue only.
- Next, the authors recommend performing the procedure as if doing a standard total ankle arthroplasty by starting with the tibial alignment and resection:
  - A standard jig or patient-specific tibial cut guide may be used per the surgeon's preference. Using standard technique according to the manufacturer's instructions, the distal tibia is cut using a sagittal saw after alignment in orthogonal planes is confirmed.

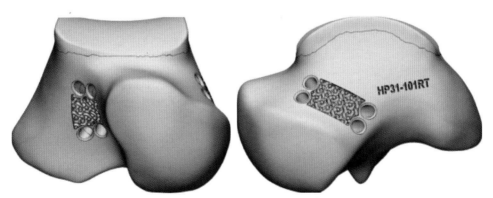

• **Fig. 8.3** Anterior and medial view of computer-aided design images of a total talus implant with eyelets for suture passage for ligament attachment. Between the eyelets, focal areas of porosity to promote soft tissue ingrowth correspond to extraarticular portions of the talus and the location of ligament attachment. (Reprinted with permission from Restor3d, Durham, NC.)

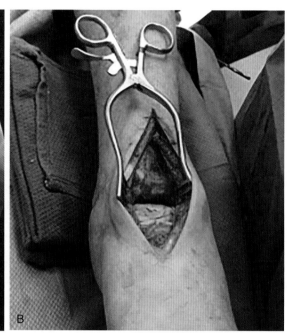

• **Fig. 8.4** (A) A 47-year-old male with an isolated open medial talus extrusion from a fall from a ladder. Subsequent wound infection occurred which required a staged reconstruction. (B) An antibiotic-impregnated cement spacer was placed and used in combination with intravenous antibiotics. Once infection was cleared, total ankle total talus replacement was performed.

• If the tibial resection is easily removed then it may be excised at this juncture, which allows for more efficient talectomy. If much difficulty is encountered, the surgeon may consider proceeding with talectomy, thereby making tibial resection easier.

• Multiple techniques have been anecdotally described to resect the talus:

- Free-hand technique: A biplanar osteotomy of the talar neck is made. The neck is then removed with sharp, precise release of soft tissue attachments using a meniscotome or scalpel. The head is removed by manually distracting the head and sharply releasing soft tissue attachments. Next the medial and lateral ligaments are released, taking care to spare superficial deltoid and calcaneal-fibular ligaments. Multiple vertical osteotomies are created from anterior to posterior using an osteotome or sagittal saw. The body can then be excised with rongeurs (Fig. 8.5).

- Patient-specific cut guide technique: The soft tissue attachments easily accessible are released sharply and all soft tissue is excised from the dorsal talar neck to ensure ideal guide placement. A guide, which is created during the preoperative planning stage, is secured to the talar neck with k-wires and position checked on fluoroscopy and compared to the preoperative plan. Under fluoroscopy, an osteotomy of the talar dome and a portion of the posterior talar body is created, taking care not to violate the subtalar joint. Additional wires are placed through the guide into the talar neck and the guide is removed. An osteotomy of the talar neck is performed using the talar neck wires as a guide

and is done so under fluoroscopy to ensure the calcaneus is not violated. The neck and head are removed by distracting with a point-to-point clamp and releasing the soft tissue attachments. The dome and posterior body are then removed in a similar manner. The tibial resection can now be easily removed with sufficient release of posterior soft tissue, which is more accessible after the talar dome and body are removed. Visualization of the remaining talar body is enhanced, thereby allowing easy and efficient excision (Fig. 8.6).

• Osteotomies of the talus may be performed with an osteotome or sagittal saw but should be completed under fluoroscopic guidance to ensure the cartilage of the calcaneal facets are not damaged.

• With either technique, use of a Steinmann pin to serve as a joystick for firmly attached aspects of the talus may be helpful. In addition, the authors recommend resection of the posterior capsule with electrocautery or scalpel. Finally, resection of osteophytes or hypertrophic bone on the dorsal navicular and anterior fibula should be performed.

• If a staged procedure is indicated, antibiotic cement should be used prior to final implant placement and the surgeon should ensure infection is cleared. Often these cases are extremely scarred and fibrotic, and this allows for improved sagittal plane ROM (see Fig. 8.4).

• After talectomy and tibial resection, the tibial component and total talus trials are utilized. Polyethylene is then trialed and sized (Fig. 8.7):

- In the authors' experience, the nominal size total talus is most commonly utilized.

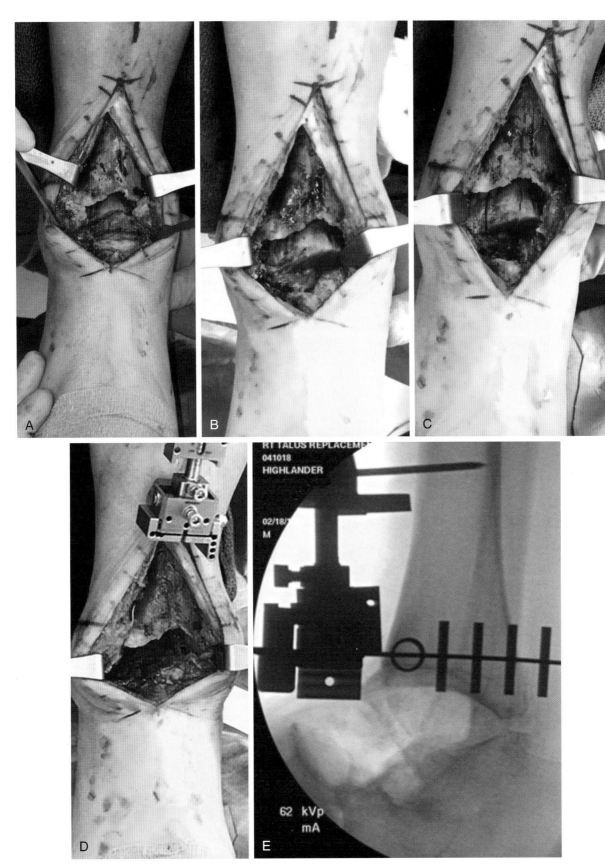

• **Fig. 8.5** Intraoperative photos demonstrating the "free-hand" talectomy technique via anterior incision. (A) Once exposure is obtained a biplanar osteotomy of the talar neck is performed. The neck can easily be removed due to the lack of soft tissue attachments. (B) The head is then distracted with a Cobb elevator and soft tissue attachments are sharply released, allowing removal. (C) Two vertical osteotomies are performed of the talar body. (D) Finally, the medial and lateral soft tissue attachments are sharply released and the talar body may be removed with rongeurs. (E) In this particular case, the tibial resection was performed after talectomy.

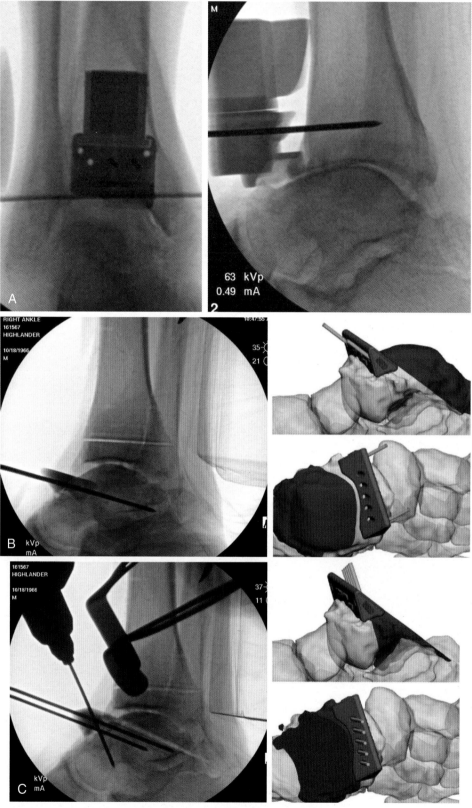

• **Fig. 8.6** Radiographs and computer-aided design images demonstrating the use of a custom cut guide for talectomy. The author (PDH) finds this technique to be most efficient by making all osteotomies then resecting the bone in a step-wise fashion. (A) In this case, a patient-specific tibial cut guide was utilized. After the tibial cuts were made, a patient-specific cut guide is placed on the dorsal talar neck and pinned to the posterior body using two 2.0-mm wires. (B) A reciprocating saw is used with the guide to perform an osteotomy of the talar dome and a portion of the posterior body. Then additional 2.0-mm wires are placed within the guide and across the talar neck in a dorsal-to-plantar direction. (C) The two wires placed into the posterior talar body are removed.

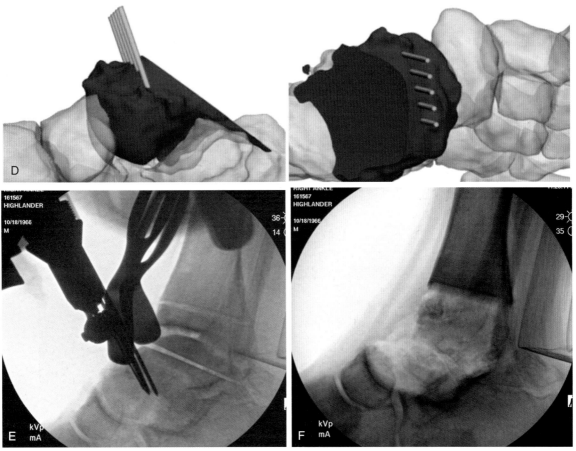

• **Fig. 8.6, cont'd** (D) The guide is slid over the talar neck wires for removal. (E) An osteotomy of the neck is performed with a sagittal saw along the wires. The head and distal neck is removed by pulling traction while releasing the soft tissue attachments. The talar dome is removed in a similar manner, which yields the posterior capsule more accessible for release of the tibial resection. (F) The remaining talar body is then easily removed with osteotomes and rongeurs.

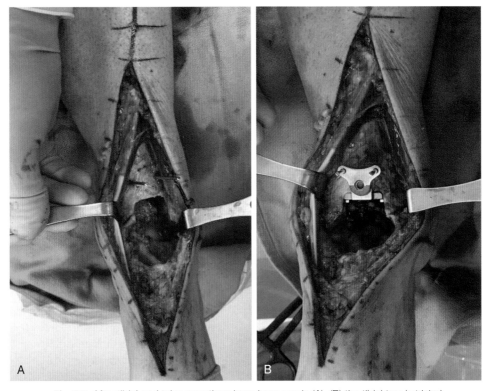

• **Fig. 8.7** After tibial and talar resections have been made (A), (B) the tibial tray is trialed.

Continued

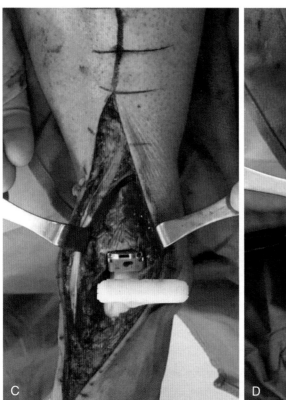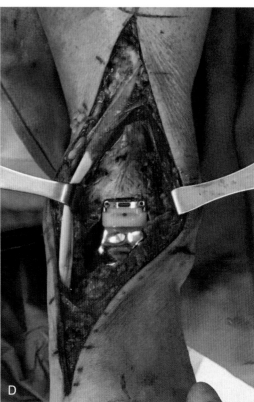

• **Fig. 8.7, cont'd** (C) The total talus trial is placed followed by the polyethylene trial. (D) Once ideal sizing is determined the trials are removed, the surgical site is irrigated, and final implants are placed.

- The surgeon should evaluate stability, ROM, and ensure physiologic tension of adjacent soft tissues are recreated. At this point, the surgeon should consider any need for soft tissue balancing, such as medial or lateral ligament repair.
- The authors prefer total talus trials impregnated with barium sulfate yielding the trial radiopaque, therefore making radiographic assessment easier (Fig. 8.8).
- All trials are removed and the final tibial component is placed. The final total talus is then placed and the polyethylene trialed again. ROM and stability are once again examined, and the final polyethylene component is placed after the proper size is determined.
- ROM and stability are closely evaluated on the table as well as under fluoroscopy. Adjunctive soft tissue–balancing procedures are then performed if indicated. The authors recommend collateral ligament stabilization (i.e., modified Broström or Broström-Evans) if >2 mm of tibiotalar gapping is observed upon stress exam. Posterior muscle group lengthening (i.e., gastrocnemius recession) is the most common adjunct soft tissue procedure used by the authors.
- The surgical site is irrigated copiously and a standard layered closure is performed. The authors recommend utilizing anterior incisional vacuum assisted closure (VAC) coverage as well. A well-padded Robert Jones cotton dressing is then applied.

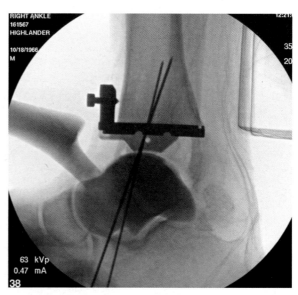

• **Fig. 8.8** For better assessment of the fit, stability, and range of motion of the total talus, the authors recommend using barium sulfate-impregnated talar trials, which yields the trial radiopaque.

Postoperative Protocol

- There are no dedicated guidelines for postoperative management for this procedure; however, the authors have experienced no significant difference with this procedure and traditional total ankle arthroplasty in terms of postoperative protocol.

- Non–weight bearing in a splint for 1 to 2 weeks or until the first postoperative appointment at which time the patient is transitioned to a cast or controlled ankle motion (CAM) boot pending incision healing and patient compliance.
- Once the incision is healed, active ROM exercise, physical therapy, and weight bearing in a CAM boot may begin. If the patient underwent concomitant procedures such as osteotomies or fusions, then the postoperative protocol is dictated by those procedures.
- At week 6, the patient may begin to transition out of the CAM boot and into a functional lace-up ankle brace with an athletic shoe.
- Weight-bearing radiographs are taken at 2 weeks, 6 weeks, 3 months, 6 months, and 1 year.

Results/Outcomes

- TAR continues to gain popularity as the preferred procedure for the management of end-stage ankle arthritis in patients looking to preserve joint motion and prevent accelerated arthritis in adjacent joints.[4-7]
- Traditionally, AVN is a contraindication for ankle arthroplasty due to a high risk of implant subsidence, migration, and eventual failure. The most common reported cause of revision surgery in TAR has been linked to talar component loosening.[8]
- Prior to the development of custom-designed 3D-printed talar implants, treatment options for both failed TAR and talar AVN were limited to arthrodesis with bulk allograft or amputation. Today, total talar implants are being used in isolation and in combination with tibial implants for ankle arthritis.

- Kanzaki et al. retrospectively reviewed 22 patients who underwent total ankle total talus replacement (TATTR) for ankle arthritis with either talar osteonecrosis, subtalar arthritis, or a flat top talus using a patient-specific alumina ceramic implant. At the final follow-up (mean: 34 months), the authors reported significant improvements in function, ROM, and pain. Complications were similar to those for TAR alone, with three patients suffering from wound-healing complications and four fractures of the medial malleolus.[9]
- Kurokawa et al. compared traditional TAR in 12 patients to TATTR in 10 patients. Indications for surgery were end-stage arthritis in the total ankle group and the same arthritis along with talar body collapse or large cyst formation in the TATTR group. They used the same patient-specific alumina ceramic implant with a fixed bearing tibial component. At final follow-up, the authors reported no significant difference in functional, pain, or disability outcome measures.[10]
- In the United States, total talus implants are patient-specific 3D-printed and metallic, either CoCr or titanium alloy. CoCr remains the material of choice for articulating (with native cartilage or polyethylene components) metallic joint-replacement components. There is a trace amount of nickel in CoCr, therefore it should be avoided in patients with a nickel sensitivity.
- The authors' collective experience in performing TATTR has been successful when using a variety of TAR implants combined with patient-specific 3D-printed CoCr total talus implants (Fig. 8.9).
  1. The tibial component design may vary, and until further research becomes available it is the authors' opinion that a fixed bearing implant provides increased stability.

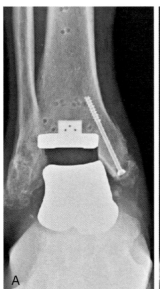
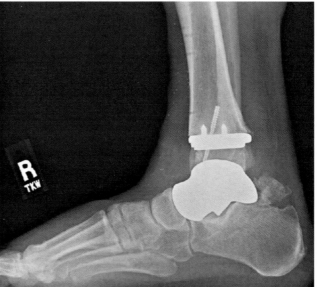

• **Fig. 8.9** The authors' combined experience has shown success in using a variety of total ankle replacement (TAR) systems when performing total ankle total talus replacement. Patient factors and the surgeon's comfort should be considered when selecting which TAR system to pair with a 3D-printed total talus replacement. These radiographs demonstrate the utility of various tibial implants on 3D-printed total tali. (A) Axiom (Kinos Medical Inc., Durham, NC).

Continued

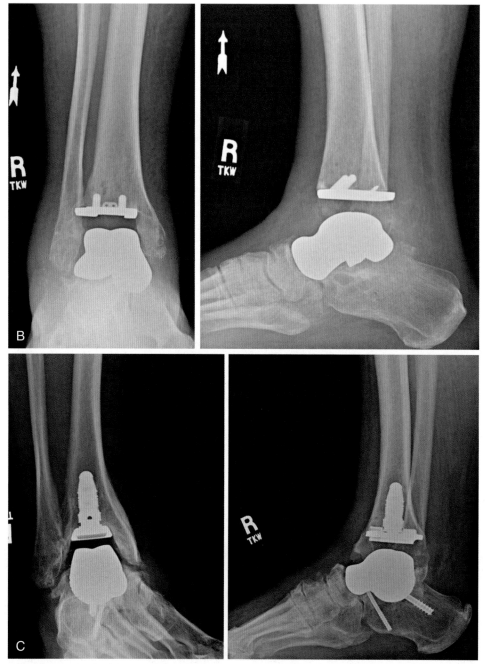

• **Fig. 8.9, cont'd** (B) Cadence (Smith & Nephew Inc., Memphis, TN). (C) InBone (Wright Medical/ Stryker, Memphis, TN).

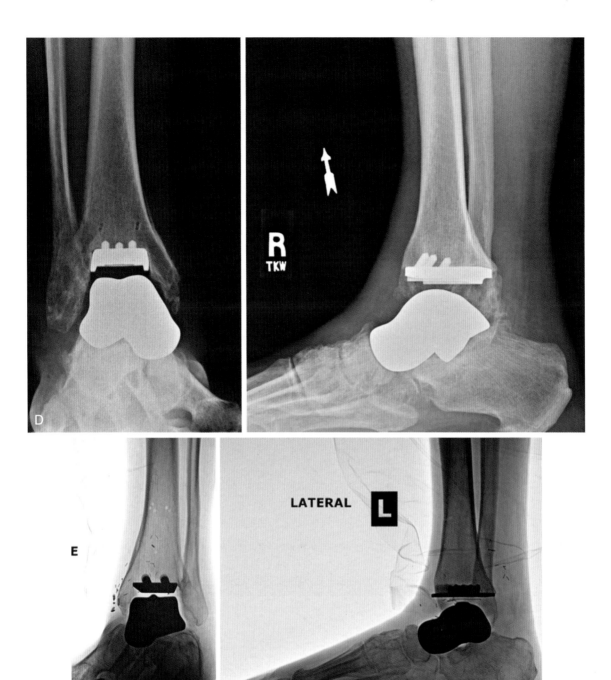

• **Fig. 8.9, cont'd (D)** Infinity (Wright Medical/Stryker, Memphis, TN). (E) STAR Ankle (Courtesy of Enovis Corporation.)

2. When deciding which total ankle system to pair with a patient-specific total talus, surgeons should make the selection based on patient factors such as bone quality, deformity, and preoperative ligament stability, as well as the surgeon's comfort and experience with a given total ankle system.

TIPS AND TRICKS

Indications	End-stage ankle arthritis with osseous deficit within the talus secondary to AVN, large cysts, fracture nonunion, prior infection
Goal of reconstruction	Restore function of the ankle joint while preventing talar subsidence and avoidance of fusion
Imaging	• MRI is best for diagnosis while CT is superior for preoperative planning
	• Preoperative bilateral CT scans are necessary for accurate implant design and should include the tibial tubercle
	• Obtaining an accurate length of the tibia, talus, and calcaneus of the unaffected limb will help determine the anatomic location of the ankle joint axis, thereby guiding the height of the talar implant
	• Follow guidelines provided by the 3D printing manufacturer
Labs/work-up	Important to rule out active infectious process
Design	• Use CT and CAD images to determine nominal implant size and optimal level of tibial resection (which may dictate talar implant sizing)
	• Request at least three talar implant sizes which may differ in total volume (i.e., ±5% to 10%) or only in talar height (±2 mm)
	• Highly polished CoCr remains the material of choice
	• Eyelets for ligament attachment and rough/porous areas for soft tissue ingrowth to add stability
	• The talar dome should mirror the polyethylene component being used
Implantation	• It appears to be most efficient to perform tibial cuts followed by talar osteotomies with patient-specific guides
	• Avoid damaging calcaneal facets and navicular cartilage when performing osteotomies
	• After all osteotomies are performed, conduct tibial resection and remove the talus in its entirety
	• Trial in succession the tibial component, the talar implant, then polyethylene
	• Ensure physiologic tension of adjacent soft tissues
	• Evaluate alignment, ROM, and stability on orthogonal radiographs
Tibial component selection	• Fixed bearing devices appear to provide added stability
	• Multiple tibial components have shown success
	• Consider patient factors: deformity, age, weight, activity, tibial bone quality, etc.
	• The surgeon's preference, experience, and comfort level should be considered

AVN, Avascular necrosis; *CAD*, computer-aided design; *CoCr*, cobalt chrome; *ROM*, range of motion.

PEARLS AND PITFALLS

Contraindications	• Active infection
	• Neuropathy
	• Severe malleolar dysplasia
	• Poor tibial bone quality not amenable to OTS tibial components
	• Severely arthritic calcaneal facets and/or navicular cartilage may require arthrodesis
Implant design	• Titanium should be avoided if possible due to higher wear of the polyethylene component
	• Special features are determined based on patient factors, particularly the need for ligament repair, corrective osteotomies, or subtalar or talonavicular joint fusion
	• Talar implant sizing options, particularly height, should be based on location of the ankle joint axis, which can reliably be determined by CT of the contralateral limb
Surgical technique	• Standard anterior ankle approach. Ensure the talonavicular joint and malleolar gutters are visible
	• Precise sharp release of soft tissue attachments onto the talus
	• Consider the tibial resection technique and use of patient-specific guides
	• Consider talectomy technique and use of patient-specific guides
	• Perform talar osteotomies under fluoroscopy to ensure preservation of calcaneal facet cartilage
	• Closely evaluate adjacent cartilage of calcaneal facets and navicular bone. Focal areas of cartilage damage may be drilled and grafted
	• Restore physiologic tension of adjacent soft tissues and perform ligament/tendon balancing as needed
	• Nominal size talar implants appear to be used most commonly
	• Recommend the use of radiopaque talar trials impregnated with barium sulfate for more efficacious radiographic evaluation

OTS, Off-the-shelf.

References

1. Haskell A. Natural history of avascular necrosis in the talus: when to operate. *Foot Ankle Clin.* 2019;24(1):35-45. doi:10.1016/j.fcl.2018.09.002.

2. Delanois RE, Mont MA, Yoon TR, Mizell M, Hungerford DS. Atraumatic osteonecrosis of the talus [published correction appears in *J Bone Joint Surg Am.* 1999 Feb;81(2):296]. *J Bone Joint Surg Am.* 1998;80(4):529-536. doi:10.2106/00004623-199804000-00009.

3. Hernigou P, Dubory A, Flouzat Lachaniette CH, Khaled I, Chevallier N, Rouard H. Stem cell therapy in early post-traumatic talus osteonecrosis. *Int Orthop.* 2018;42(12):2949-2956. doi:10.1007/s00264-017-3716-7.

4. Stavrakis AI, SooHoo NF. Trends in complication rates following ankle arthrodesis and total ankle replacement. *J Bone Joint Surg Am.* 2016;98(17):1453-1458. doi:10.2106/JBJS.15.01341.

5. SooHoo NF, Zingmond DS, Ko CY. Comparison of reoperation rates following ankle arthrodesis and total ankle arthroplasty. *J Bone Joint Surg Am.* 2007;89(10):2143-2149. doi:10.2106/JBJS.F.01611.

6. McKenna BJ, Cook J, Cook EA, et al. Total ankle arthroplasty survivorship: a meta-analysis. *J Foot Ankle Surg.* 2020;59(5):1040-1048. doi:10.1053/j.jfas.2019.10.011.

7. Haddad SL, Coetzee JC, Estok R, Fahrbach K, Banel D, Nalysnyk L. Intermediate and long-term outcomes of total ankle arthroplasty and ankle arthrodesis. A systematic review of the literature. *J Bone Joint Surg Am.* 2007;89(9):1899-1905. doi:10.2106/JBJS.F.01149.

8. Gross C, Erickson BJ, Adams SB, Parekh SG. Ankle arthrodesis after failed total ankle replacement: a systematic review of the literature. *Foot Ankle Spec.* 2015;8(2):143-151. doi:10.1177/1938640014565046.

9. Kanzaki N, Chinzei N, Yamamoto T, Yamashita T, Ibaraki K, Kuroda R. Clinical outcomes of total ankle arthroplasty with total talar prosthesis. *Foot Ankle Int.* 2019;40(8):948-954. doi:10.1177/1071100719847135.

10. Kurokawa H, Taniguchi A, Morita S, Takakura Y, Tanaka Y. Total ankle arthroplasty incorporating a total talar prosthesis: a comparative study against the standard total ankle arthroplasty. *Bone Joint J.* 2019;101-B(4):443-446. doi:10.1302/0301-620X.101B4.BJJ-2018-0812.R2.

9

Custom Constrained 3D Total Talus/ Navicular Replacement

JASON NOWAK, GARRET STRAND

Definition

- The utilization of 3D printing technology for combined total talus and navicular replacement with incorporation of subtalar joint fusion and total ankle replacement.

Indications[1-11]

- Talar avascular necrosis
- Aseptic talar body collapse
- Failure of total ankle arthroplasty with talar subsidence/ collapse
- Nonunion of talar fracture following open reduction and internal fixation (ORIF)
- Failed nonoperative management

Patient History and Physical Exam

- Detailed patient history must include history of trauma, arthritis, prior surgeries, and postoperative course.
- Duration, degree of dysfunction, and intensity of pain should be documented.
- Pain is predominately isolated to the ankle and hindfoot.
- Range of motion (ROM) should be assessed. Typically, the patient's ankle and subtalar joint ROM is severely limited due to pain and crepitus (Fig. 9.1).
- Clinical alignment is determined with the patient weight bearing. The surgeon should note any deformities including equinus and varus/valgus malpositioning.
- The soft tissue envelope is examined for prior incisions, preulcerative lesions, global swelling, and signs of infection.
- Examine the neurovascular status for signs of neuropathy or vascular impairment.

Imaging and Other Testing

- Standard plain film weight-bearing radiographs should be obtained of the foot and ankle including anteroposterior (AP),

mortise ankle views, as well as AP, oblique, and lateral ankle/foot views (Fig. 9.2).
- Advanced imaging is required for preoperative planning as well as engineering of the proposed custom implant. Bilateral CT scans should be obtained of both ankles. The custom implant is constructed based on the patient's contralateral nonpathologic talus (Fig. 9.3).
- Infection must be ruled out and may be done so with laboratory studies, advanced imaging such as CT or MRI, joint aspiration, and bone biopsy.

Nonoperative Management[1-11]

- Bracing
- Nonsteroidal antiinflammatory medications
- Shockwave therapy
- Intra-articular injections

Traditional Surgical Management[1-11]

- Bone-block pantalar arthrodesis
- Total talus replacement (TTR)
- Below-knee amputation

3D-Printed Implant Design Specifications and Considerations

- Titanium alloy implant was designed and manufactured utilizing 3D printing technology incorporating a total talus and navicular bone into one combined custom implant. The size and dimensions of the implant were based on the contralateral, unaffected ankle, and hindfoot.
- Modifications were made in order to accommodate fixation through the custom implant with screws and staples.
- The fixation was designed to accept 5.5- to 6.5-mm headed screws and high-strength nitinol compression staples.

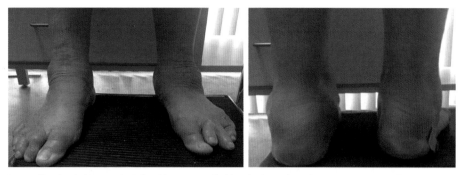

• **Fig. 9.1** On physical exam, the left ankle presented with pain throughout the range of motion. There was moderate global swelling around the ankle joint. The patient had pain to palpation to the medial and lateral gutters of the ankle as well as over the sinus tarsi and dorsal navicular regions. Her heel alignment was neutral with a plantigrade foot. She was neurovascularly intact. Her skin was warm, dry, and well perfused with well-healed incisions.

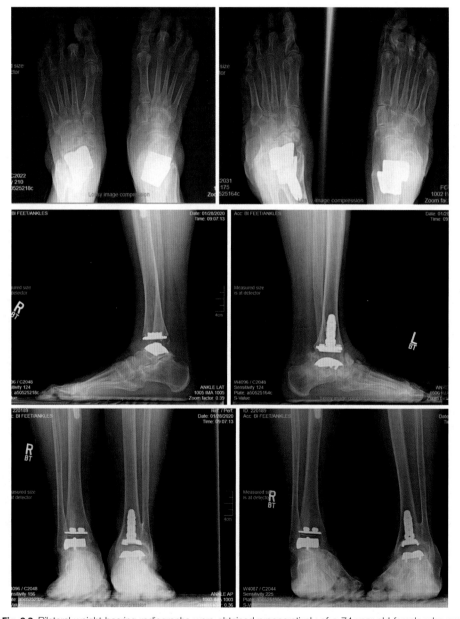

• **Fig. 9.2** Bilateral weight-bearing radiographs were obtained preoperatively of a 74-year-old female who presented to the clinic with worsening left ankle pain. She had initially undergone bilateral total ankle arthroplasty with a mobile bearing implant. The left ankle implant failed and the patient underwent a revision total ankle arthroplasty with a fixed bearing implant utilizing a stemmed tibial component. One year later, the patient was referred to our office after postoperative radiographs revealed talar body aseptic collapse. Radiographs demonstrated severe loss of height of the left ankle. The talar component had completely subsided, resting on the superior aspect of the calcaneus. There was also fragmentation of the navicular bone and lateral gutter impingement.

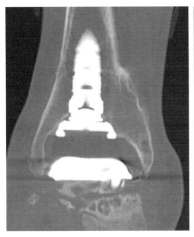
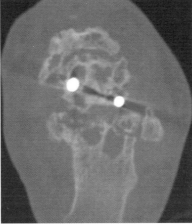
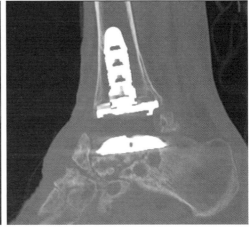

• **Fig. 9.3** Preoperative ankle CT scan demonstrated complete talar subsidence with severe collapse of the talar component, severe subchondral cystic changes, as well as degeneration and fragmentation of the navicular bone. The tibial stemmed component was stable without signs of periprosthetic lucency.

• The inferior aspect of the talar component and the distal aspect of the navicular component was engineered with plasma-coated lattice surfaces to aid in bony ingrowth at the proposed arthrodesis sites.

Surgical Management With 3D-Printed Technology

• Proper stable positioning is vital during this procedure. The authors recommend a flat radiolucent operating table. A towel or bean bag hip bump is placed under the ipsilateral hip, maneuvering the operative lower extremity from an externally rotated position into a neutral position.
• A stack of blankets is placed under the operative lower limb prior to prepping and draping, elevating it above the contralateral leg, thus decreasing superimposition with the contralateral limb during lateral intraoperative fluoroscopic imaging.
• A standard large C-arm is recommended along with a thigh pneumatic tourniquet while the leg is prepped and sterilely draped above the level of the tibial tuberosity.
• Proper positioning allows for consistent intraoperative fluoroscopic images—AP ankle, mortise ankle, AP foot, Saltzman, and lateral foot/ankle views.
• Approach:
  • A standard anterior ankle incision approach utilizing a 16-cm linear incision lateral to the tibialis anterior tendon.
  • A superficial peroneal nerve is identified and retracted throughout the procedure.
  • An interval is established between the extensor hallucis longus and the tibialis anterior tendon. It is important to preserve the tibialis anterior tendon sheath (Fig. 9.4).
  • The capsule is dissected, exposing the ankle implant.

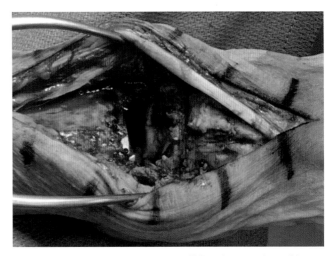

• **Fig. 9.4** Intraoperative exposure utilizing the anterior ankle approach between the extensor hallucis longus and tibialis anterior tendons.

• Removal of preexisting implants and nonviable bone:
  • The talar implant is removed, exposing the talar avascular necrotic bone. Osteotomes are useful for removing the talar implant component.
  • The necrotic talus and navicular bones are removed using a double-action rongeur. Other instruments including pituitary rongeurs, osteotomes, and periosteal elevators are useful to remove the remaining necrotic bone and soft tissue. Often, a sagittal saw is useful to transect the talar neck, allowing easier removal of the talar head, followed by removal of the remaining talar body (Figs. 9.5 and 9.6).
  • Evaluate for any loose bodies that would impede proper placement of the implant (Fig. 9.7.)
• Trial implant and joint preparation:
  • A 3D-printed trial implant is then placed. A trial polyethylene component is also placed into the tibial

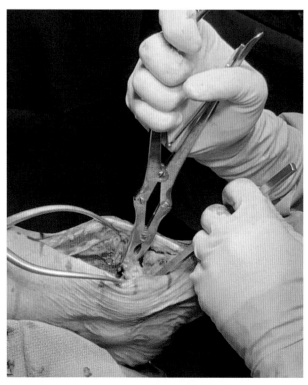

• **Fig. 9.5** The avascular talus and navicular are resected using rongeurs, osteotomes, and a sagittal saw.

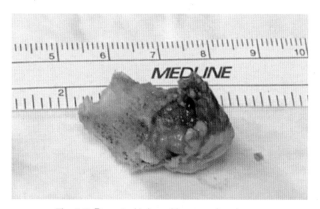

• **Fig. 9.6** Resected talus with avascular changes.

implant component to help assess fit, ROM, and coronal stability (Fig. 9.8).

- The size of the custom talar implant is then determined. It is valuable to trial multiple sizes to determine ideal fit.
- Preemptively examine the potential placement of the screw/staple fixation while determining the size of the implant.
- The superior aspect of the calcaneus and the proximal surfaces of the cuneiforms are prepared in the usual fashion—denuding all remaining cartilage, penetrating the subchondral plate with a 4.0-mm round cutting bur until bleeding medullary bone is exposed, and fenestrating using a solid drill bit (Fig. 9.9).
- Final implantation and fixation:
  - Prepare the final 3D-printed implant's porous surfaces for fusion by packing with bone allograft and biologics per the surgeon's preference (Fig. 9.10). The implant is then placed.
  - The custom metallic implant is designed to allow for placement of the hardware through the implant, across the planned arthrodesis sites, and once the desired placement is obtained the implant is pinned with guidewires (Fig. 9.11).
  - After the implant is fixated, trial polyethylene components are again placed. ROM and soft tissue balancing is again examined to determine final polyethylene size. Soft tissue rebalancing may be performed as necessary (Figs. 9.12 and 9.13).
- Ancillary procedures and closure:
  - The ankle is placed through ROM while being flushed with normal saline (Fig. 9.14).
  - The authors recommend assessing ROM and stability with fluoroscopy to determine the necessary ancillary procedures (Fig. 9.15).
  - The wound is closed in a layered fashion while the foot is held in a slightly dorsiflexed position in order

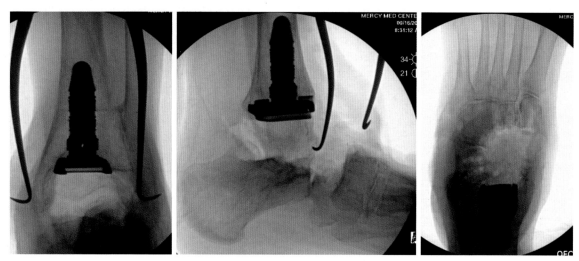

• **Fig. 9.7** Intraoperative images confirming that the necrotic talus and navicular bones are removed appropriately.

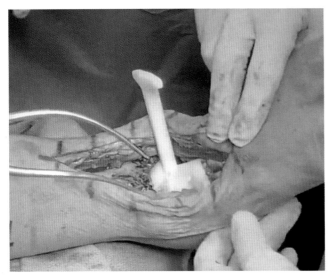

• **Fig. 9.8** 3D-printed trials are placed with the polyethylene trial to determine ideal fit, range of motion, and stability.

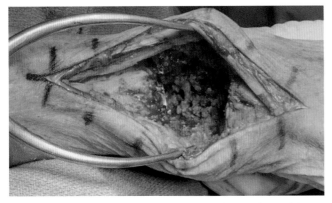

• **Fig. 9.9** The trial implants are removed and the calcaneal facets and cuneiforms are prepared for fusion. Copious irrigation is recommended to ensure all debris has been removed prior to final implantation.

to decrease tension over the incision site and prevent bowstringing of the extensor tendons.

- We begin our closure at the ankle joint capsule, followed by the extensor retinaculum using 3-0 Vicryl sutures in a running baseball stitch.
- We then perform interrupted subcutaneous closure using 3-0 Vicryl. Skin is closed in a horizontal mattress suture technique using 3-0 nylon.
- A sterile postoperative dressing is placed on the incisions using a triple antibiotic ointment and a nonadherent dressing. The patient is then placed into a well-padded posterior/sugar tong splint with the foot and ankle at a neutral or slightly dorsiflexed position.

Postoperative Protocol

- The patient is maintained in their posterior splint for 2 weeks, in a non–weight-bearing status. They are encouraged to ice and elevate the operative ankle.
- Sutures are routinely removed at 2 weeks if incisions are well coapted. X-rays are also obtained of the operative foot and ankle at this appointment.
- Due to the fusion healing process, the patient is then placed into a short-leg cast and maintained non–weight bearing for an additional 4 weeks.
- At 6 weeks postoperatively, repeat X-rays are obtained of the operative foot and ankle. If there is good bony consolidation at the fusion site(s), the patient is transitioned into a controlled ankle motion (CAM) walker boot with an arch support placed into the boot. Gradual protected weight bearing and physical therapy is initiated at this point.
- At 12 weeks postoperatively, repeat X-rays are again obtained of the operative foot and ankle. If osseous healing is maintained, the patient is transitioned into a tennis

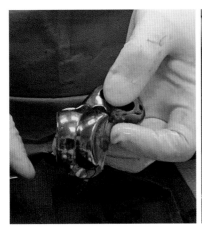
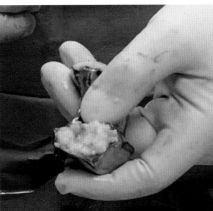
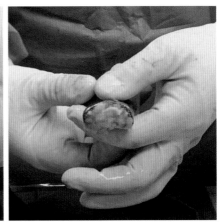

• **Fig. 9.10** In this case example, a custom metallic implant to replace both the avascular talus and navicular bones was utilized. Since this is meant to be a constrained implant, the metal-bone interfaces are designed with a porous lattice surface. The lattice surfaces are designed to allow for bony ingrowth at the arthrodesis sites. The lattice surfaces are packed with bone allograft of the surgeon's preference.

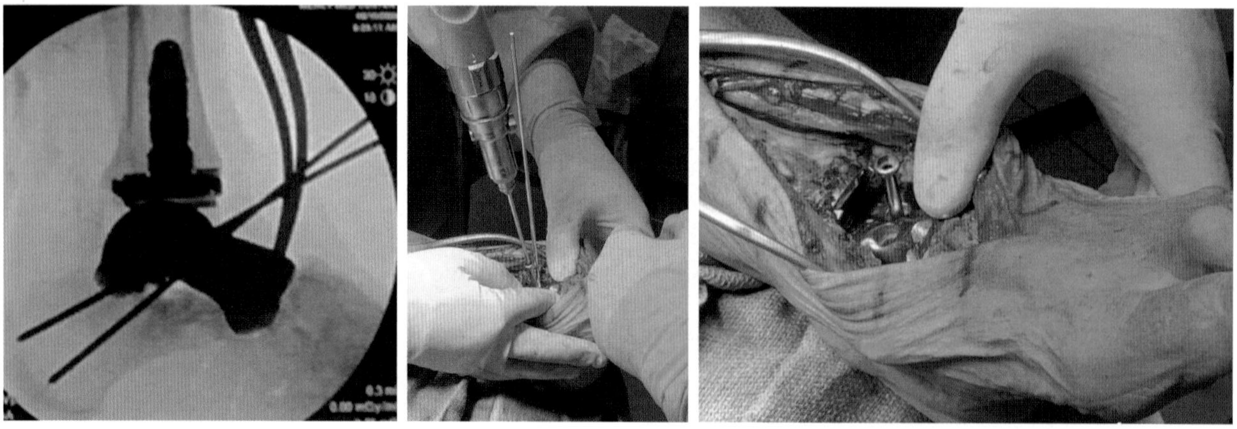

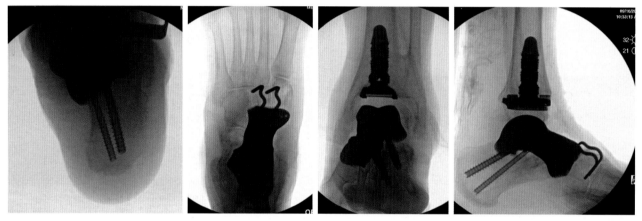

• **Fig. 9.11** In this case, the custom implant was designed to allow for screw fixation across the subtalar joint arthrodesis site, and staple fixation across the naviculocuneiform joint arthrodesis site. Guidewires were first placed through the custom implant and the position was confirmed with fluoroscopic imaging.

• **Fig. 9.12** Intraoperative fluoroscopic images showing final placement of the custom implant and hardware.

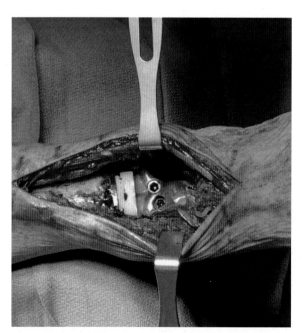

• **Fig. 9.13** Intraoperative photo of the final talar/navicular implant and fixation with the final polyethylene component.

shoe with arch support and allowed to return to normal low-impact activities.
• We routinely evaluate our total ankle arthroplasty and TTR patients, both clinically and radiographically, on an annual basis (Fig. 9.16).

Conclusion

This case study highlights a 74-year-old female with severe talar and navicular collapse after failed revision total ankle arthroplasty. The patient underwent a successful custom constrained 3D total talus/navicular replacement while the stable tibial total ankle component was maintained. The implant was fixated with high compression nitinol staples as well as partially threaded headed screws. The patient was appropriately managed postoperatively, transitioning to a partial weight-bearing status at 6 weeks. The patient then eventually transitioned to her daily activities while maintaining a stable implant.

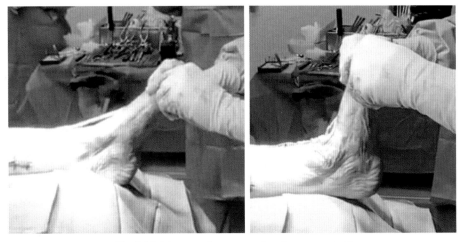

• **Fig. 9.14** Intraoperative range of motion assessment.

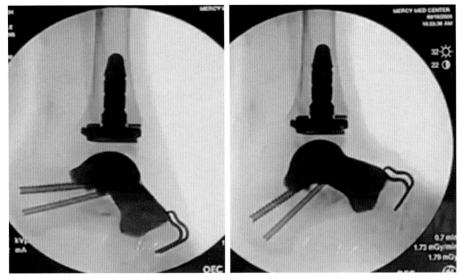

• **Fig. 9.15** A gastrocnemius recession was also incorporated into this case to increase dorsiflexion. These intraoperative images depict end range of motion following final placement of the custom implant and hardware, followed by gastrocnemius recession.

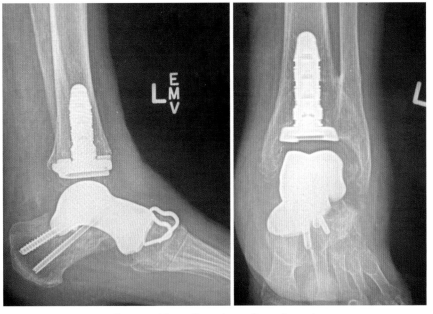

• **Fig. 9.16** 12-month postoperative radiographs.

TIPS AND TRICKS

Indication and preoperative considerations	Determining the cause of talar collapse is important, especially after a total ankle arthroplasty or talus ORIF. The surgeon must rule out infectious processes. Laboratory studies, advanced imaging, joint aspiration, and bone biopsy may be helpful in determining infection
Approach and exposure	If the patient presents with a prior anterior ankle incision approach, scar tissue is likely observed while performing dissection. Care must be taken to avoid iatrogenic neurovascular injury. While removing talar implants and necrotic bone, the surgeon should be cognizant not to damage or disrupt the stable tibial component
Joint preparation	Overly aggressive joint preparation without maintaining native anatomic contour will decrease the contact area between the bone and implant. The surgeon should follow the contour of the surrounding osseous structures while prepping for the fusion
Fixation and alignment	Temporary fixation is important during this portion of the procedure. The hindfoot and midfoot position should be properly aligned clinically and radiographically prior to final fixation. It is difficult to correct a malpositioned hindfoot once the final implant is inserted. This should be checked during the trial phase
Ancillary procedures	Without correcting the equinus position, the patient will be susceptible to overloading at the bone–implant interfaces. Specifically at the midfoot level, this could lead to decreased bony ingrowth or even broken hardware

ORIF, Open reduction and internal fixation.

References

1. Harnroongroj T. The talar body prosthesis: results at ten to thirty-six years of follow-up. *J Bone Joint Surg Am.* 2014; 96(14):1211-1218.
2. Tonogai I, Hamada D, Yamasaki Y, et al. Custom-made alumina ceramic total talar prosthesis for idiopathic aseptic necrosis of the talus: report of two cases. *Case Rep Orthop.* 2017;2017:8090804.
3. Kadakia R, Akoh C, Chen J, Sharma A, Parekh S. 3D printed total talus replacement for avascular necrosis of the talus. *Foot Ankle Int.* 2020;41(12):1529-1536. doi:10.1177/1071100720948461.
4. Lachman J, Parekh S. Total talus replacement for traumatic bone loss or idiopathic avascular necrosis of the talus. *Tech Foot Ankle Surg.* 2019;18(2):87-98. doi:10.1097/btf.0000000000000203.
5. Akoh C, Chen J, Adams S. Total ankle total talus replacement using a 3D printed talus component: a case report. *J Foot Ankle Surg.* 2020;59(6):1306-1312. doi:10.1053/j.jfas.2020.08.013.
6. Trovato A, El-Rich M, Adeeb S, Dhillon S, Jomha N. Geometric analysis of the talus and development of a generic talar prosthetic. *Foot Ankle Surg.* 2017;23(2):89-94.
7. Tracey J, Arora D, Gross C, Parekh S. Custom 3D-printed total talar prostheses restore normal joint anatomy throughout the hindfoot. *Foot Ankle Spec.* 2019;12(1):39-48.
8. Wagener J, Gross C, Schweizer C, Lang T, Hintermann B. Custom-made total ankle arthroplasty for the salvage of major talar bone loss. *Bone Joint J.* 2017;99-B(2):231-236.
9. Tsukamoto S, Tanaka Y, Maegawa N, et al. Total talar replacement following collapse of the talar body as a complication of total ankle arthroplasty. *J Bone Joint Surg Am.* 2010;92(11):2115-2120.
10. Scott D, Parekh S. Outcomes following 3D printed total talus arthroplasty. *Foot Ankle Orthop.* 2018;3(3):2473011418S0041. doi:10.1177/2473011418s00419.
11. Taniguchi A, Takakura Y, Tanaka Y, et al. An alumina ceramic total talar prosthesis for osteonecrosis of the talus. *J Bone Joint Surg Am.* 2015;97(16):1348-1353.

10

3D-Printed Solutions for Avascular Necrosis of the Talonavicular Joint

COLEMAN OLIVER CLOUGHERTY, MARK RAZZANTE, PAUL R. LEATHAM, SARAH MESSINA

Definition

- Excision of the talus and navicular in total, which is then replaced with a metallic, patient-customized 3D-printed implant.

Indications

- Avascular necrosis (AVN) of the talus and/or the navicular.
- Comminuted fracture of talus and navicular.
- Post-traumatic arthritis with poor bone quality and cystic formation.
- Osteolysis or bone resorption secondary to an infection.

Anatomy

- The talonavicular joint (TNJ) is a ball and socket type of joint that consists of the articulation between the concavity produced by the proximal posterior aspect of the navicular and the convex, ellipsoid surface of the talar head.[1]
- The articulation of the TNJ is maintained by various ligaments, including the talonavicular ligament, the bifurcate ligament, and the calcaneonavicular (spring) ligament.[2]
- The TNJ composes the transverse tarsal joint and is an essential joint in the medial column, forming a portion of the medial longitudinal arch.[3]
- The primary plane of motion for the TNJ is from dorsal lateral to plantar medial. Its primary function is as part of the transverse tarsal joint along with the calcaneocuboid joint, which acts in unison with the subtalar and ankle joint during gait.[1]
- Talonavicular motion and function is closely paired with the subtalar joint. Fusion of either joint tremendously affects the other in terms of remaining functional motion.[4]
- Vascular supply of the talus and navicular is delicate, with the predominant vascular supply coming from two main suppliers, the dorsalis pedis and the medial branch of the posterior tibial artery.[3,5-8]

Pathogenesis

- AVN is characterized by osseous cell death secondary to vascular compromise. AVN can result from a variety of causes, including corticosteroid use, trauma, osteomyelitis, septic arthritis, alcoholism, sickle cell disease, diabetes, and systemic lupus erythematosus (SLE).[9,10]
- Spontaneous osteonecrosis of the navicular and talus (SONNT) is an idiopathic disease that is characterized by symptomatic osteonecrosis of both the navicular and talus simultaneously with associated osteoarthritis of the TNJ. While the cause of SONNT is unknown, possible atraumatic causes are insufficient blood supply and developmental reasons.[11]
- Comminuted fractures frequently occur after high-impact trauma and can result in the splintering of bone into multiple fragments as well as the disruption of vascular supply.[12]

Patient History and Physical Exam Findings

- A typical presentation of this injury involves an inability to bear weight and an inability to tolerate midtarsal range of motion, along with pain on ambulation.
- Patients often complain of point tenderness over the navicular or TNJ with or without erythema, edema, or temperature increase.
- Patients may have an antalgic gait with increased weight bearing to the lateral aspect of their foot.
- Previous history of trauma to the TNJ or rheumatoid arthritis is common among these patients, especially with risk factors that could cause AVN (Figs. 10.1 and 10.2).

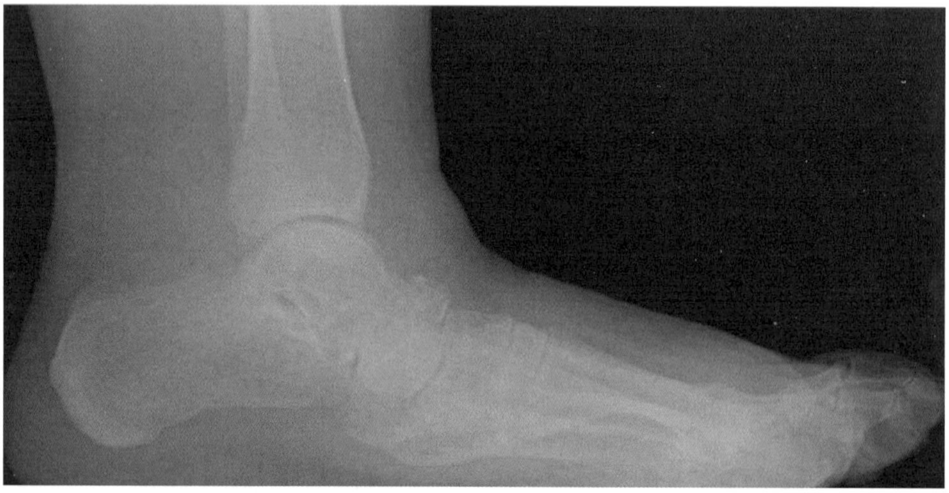

• **Fig. 10.1** Anteroposterior view of the surgical foot preoperatively.

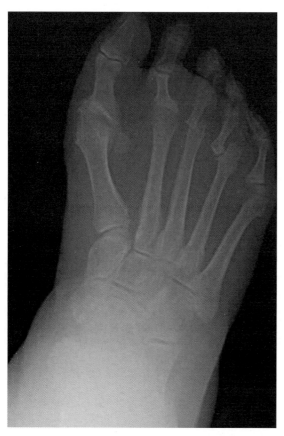

• **Fig. 10.2** Lateral view of the surgical foot preoperatively.

• Frequently patients will have a history of failing conservative treatment methods such as casts, boots, and a series of corticosteroid injections.[13]

• In longstanding TNJ injuries you will see a progressive valgus deformity as the longitudinal arch continues to collapse, resulting in an alteration of subtalar joint motion.[1]

Imaging and Other Diagnostic Testing

• Radiographs often demonstrate initial minor osteopenia, patchy sclerosis with rim calcification of affected bones,

possible subchondral cyst formation, late cortex collapse with "crescent sign," and associated soft tissue edema.[13]

• If there is any suspicion of AVN, MRI and CT scans are indicated to allow for appropriate preoperative evaluation of the extent of the AVN.

• If 3D printing technology is being utilized, CT is the preferred imaging modality.[14]

• Vascular studies to ensure that the patient has adequate blood supply to the anterior ankle angiosomes are required with the anterior ankle incisional approach due to the nature of this incision having issues with healing.

Treatment Options

• Nonoperative management includes:
  • Conservative treatment is suggested prior to consideration for surgical intervention; however, frequently patients will experience no relief and AVN will progress.[13]
    • Prolonged non–weight bearing through the use of casting or controlled ankle motion (CAM) boots.
    • Activity modification.
    • Custom orthotics.
    • Bracing.
    • Corticosteroid injections.
    • Extracorporeal shockwave therapy.
    • Electrical bone stimulation using a pulsed electromagnetic field.

Traditional/Alternative Surgical Management

• Vascularized bone graft with a plate fixation technique.[15,16]

• Talus removal with a tibiotalocalcaneal (TTC) arthrodesis technique utilizing an osseous graft.[15]

• Core decompression of the talus and navicular technique.[15,17]

• Conservative care and other midfoot and/or hindfoot fusions.

- By utilizing more traditional options, such as those listed here, you are eliminating the possibility for a revisional surgery down the line by early fusion of multiple joints or utilizing autologous or allograft bone.[18]

3D-Printed Implant Design Specifications and Considerations

- A 3D-printed implant comprising both the talus and navicular for total TNJ replacement allows for precise restoration of medial column length but also avoids ankle arthrodesis by restoring the articular surface of the talar dome (Figs. 10.3 to 10.6).
- A CT scan should be obtained to help create and design implants. If there is any collapse or significant deformity at the TNJ, a contralateral CT can be obtained in order to create inverted variants for nominal anatomy of the affected TNJ.
- The implant material may vary according to the surgeon's preference. The implant featured in this chapter is made from titanium alloy (Ti6Al4V). Cobalt chromium (CoCr) is also a common 3D-printed material. The implant can contain multiple-sized honeycomb lattice–shaped pores, which are also made up of CoCr (see Figs. 10.1 and 10.2). This is the senior author's preference, as this specific pattern has been shown to allow for better ingrowth than the roughened surface of the implant alone. Larger diameter pores are located plantarly and smaller diameter pores are located on the medial aspect of the talonavicular implant.
- The shape of the implant was in the form of a fused talus and navicular bone. The senior author prefers the implant

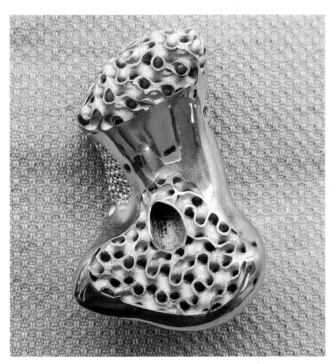

• **Fig. 10.3** Plantar view of the talonavicular implant.

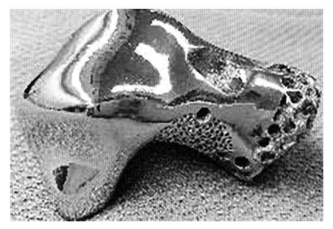

• **Fig. 10.4** Lateral view of the talonavicular implant.

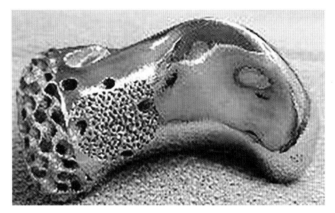

• **Fig. 10.5** Medial view of the talonavicular implant.

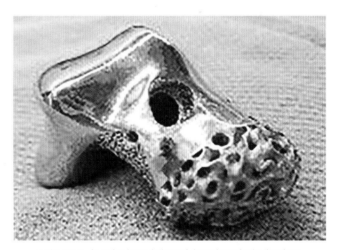

• **Fig. 10.6** Anterior-lateral view of the talonavicular implant.

to be shaped like a truncated cone that is wider anteriorly than posteriorly, with an extension off the distal aspect in the shape of a boat that allows for seamless integration with the medial, intermediate, and lateral cuneiform.
- Polished surfaces were located on the dorsal aspect of the implant extending from the articular surface of the talus distal to the navicular cuneiform joint.
- Rough surfaces with a porous lattice were located on both the distal navicular portion and the plantar aspect

of the talonavicular implant to promote osseous ingrowth.

- Holes should be designed within the implant to allow fixation into the calcaneus and individual cuneiforms. The holes can be designed to accommodate screw or staple fixation.
- Fixation of the implant to the intended arthrodesis sites can also vary according to preference; however, the authors' experience includes utilizing multiple types of fixations from the implant across the cuneiforms. This includes individual staples into respective cuneiforms and multiple screws in divergent patterns from the implant into the cuneiforms. Screws should be headed to allow for contact with the implant. Screw sizes can vary based on availability and surgeon preference; however, 4.0 and 7.0 mm into the cuneiform and calcaneus, respectively, have worked well.
- In regard to fixating the subtalar arthrodesis, there are multiple options. Larger diameter fixation with a screw seems optimal. The plantar surface can be designed according to the native contour of the contralateral talus, or another available option in design is building a convex surface to the plantar aspect of the talar portion of the implant. When prepping the subtalar joint, utilizing an acetabular reamer allows an increased surface area of implant to bone interface. In addition, the convex-concave relationship allows for rotation of the calcaneus for any potential need for deformity correction. If the convex portion is pursued in implant design, ensure the same sized reamer is used as the implant.
- Areas for intended arthrodesis should be designed to be rough, trabecular, and porous to promote bony ingrowth.
- Articulating portions of the implant, specifically the talar dome, should be smooth and highly polished.
- Certain designs for potential soft tissue reattachment can be incorporated with rough surfaces and additional eyelet anchor sites.
- There is a fine balance to be achieved when incorporating an increased amount of fixation options for a stable construct, as a higher number of clearances designed into the implant decrease the opportunity for bony ingrowth that facilitates implant adherence.
- Although there are varying concomitant procedures that are ultimately up to the surgeon's preference, it is the senior author's recommendation to incorporate arthrodesis of the subtalar and cuneiform interface to increase the stability of a large sized total implant.
- Small loops can be incorporated into the device designs to allow for reattachment of ligament and tendon insertions, specifically the posterior tibial (PT) tendon.
- To account for variations in sizing intraoperatively, the senior author prefers to have three different sizes of the implant available, which range from nominal and ±5% to 10% of the length of the nominal-sized implant. The size of the implant used is determined by press fitting it into the operative site.

- Trial guides are used to confirm which size of the implant fits optimally in an intraoperative setting. Trial guides can be made from radiopaque material, which eases visualization prior to implantation.
- Harvested bone autograft can be morselized and packed into porous surfaces at the intended fusion implant interface.

Surgical Management With 3D-Printed Devices

- All surgical planning was performed with an engineering design team from the product manager and included multiple options for this specific patient as well as adjunct fixation options due to the less than ideal quality of the patient's bone for fusion.
- The surgeon's preference is general anesthesia with a preoperative regional nerve block.
- The surgical approach is best achieved through the supine position with a hip bump.
- Incision planning should be well planned in accordance with the adjunctive procedures that are to be performed. However, direct visualization of the talus and navicular is vital to the procedure. An incision interval for anterior ankle exposure is used. The incision starts approximately 5 cm proximal to the ankle joint lateral to the tibialis anterior tendon, and then continues distal along the tendon but then medially deviates towards the extensor hallucis longus tendon as the incision extends to its completion distal to the ankle joint. The incision should end distal to the level of the cuneiform metatarsal joint to allow for complete exposure (Fig. 10.7A,B).
- The authors recommend the use of a bone saw with osteotomes for the excision of native talus and navicular. A bone rongeur can assist with the removal of smaller osseous fragments to ensure entire removal of the talus and navicular (Figs. 10.8 and 10.9). Careful attention is required to appropriately retract and protect the surrounding soft tissues, extensor hallucis longus, tibialis anterior, and close neurovascular structures, including the dorsalis pedis artery and deep peroneal nerve.
- Sizing trial guides can be manufactured from a polymer, with barium sulfate allowing for precise visualization on intraoperative fluoroscopy.
- Caution is required in order to select an appropriately sized implant, finding the correct balance between stability but also allowing range of motion at the ankle joint. If an implant is selected that is too small this may result in additional motion of the implant, which may contribute to failure. On the other hand, if an implant is too large, it may reduce motion at the ankle joint.
- A trabecular lattice including the pegs is packed with morselized bone autograft. The implant is then carefully tamped into position (Fig. 10.10).

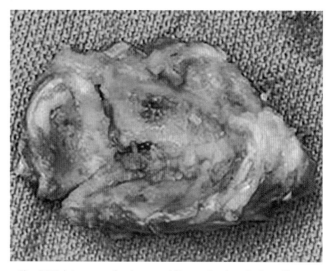

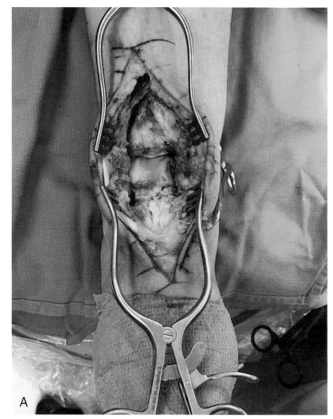

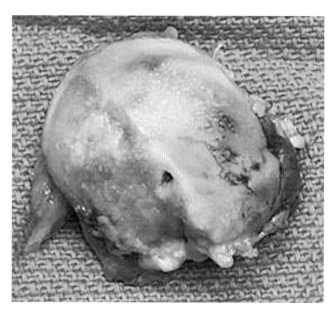

• **Fig. 10.8** Intra-operative image of the excised navicular with gross avascular changes.

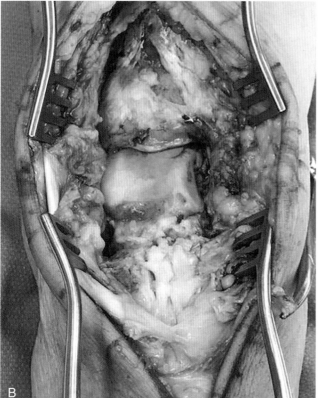

• **Fig. 10.9** Intra-operative image of the excised talar head with gross avascular changes.

• Once the desired position is confirmed on radiographs, screw holes are drilled carefully through the implant for screw and staple fixation.
• The screws and staples are then inserted, and the final position can be confirmed once all fixation has been placed.
• Common adjunctive procedures are variable based on the patient's presentation and can include first tarsometatarsal joint arthrodesis and a calcaneal slide osteotomy.

Postoperative Protocol

• The patient is initially placed into a well-padded, non–weight-bearing posterior splint.

• **Fig. 10.7** (A and B) Anterior approach to the ankle and talonavicular joints.

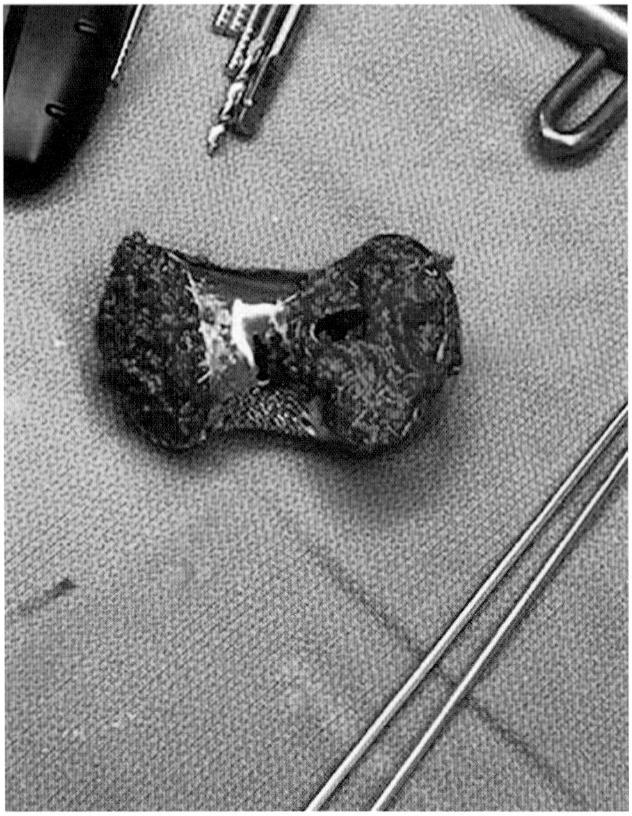

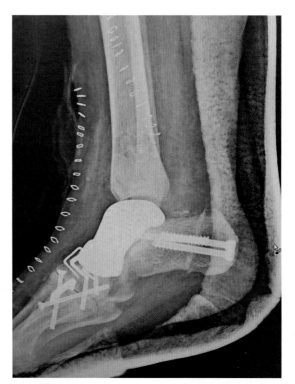

• **Fig. 10.11** Post-operative lateral radiograph demonstrating the fixation construct.

• **Fig. 10.10** Prior to implantation the porous aspects of the implant are packed with bone graft.

- At 1-week follow-up the patient is placed into a short leg cast, followed by transition to a CAM boot at week 3 while maintaining non–weight-bearing status.
- Weight bearing may begin at 8 weeks postoperatively in a CAM boot.
- At the 12-week follow-up the patient transitions to normal shoe gear, with assistance of an ankle foot orthosis (AFO), without higher impact/demanding activities.
- 6 months postoperatively it is acceptable to begin to transition to higher demand activities, that is, a longer period of standing/prolonged walking.
- Radiographs are obtained at every postoperative visit with the exception of the first postoperative visit (Figs. 10.11 to 10.14).
- Postoperative CT scans can be obtained immediately postoperatively, and at 3, 6, and 12 months. This is used to evaluate bony ingrowth and incorporation of the implant.

Results/Outcomes

- The patient was able to begin weight bearing with minimal pain as per the protocol given earlier, and then transitioned into full unassisted weight bearing at 6 months following a small postoperative dehiscence, which was resolved with local wound care and a skin graft.
- No peer-reviewed reports have been published at the time of writing this chapter.

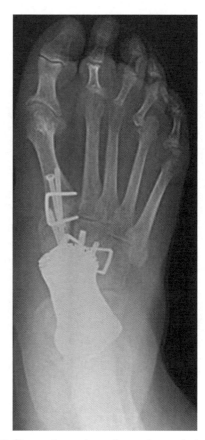

• **Fig. 10.12** Six-month postoperative anteroposterior radiograph demonstrating preserved alignment and stable fixation.

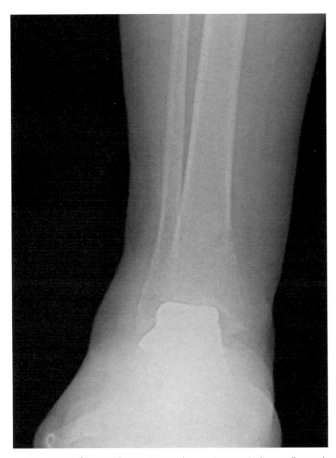

• **Fig. 10.13** Six-month postoperative anteroposterior radiograph demonstrating the implant articulation with the tibia and fibula.

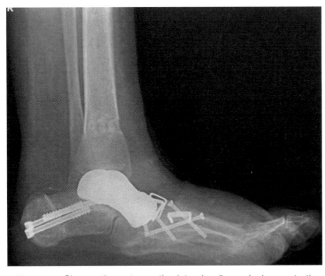

• **Fig. 10.14** Six-month postoperative lateral radiograph demonstrating preserved alignment and stable fixation.

• Possible complications include failure of the arthrodesis site, postoperative hardware infection, and surgical site dehiscence.

• Multiple factors went into the decision to proceed with a total talonavicular implant. The patient was given multiple options including talus removal with fusion, a free osseous graft with fusion, conservative care, and other midfoot and hindfoot fusions. She was given these options and chose to avoid fusions at all costs. Technically, the authors feel that an anterior incisional approach is the most efficient for removing the talus and navicular, and allows for the easiest exposure for implantation and joint preparation, as well as adjunct fixation placement. The postoperative course appeared to be appropriate and beneficial to getting the patient back into her weight bearing without pain status.

• Pitfalls all occurred within the postoperative course, as the patient had a minor wound dehiscence, which put her rehabilitation on hold for about 3 weeks. The patient's dehiscence was accounted for by being placed back onto her rheumatoid arthritis medications, and shortly after this her complications arose. Once these were stopped in agreement with her rheumatologist, her skin was able to heal and she was able to progress back into her postoperative protocol.

TIPS AND TRICKS

Indications	Avascular necrosis of the talus and/ or navicular
	Osteolysis or bone resorption secondary to an infection
	Comminuted fracture of the talus and/or navicular
Contraindications	Active infection
Implant design	The implant itself is composed of cobalt chromium with multiple sizes of honeycomb lattice– shaped pores on surfaces where arthrodesis is to happen. An inverted variant was created from a CT scan of the contralateral foot and utilized for implant design. Morselized harvested bone graft and putty can be packed into the honeycomb lattice–shaped pores to help promote bony ingrowth
Surgical technique	Ensure all compromised bone is removed
	Ensure adequate joint preparation has taken place prior to implant placement
	Implant placement should allow for the restoration of medial column length without compromising neurovascular structures
Goal of reconstruction	Restore medial column length and function, reduction in pain
Imaging	CT scan of bilateral feet
Labs/work up	A thorough presurgical vascular workup is important to ensure adequate vascular supply to the affected foot to facilitate its ability to heal

Implantation	Technically the authors feel that an anterior incisional approach allows the easiest exposure for implantation and joint preparation, as well as adjunct fixation placement
Fixation	The authors recommend direct fixation utilizing three screws and two staples that promote arthrodesis of both the subtalar joint and naviculocuneiform joints
Possible complications	Failure of the arthrodesis site, postoperative hardware infection, and surgical site dehiscence

References

1. Sammarco VJ. The talonavicular and calcaneocuboid joints: anatomy, biomechanics, and clinical management of the transverse tarsal joint. *Foot Ankle Clin.* 2004;9(1):127-145. doi:10.1016/s1083-7515(03)00152-9.
2. DiGiovanni CW. Fractures of the navicular. *Foot Ankle Clin.* 2004;9(1):25-63.
3. Rosenbaum AJ, DiPreta JA, Tartaglione J, Patel N. Acute fractures of the tarsal navicular. *JBJS Rev.* 2015;3(3):e5.
4. Astion DJ, Delannd JT, Otis JC, Kenneally S. Motion of the hindfoot after simulated arthrodesis. *J Bone Joint Surg Am.* 1997;79(2):241-246.
5. Golano P, Farinas O, Saenz I. The anatomy of the navicular and periarticular structures. *Foot Ankle Clin.* 2004;9(1):1-23.
6. Gelberman RH, Mortensen WW. The arterial anatomy of the talus. *Foot Ankle.* 1983;4(2):64-72.
7. Prasarn ML, Miller AN, Dyke JP, Helfet DL, Lorch DG. Arterial anatomy of the talus: a cadaver and gadolinium-enhanced MRI study. *Foot Ankle Int.* 2020;31(11):987-993.
8. Haliburton RA, Sullivan CR, Kelly PJ, Peterson LFF. The extra-osseous and intra osseous blood supply of the talus. *J Bone Joint Surg Am.* 1958;40(5):1115-1120.
9. Dhillon MS, Rana B, Panda I, Patel S, Kumar P. Management options in avascular necrosis of talus. *Indian J Orthop.* 2018;52(3):284. doi:10.4103/ortho.ijortho_608_17.
10. Buchan CA, Pearce DH, Lau J, White LM. Imaging of postoperative avascular necrosis of the ankle and foot. *Semin Musculoskelet Radiol.* 2012;16(3):192-204. doi:10.1055/s-0032-1320060.
11. Vaishya R, Kumar V, Agarwal AK, Vijay V. Spontaneous osteonecrosis of navicular and talus (SONNT). *J Clin Orthop Trauma.* 2016;7:83-87. doi:10.1016/j.jcot.2016.06.005.
12. Katsui R, Takakura Y, Taniguchi A, Tanaka Y. Ceramic artificial talus as the initial treatment for comminuted talar fractures. *Foot Ankle Int.* 2020;41(1):79-83. doi:10.1177/1071100719875723.
13. Haskell A. Natural history of avascular necrosis in the talus. *Foot Ankle Clin.* 2019;24(1):35-45. doi:10.1016/j.fcl.2018.09.002.
14. Dekker TJ, Steele JR, Federer AE, Hamid KS, Adams SB Jr. Use of patient-specific 3D-printed titanium implants for complex foot and ankle limb salvage, deformity correction, and arthrodesis procedures. *Foot Ankle Int.* 2018;39(8):916-921.
15. Gross CE, Sershon RA, Frank JM, Easley ME, Holmes GB. Treatment of osteonecrosis of the talus. *JBJS Rev.* 2016;4(7):e2.
16. Kodama N, Takemura Y, Ueba H, Imai S, Matsusue Y. A new form of surgical treatment for patients with avascular necrosis of the talus and secondary osteoarthritis of the ankle. *Bone Joint J.* 2015;97-B(6):802-808. doi:10.1302/0301-620x.97b6.34750.
17. Sultan AA, Mont MA. Core decompression and bone grafting for osteonecrosis of the talus: a critical analysis of the current evidence. *Foot Ankle Clin.* 2019;24(1):107-112. doi:10.1016/j.fcl.2018.11.005.
18. Lachman JR, Adams SB. Tibiotalocalcaneal arthrodesis for severe talar avascular necrosis. *Foot Ankle Clin.* 2019;24(1):143-161. doi:10.1016/j.fcl.2018.11.002.

11

Tibiotalocalcaneal Fusion With Talar Cage for Hindfoot Reconstruction

DANIEL J. TORINO, HUI ZHANG, GERARD J. CUSH Jr.

Definition

- Tibiotalocalcaneal (TTC) fusion is a salvage procedure for patients with substantial ankle and subtalar arthritis or severe malalignment of the ankle-hindfoot complex. In many cases, this procedure is the only option available to provide patients with a stable, painless, plantigrade foot for ambulation. General indications for TTC include severe symptomatic hindfoot and ankle deformity or combined ankle and hindfoot arthritis for which nonsurgical management has failed. What makes this treatment modality even more challenging is the often-associated bone loss, especially in cases of neuropathic arthropathy or Charcot arthropathy. As the indications for TTC fusion expand, the number of procedures performed continues to rise.[1–3]

Diagnosis

- Specific conditions for which such fusion is commonly indicated include inflammatory arthropathies; congenital deformity; neuropathic arthritides secondary to diabetes mellitus or inherited polyneuropathies; failed total ankle arthroplasty; severe pes planovalgus deformity; fracture malunion and nonunion; and bone loss and collapse secondary to trauma, tumor, osteonecrosis, Charcot arthropathy, or infection.[1]
- Patient factors that have been shown to affect outcomes of TTC fusion include medical comorbidities such as diabetes mellitus, previous ulcerations, peripheral vascular disease, renal disease, immunosuppression, chronic steroid use, rheumatologic disease, malnutrition, and smoking. In addition, a history of surgical intervention, particularly with postoperative complications (e.g., deep infection, problems with wound healing), may affect postoperative outcomes. In several studies of TTC arthrodesis, 20% to 40% of patients had a history of diabetes mellitus or smoking, resulting in poorer than average outcomes in these patients.[2,3]

Anatomy

- The ankle joint is a ginglymus (hinge) joint involving the tibia, talus, and fibula. The talar dome is biconcave with a central talar sulcus. Viewed axially, the joint is trapezoidal and wider anteriorly than posteriorly. The talus is the only tarsal bone without muscular or ligamentous insertions.
- The syndesmosis is the tibiofibular articulation composed of the tibial incisura fibularis and its corresponding fibular facet. It has three ligamentous structures that are variably responsible for its support: the anterior inferior tibiofibular ligament, the interosseous ligament, and the posterior tibiofibular ligament.
- The subtalar joint has three facets: posterior, middle, and anterior. The posterior facet is the largest, the middle facet rests on the sustentaculum of the calcaneus and is located medially. The anterior facet is often continuous with the talonavicular joint.
- The transverse tarsal joint (Chopart joint) is composed of the talonavicular and calcaneocuboid joints and acts in concert with the subtalar joint to control foot flexibility during gait. The talonavicular joint is supported by the spring ligament complex, which has two separate components: the superior medial calcaneonavicular ligament and the inferior calcaneonavicular ligament. The calcaneocuboid joint is saddle-shaped. It is supported plantarly by the inferior calcaneocuboid ligaments (superficial and deep) and superiorly by the lateral limb of the bifurcate ligament.[4]

Biomechanics

- The ankle joint's primary motion is dorsiflexion and plantarflexion. With the foot fixed, dorsiflexion is accompanied by internal tibial rotation and plantar flexion is accompanied by external tibial rotation. The bimalleolar axis runs obliquely at 82 degrees ± 4 degrees in the coronal plane and defines the main motion of the ankle.

The talus is wider anteriorly than posteriorly, and the contact area of the dome of the talus increases and moves anteriorly with dorsiflexion. Increased load transmission in the malleoli also occurs with dorsiflexion. The fibula transmits approximately 10% to 15% of the axial load. The tibiofibular syndesmosis allows rotation and proximal and distal migration of the fibula with the tibia but little motion in the sagittal or coronal planes.

- The subtalar and Chopart joint act through a series of coupled motions to create inversion and eversion of the hindfoot and to lock and unlock the midfoot. Inversion of the subtalar joint locks the transverse tarsal joint; eversion unlocks the joint. The joints are parallel during heel strike when the calcaneus is in eversion, allowing the midfoot to be flexible for shock absorption as the foot accepts the body's weight. The joint axes are deviated as the subtalar joint moves to inversion (e.g., during push-off), making the foot inflexible so that it provides a rigid lever arm for push-off.[4]

Pathogenesis

- The hindfoot articulations include the subtalar, talonavicular, and calcaneocuboid joints. Arthritides of the hindfoot are most often posttraumatic in origin but can also develop from inflammatory arthritis, primary osteoarthritis (OA), end-stage tibialis posterior tendon disorders, tarsal coalitions, or neurologic disorders including Charcot arthropathy.
- The pathogenesis of Charcot arthropathy (also termed Charcot foot) has been explained using two major theories—neurotraumatic and neurovascular:
  - The neurotraumatic theory attributes bond destruction to the loss of pain sensation and proprioception, combined with repetitive and mechanical trauma to the foot.
  - The neurovascular theory suggests that joint destruction is secondary to an autonomic stimulated vascular reflex causing hyperemia and periarticular osteopenia with contributory trauma.
  - There is a growing body of evidence that dysregulation of inflammatory and bone metabolism pathways, with upregulation of receptor activator of nuclear factor-kappa B ligand (RANK-L), lead to osteoclast overactivation and bone resorption.[5-7]
- Clinically, midfoot osteoarthropathy manifests as a noninfectious, osteolytic process that may ultimately result in profound deformity and instability from bone and joint collapse.[8] Deformity with neuropathy may lead to ulceration and potentially to a limb-threatening condition.
- In 1966, orthopedic surgeon Sidney N. Eichenholtz published clinical, radiographic, and pathologic data used to define three stages of Charcot arthropathy based on the natural history of the condition.[9] The three stages he described were (I) development; (II) coalescence; and (III) reconstruction and reconstitution.
- Clinical signs (such as swelling, warmth, and erythema) regularly precede the radiographic findings seen with

TABLE 11.1 Eichenholtz Classification of Charcot Arthropathy Based on the Natural Progression of the Condition

Stage	Characteristics
0: Acute inflammatory phase[a]	Foot is swollen, erythematous, warm, hyperemic; radiographs reveal periarticular soft tissue swelling and varying degrees of osteopenia
I: Developmental or fragmentation	Periarticular fracture and joint subluxation with risk of instability and deformity
II: Coalescence stage; subacute	Resorption of bone debris and soft tissue homeostasis
III: Consolidation or reparative stage; chronic	Restabilization of the foot with fibrous or bony arthrodesis of the involved joints

[a]The staging system was amended to include a prodromal stage zero phase by Shibata et al.[8]
Rosenbaum, A.J., DiPreta, J.A. Classifications in Brief: Eichenholtz Classification of Charcot Arthropathy. Clin Orthop Relat Res 473, 1168–1171 (2015). https://doi.org/10.1007/s11999-014-4059-y and Eichenholtz SN. Charcot Joints. Springfield, IL, USA: Charles C. Thomas; 1966.

Eichenholtz stage I arthropathy.[10] As such, in 1990 Shibata et al. added a fourth stage, stage 0, to the conventional Eichenholtz classification (Table 11.1).[8]

Patient History and Physical Exam Findings

- An examination of the skin and the presence of ulceration or impending ulceration is to be noted and considered in procedure selection.
- Vascular examination should include palpation of pedal pulses, the presence or absence of pedal hair, and degree of swelling. If there is any question about the vascular status of the limb in which TTC fusion is being considered, further workup is warranted and may include vascular studies or consultation with a vascular surgeon.
- A neurologic evaluation should include sensation testing with a 5.07-gauge monofilament, a tuning fork, or pin-prick test. Further, Achilles reflexes should also be tested.
- Alignment while standing and walking is of particular importance. Deformity and instability in the sagittal and coronal planes of the ankle, hindfoot, and forefoot should be assessed in detail. To assess the need for forefoot correction, the hindfoot can be held in the corrected position while the clinician assesses the position of the forefoot in the coronal plane relative to the long axis of the tibia while the patient is seated.
- Bony prominences, rocker-bottom deformity, and potential areas of increased pressure are prone to ulceration and must be addressed.

Imaging and Other Diagnostic Testing

- Weight-bearing radiographs of the ankle and foot are mandatory in the evaluation for TTC fusion.
- Radiographic evidence of arthrosis, bone loss, shortening, existing implants from prior surgeries (particularly broken screws), and deformity should be noted.
- Weight-bearing anteroposterior (AP) views of both ankles gives an excellent indication of the degree of actual or functional shortening caused by bone loss or malalignment.
- CT may be indicated in patients with substantial disruption of the normal bone architecture of the foot and ankle, and is useful in revision arthrodesis for determining the status of a previous fusion.
- MRI may be used in select cases to evaluate the extent of osteonecrosis in a foot and ankle being considered for TTC fusion.

Nonoperative Management

- Nonsurgical treatment of arthritis of the ankle and foot include nonsteroidal anti-inflammatories (systemic or topical), activity modification, corticosteroid injections, shoe modifications, and bracing.
- Most cases of acute Charcot arthropathy can be treated effectively with pressure-relieving methods such as total contact casting.
- Chronic and/or unstable ankle and hindfoot Charcot deformities are prone to fail nonsurgical treatment.

Traditional Surgical Management

- A transfibular approach is most often used for TTC fusion. Prior surgical incisions or soft tissue flaps may dictate variations in the location of the incision for such an approach. Occasionally, if the lateral skin is compromised and a lateral approach cannot be used, a posterior approach may be used to access both the subtalar and ankle joints.[11]
- Traditional TTC fixation methods include external fixation, cannulated versus solid screws, intramedullary nailing, and plating. Currently, there is no accepted standard technique for this procedure, with the type of implant typically being determined by the discretion or familiarity of the surgeon.[12]
- Autograft sources for TTC fusion grafts include the iliac crest for cancellous and corticocancellous bone, the tibia or femur for cancellous bone harvested with a reamer-irrigator aspirator device, and the fibula for interpositional struts.
- Allograft options include cancellous chips, bulk allograft obtained from the femoral head, and struts of corticocancellous bone from the iliac crest or the fibula.
- The use of a femoral head allograft to span bone defects has recently gained popularity since it can restore normal limb length and offer a conduit for fusion. However, this technique has led to mixed results, with reported rates of successful arthrodesis as low as 50%. There is also an infection risk with the use of a large bulk allograft and the potential for graft subsidence or collapse.[13]
- In patients at high risk of complications after TTC fusion, augmentation with bone marrow aspirate, platelet-rich plasma, or an orthobiologic material may be used.

3D-Printed Implant and Instrumentation Considerations

- Materials: all implants are fabricated via laser powder bed fusion (L-PBF) of medical-grade titanium alloy (Ti6Al4V ELI).
- Polished versus rough surfaces: after printing, the implants undergo multiple postprocessing steps before being delivered for surgery. The first of these steps is known as hot isostatic pressing (HIP, "hipping"), a process during which the implants are subjected to both high temperature and pressure to relieve the implants of residual thermal stresses and close any internal voids. Next, the parts undergo microblasting, during which titanium powder is blown at the implant surface under high pressure to remove any partially adhered particles of powder. Finally, the implants are subjected to a chemical passivation process which results in a thin surface oxide layer that improves the corrosion resistance of the implants.
- Shape: the implants are typically spherical with or without modifications. This geometry was selected after proving to offer significant intraoperative flexibility in terms of repositioning. Modification to the spherical implant shape may be considered, for example, a flattened lateral implant surface can aid in soft tissue closure (Fig. 11.1).
- Sizing: the surgeon's preference is nominal ±5% to 10%.
- The implant's size, shape, and special modifications may be influenced by corresponding off-the-shelf (OTS) fixation. The senior author's preference is to use a TTC fusion nail in 10 or 12 mm-diameter options. To accommodate intramedullary fixation, cages are designed with 14-mm cannulation to allow for intraoperative flexibility (Fig. 11.2).
- Patient-specific instrumentation provided for these cases generally includes a reaming guide, trials, an inserter, and an impactor (Fig. 11.3). The guides are designed to register to the preoperative tibia and designate an implant's spherical center. This center position is marked by a k-wire and the guide is then pulled off over the k-wire. A male metatarsal-phalangeal joint fusion reamer is then used over the wire to form a notch in the anatomy, which will allow for a greater amount of control when using the acetabular reamers to contour the anatomy.
- Trials corresponding to each implant size are provided and designed to be similarly cannulated. These trials are printed using a barium sulfate–doped biocompatible polymer, which provides clear visibility of the cannulation under fluoroscopy and allows for precision when reaming for the TTC fusion nail.

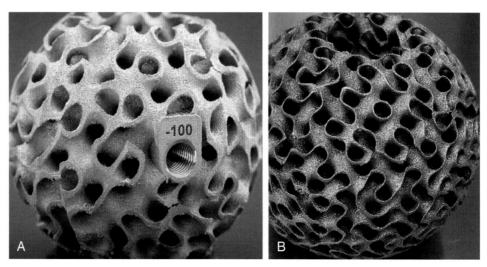

• **Fig. 11.1** Implant shape may be patient or surgeon specific. (A) The base implant shape is spherical; however, (B) a flattened lateral surface can allow easier soft tissue closure.

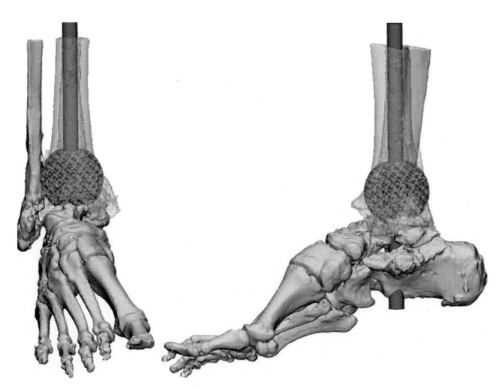

• **Fig. 11.2** Preoperative computer-aided design images depicting the fixation trajectory and proposed talar implant. (Reprinted with permission from restor3d, Inc, Durham, NC.)

- A threaded inserter that mates with the lateral face of the implant is provided to improve handling and control during implant placement and also allows for fine tuning of the implant's orientation after it has been placed.
- Finally, a polymer impactor is supplied to offer a safe material and implant-specific option in the case that additional force is needed to place the implant into the anatomy.

Surgical Management of 3D-Printed Devices

- Preoperative assessment includes physical examination, radiographs, CT scan, and recording of any pertinent patient-outcome measures (Fig. 11.4).
- General anesthesia with laryngeal mask versus endotracheal intubation.

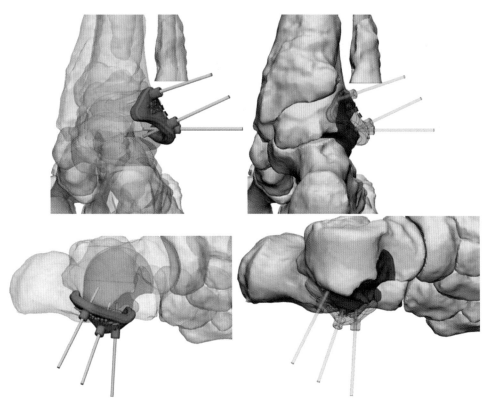

• **Fig. 11.3** Patient-specific instrumentation may include a reaming guide. After the fibular malleolus is excised, the guide is pinned to the corresponding anatomy with three wires. In this computer-aided design image, the posterior and middle wires are removed, followed by the guide. The remaining anterior wire is now in the ideal trajectory. A conical male-end metatarsophalangeal joint fusion reamer is used over the wire. The wire is removed and reaming continues with an acetabular reamer. (Reprinted with permission from restor3d, Inc, Durham, NC.)

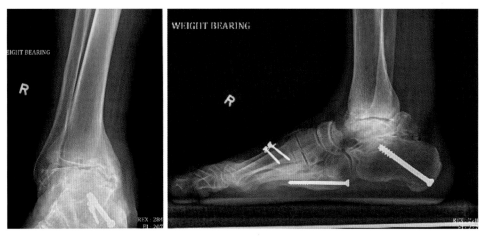

• **Fig. 11.4** Preoperative radiographs depicting avascular necrosis of the talus with collapse, adjacent joint arthritis, and deformity.

- Lateral decubitus or supine position.
- Hemostasis provided by a thigh tourniquet at 250 mmHg.
- A transfibular approach is performed with an osteotomy through the fibula with a chisel, which allows access to the distal tibia, talus, and subtalar joint. The removed portion of the fibula is taken to the back table and morselized for use as a local autograft. A 30-cc bone marrow aspiration is performed from the proximal tibia and added to the fibular autograft in combination with the allograft.
- The subtalar and tibiotalar joints are assessed for cage implantation. A custom guide is pinned in place into the lateral aspect of the talus. Sequential reamers are then utilized under fluoroscopic guidance to prepare an area for the cage (see Fig. 11.3).

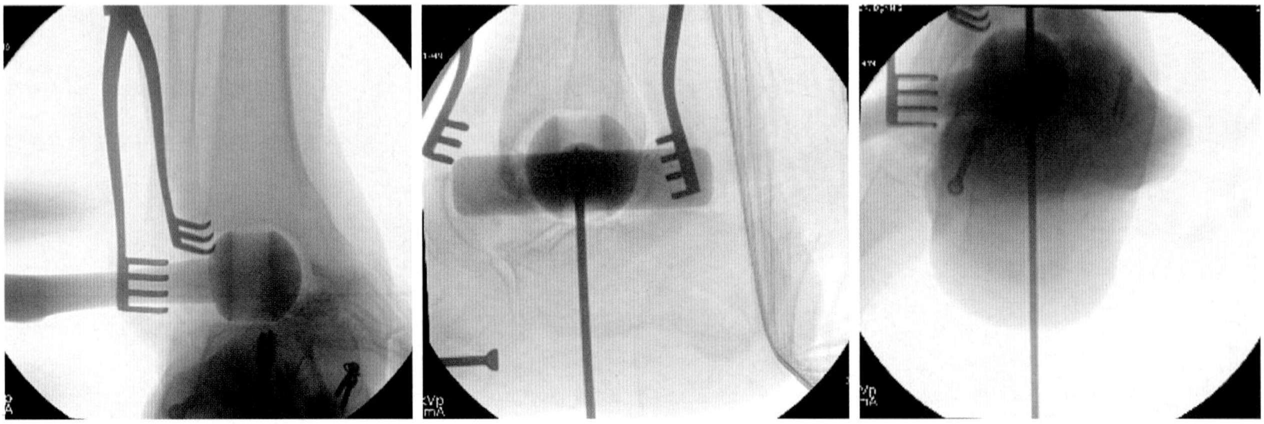

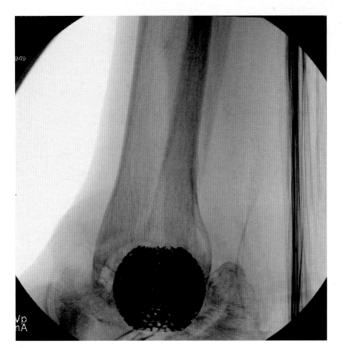

• **Fig. 11.5** Intraoperative radiographs depicting placement of the reaming guide pin through the radio-opaque trial. The authors recommend keeping the trial in place during the reaming process.

• Trial implant is sized and impacted. The ankle is then positioned in appropriate coronal and sagittal alignment for fusion in preparation for intramedullary nail placement. A guide pin is advanced from the plantar aspect of the calcaneus across the remaining talus and subtalar joint, traversing the cage trial and into the distal tibia (Fig. 11.5). This is confirmed on fluoroscopic images.

• An opening reamer is first advanced into the calcaneus up into the tibia and the guide pin is replaced with a ball tip guidewire. The position of the guide pin is confirmed with fluoroscopy and then sequential reaming is performed to 2 mm over the final measured nail size. The bone reaming is added to the bone graft mixture and manually packed into the final cage construct as well as the fusion site.

• The trial is removed and the permanent talar cage packed with bone graft is impacted (Fig. 11.6). The nail is inserted,

traversing the custom cage while maintaining appropriate fusion alignment (Fig. 11.7). Two distal interlocking screws are placed through the jig and confirmed with fluoroscopy. Manual and, if available, dynamic compression (i.e., nitinol) is applied and the nail is locked proximally with two screws through the jig.

• Deformity correction of the hindfoot and the position of the tibiotalar calcaneal fusion with the restoration cage is confirmed on orthogonal fluoroscopic images.

• After irrigation, the incisions are closed in layers and local anesthetic is administered. The operative extremity is placed in a well-padded short-leg splint.

Postoperative Protocol

• Soft tissue inspection and suture removal are performed at 2 weeks postoperatively.

• Non-weight bearing is prescribed for 12 weeks total. During the initial 6 weeks the operative extremity is kept in a short-leg splint or cast and is then transitioned to a controlled ankle motion (CAM) boot for an additional 6 weeks.

• Radiographs are evaluated at 6 weeks, 3 months, 6 months and 1 year postoperatively (Fig. 11.8).

• Physical therapy and progression to full weight bearing may begin at 3 months. Additionally, an ankle foot orthosis (AFO) or other rigid ankle brace may be considered for additional support.

Results/Outcomes

• Complication rates as high as 60% have been reported with TTC fusion, with the most common complications including nonunion, malunion, infection, and implant-related problems.[1-3] Pitts et al.'s retrospective review of 101 patients who underwent primary TTC fusion identified several factors associated with a significantly increased risk of nonunion ($P = 0.006$), including patients with preoperative diagnosis of Charcot arthropathy, primary OA, diabetes, and chronic kidney disease.[2] Additionally, patients over 60 years of age with a preoperative diagnosis of Charcot arthropathy and primary OA

• **Fig. 11.6** Intraoperative radiograph depicting placement of the talar implant.

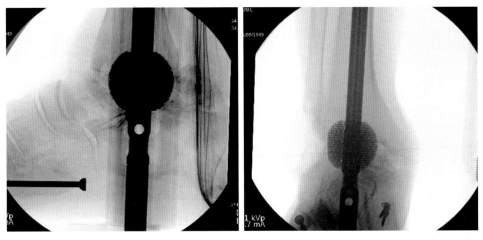

• **Fig. 11.7** Intraoperative radiograph depicting placement of the intramedullary fixation through the talar implant. It is recommended to select an intramedullary nail with two points of fixation in the calcaneus.

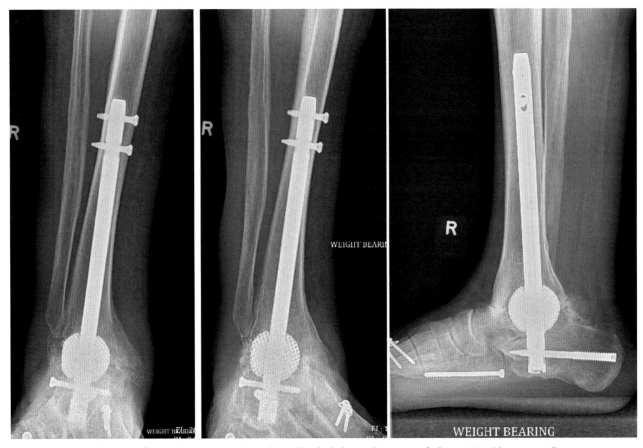

• **Fig. 11.8** Six-month postoperative radiographs depicting maintenance of alignment and bony consolidation into and around the talar implant.

had a significantly higher rate of postoperative rate of infection ($P = 0.002$).[14] The rate of amputation after TTC fusion is reported to be as high as 20%.[15] Risk factors for higher rates of complication include advanced age, neuroarthropathy, diabetes mellitus, and smoking.[16,17] In addition, wound sloughing has been reported with the correction of substantial deformities in the coronal plane and restoration of height.[18] Neurovascular structures at risk of injury with intramedullary (IM) nailing include the lateral plantar nerve and artery and the flexor hallucis longus tendon. The formation of a painful neuroma can be minimized with careful planning of the incision for TTC fusion and meticulous dissection and retraction.

- A limited number of prior studies have looked at the efficacy of 3D-printed cage/nail fusion constructs for TTC fusion. One study in 2020 by Steele et al. compared a group of eight patients treated with 3D-printed cage/nail constructs and a group of seven patients treated with a bulk femoral head allograft. They found a statistically significantly higher rate of union in the 3D-printed cage/nail construct group (92%) versus the bulk femoral head allograft group (62%).[3] Another study looked at 15 consecutive patients using patient-specific 3D–printed implants for limb salvage and found a success rate of 87% (13 out of 15 patients).[4]

- To combat the complications associated with large bulk allografts, TTC arthrodesis with custom 3D-printed titanium implants has been performed in the setting of large bony defects. There have been case reports and small case series detailing the successful use of custom 3D-printed implants in a variety of settings for hindfoot fusions, deformity corrections, and trauma.[19-21] A spherical implant has advantages over highly conforming implants. First, once implanted, the surgeon can rotate the foot around the spherical implant to achieve the desired amount of varus/valgus and dorsiflexion/plantar flexion of the foot in relation to the tibia. 2nd, if using an intramedullary nail for TTC arthrodesis, the cannulated spherical implant can rotate in situ to allow the passage of the nail in the correct trajectory. Moreover, these patient-specific 3D-printed implants have potential benefits over femoral head allografts, including patient-specific custom sizes, no graft collapse, stronger mechanical properties, and coatings to promote bone growth and prevent infection. Steele et al. demonstrated a statistically higher rate of total fused articulations when comparing 3D-printed sphere devices to femoral head allografts.[3]

- Our institution's experience with 3D-printed cage/nail implants for TTC fusion has been favorable thus far. While more study is needed, and longer-term results need to be followed, between 2018 and 2020, 13 patients were treated with cage/nail fusions. Ten of the 13 had Charcot arthropathy. With an average follow-up of 323 days, 11 out of 13 (85%) patients had functional limb salvage, with 2 out of 13 patients undergoing subsequent below-knee amputation (BKA, 15%). Both patients who underwent BKA had Charcot arthropathy. Interestingly, both patients who underwent BKA when asked reported that they would have still chosen the same limb-salvage pathway, despite it not being successful for them.

TIPS AND TRICKS

Preoperative planning	CT scan of the affected limb is needed for customization of the 3D-printed cage May utilize the contralateral limb as a model if needed owing to advanced collapse and deformity
Surgical approach	Use the transfibular approach and save the excised fibula as a morselized autograft Sequentially ream until adequate space is created for the custom cage and save quality viable reamings as autografts
Implant design	Spherical cages allow extra degrees of freedom for final positioning of the cage to accommodate limb alignment and nail insertion Cages with a flattened lateral wall offer less bulk and ease of soft tissue closure with less tension laterally
Implant choice	Have an available true-to-portion-size implant, a 5%–10% downsized implant, and a 5%–10% upsized implant to ensure options maximized for best fit Will often utilize a downsized implant due to soft tissue contraction with chronic talus/hindfoot collapse

References

1. Asomugha EU, Den Hartog BD, Junko JT, Alexander IJ. Tibiotalocalcaneal fusion for severe deformity and bone loss. *J Am Acad Orthop Surg.* 2016;24(3):125-134. doi:10.5435/JAAOS-D-14-00102.

2. Pitts C, Alexander B, Washington J, et al. Factors affecting the outcomes of tibiotalocalcaneal fusion. *Bone Joint J.* 2020; 102-B(3):345-351. doi:10.1302/0301-620X.102B3.BJJ-2019-1325.R1.

3. Steele JR, Kadakia RJ, Cunningham DJ, Dekker TJ, Kildow BJ, Adams SB. Comparison of 3D printed spherical implants versus femoral head allografts for tibiotalocalcaneal arthrodesis. *J Foot Ankle Surg.* 2020;59(6):1167-1170. https://doi.org/10.1053/j.jfas.2019.10.015.

4. Lieberman JR, American Academy of Orthopaedic Surgeons. *AAOS Comprehensive Orthopaedic Review.* Rosemont, IL: American Academy of Orthopaedic Surgeons; 2020.

5. Hingsammer AM, Bauer D, Renner N, Borbas P, Boeni T, Berli M. Correlation of systemic inflammatory markers with radiographic stages of Charcot osteoarthropathy. *Foot Ankle Int.* 2016;37(9):924-928.

6. Sinacore DR, Bohnert KL, Smith KE, et al. Persistent inflammation with pedal osteolysis 1 year after Charcot neuropathic osteoarthropathy. *J Diabetes Complications.* 2017;31(6):1014-1020.

7. Zhao HM, Diao JY, Liang XJ, Zhang F, Hao DJ. Pathogenesis and potential relative risk factors of diabetic neuropathic osteoarthropathy. *J Orthop Surg Res.* 2017;12(1):142.

8. Shibata T, Tada K, Hashizume C. The results of arthrodesis of the ankle for leprotic neuroarthropathy. *J Bone Joint Surg Am.* 1990;72:749-756.

9. Eichenholtz SN. *Charcot Joints.* IL, USA: Springfield; 1966.

10. Classen JN, Rolley RT, Carneiro R, Martire JR. Management of foot conditions of the diabetic patient. *Am Surg.* 1976;42:81-88.

11. Ahmad J, Pour AE, Raikin SM. The modified use of a proximal humeral locking plate for tibiotalocalcaneal arthrodesis. *Foot Ankle Int.* 2007;28(9):977-983.

12. Thomas RL, Sathe V, Habib SI. The use of intramedullary nails in tibiotalocalcaneal arthrodesis. *J Am Acad Orthop Surg.* 2012; 20(1):1-7.

13. Jeng CL, Campbell JT, Tang EY, Cerrato RA, Myerson MS. Tibiotalocalcaneal arthrodesis with bulk femoral head allograft for salvage of large defects in the ankle. *Foot Ankle Int.* 2013;34 (9):1256-1266.

14. Jehan S, Shakeel M, Bing AJ, Hill SO. The success of tibiotalocalcaneal arthrodesis with intramedullary nailing: a systematic review of the literature. *Acta Orthop Belg.* 2011;77(5):644-651.

15. Bussewitz B, DeVries JG, Dujela M, McAlister JE, Hyer CF, Berlet GC. Retrograde intramedullary nail with femoral head allograft for large deficit tibiotalocalcaneal arthrodesis. *Foot Ankle Int.* 2014;35: 706-711. https://doi.org/10.1177/1071100714531231.

16. DeVries JG, Berlet GC, Hyer CF. Predictive risk assessment for major amputation after tibiotalocalcaneal arthrodesis. *Foot Ankle Int.* 2013;34(6):846-850.

17. Cooper PS. Complications of ankle and tibiotalocalcaneal arthrodesis. *Clin Orthop Relat Res.* 2001;391:33-44.

18. Den Hartog BD, Palmer DS. Femoral head allografts for large talar defects. *Tech Foot Ankle Surg.* 2008;7(4):264-270.

19. Dekker TJ, Steele JR, Federer AE, Hamid KS, Adams SB Jr. Use of patient-specific 3D printed titanium implants for complex foot and ankle limb salvage, deformity correction, and arthrodesis procedures. *Foot Ankle Int.* 2018;39:916-921. https://doi.org/10.1177/1071100718770133.

20. Hamid KS, Parekh SG, Adams SB. Salvage of severe foot and ankle trauma with a 3D printed scaffold. *Foot Ankle Int.* 2016;37:433-439. https://doi.org/10.1177/1071100715620895.

21. Hsu AR, Ellington JK. Patient-specific 3-dimensional printed titanium truss cage with tibiotalocalcaneal arthrodesis for salvage of persistent distal tibia nonunion. *Foot Ankle Spec.* 2015;8:483-489. https://doi.org/10.1177/1938640015593079.

12

Distraction Subtalar Joint Fusion Using a Custom 3D-Printed Implant

DAVID VIER, J. KENT ELLINGTON

Definition

- A patient-specific custom 3D–printed porous titanium implant for subtalar joint fusion to restore height, length, and alignment of the hindfoot.

Indications

- Calcaneus malunion/nonunion
- Subtalar fusion malunion.

Anatomy and Pathogenesis

- The subtalar joint is comprised of the talocalcaneal joint and the talocalcaneonavicular joints.[1]
- The subtalar joint allows for inversion and eversion of the hindfoot but also has a rotational component, allowing the talar head to internally rotate and drop down during eversion.[1-4]
- Calcaneal malunion after a calcaneus fracture typically treated nonoperatively can lead to loss of height, length, varus malposition, widening of the heel, and joint incongruity.[5]
- Posterior facet and articular surface malreduction can lead to subtalar arthritis.
- Lateral wall blowout leads to increased heel width.
- Loss of talar declination due to decreased calcaneal height leads to anterior ankle impingement.
- Varus malposition of the calcaneus leads to lateral column overload.
- Calcaneal malunion after calcaneus open reduction and internal fixation (ORIF) can cause similar issues as nonoperative treatment of calcaneus fractures. Although calcaneus fractures can be very challenging cases, not restoring appropriate heel alignment (out of varus) and calcaneal height and width, and restoring the articular surface can result in similar clinical findings as above.[5-7]

- Peroneal dislocation is also commonly missed after calcaneus fractures.[5]

Patient History and Physical Exam Findings

- A history of calcaneus fracture treated nonoperatively or operatively.
- Pain and instability walking on uneven surfaces; pain along the sinus tarsi.
- Anterior ankle impingement pain.[8]
- Pain/subluxation of peroneal tendons and with resisted eversion.
- Issues fitting into shoes due to heel width as well as subfibular impingement.

Imaging and Other Diagnostic Testing

- Radiographs in the setting of malunion will demonstrate decreased talar declination, decreased hindfoot height, subtalar arthrosis, and varus heel position with increased calcaneus width on axial views, as seen in Fig. 12.1.
- Nonunion will demonstrate lack of callus or bony consolidation across the fracture site as well as subluxation of the subtalar joint or change in alignment.
- MRI can be useful to look at the soft tissue etiology of the pain, including peroneal tendonitis/dislocation as seen in Fig. 12.2, cartilage injury in ankle and subtalar arthrosis, as well as bony edema resulting from impingement.
- CT is typically more useful in analyzing arthrosis and union/malunion. Weight-bearing CT allows for additional assessment of more accurate hindfoot alignment as well as impingement. There is even some, although limited, information about the soft tissue that can be learned from the CT scan such as dislocated peroneals with a soft tissue window.

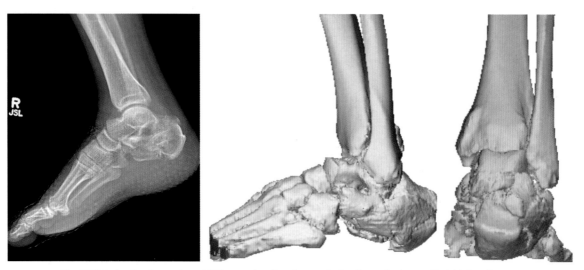

• **Fig. 12.1** Lateral radiograph and CT reconstruction demonstrating loss of calcaneal height, length, varus alignment, as well as anterior ankle impingement.

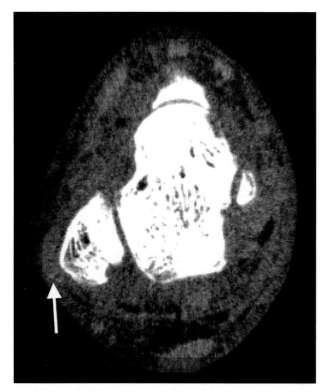

• **Fig. 12.2** Axial CT slice with soft tissue window demonstrates dislocated peroneal tendons *(white arrow)* from the fibular groove

- CT also is the imaging modality of choice for 3D-printing technology.
- Bony metabolic workup should be initiated in cases of nonunion including vitamin D, parathyroid hormone (PTH), and thyroid stimulating hormone (TSH).

Nonoperative Management

- Shoe modification with a wide heel
- Orthotics, such as a solid ankle cushion heel (SACH)

- Bracing
- Oral and topical antiinflammatories
- Corticosteroid injections
- Physical therapy.

Traditional Surgical Management

- Malunion/nonunion revision ORIF: typically not useful, likely due to already rapidly accelerated subtalar arthritis as well as difficulty in restoring alignment.
- In situ subtalar arthrodesis: fusion can relieve pain from subtalar arthritis but does not restore alignment and height, resulting in similar problems as calcaneal malunion such as anterior ankle impingement, subfibular impingement, and lateral column overload.[6,7,9]
- Subtalar distraction osteogenesis: useful in restoring alignment but inconvenient for patients due to prolonged use of the external fixator.
- Subtalar distraction bone block arthrodesis with autograft/allograft: improves anterior ankle impingement by regaining height, and restores hindfoot alignment out of varus. Overall good radiographic and clinical outcomes but very technically difficult, with increased nonunion rates.[9-18]
- Subtalar distraction arthrodesis with trabecular metal augment: a titanium wedge has equivalent outcomes but possibly stronger and better bony incorporation compared to autograft/allograft.[19-21]

3D-Printed Implant and/or Instrumentation Considerations

- The main advantage in using a 3D-printed implant is the ability to preoperatively plan an already very challenging and technically difficult procedure. The hindfoot alignment correction can be dialed in using appropriate cuts and patient-specific custom wedges.

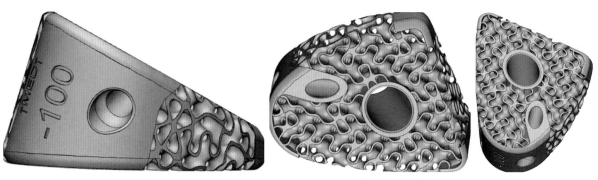

• **Fig. 12.3** Proposed custom subtalar wedge featuring a porous gyroid structure as well as planned fixation with a 7 × 70-mm DynaMini hindfoot nail and a 4.0-mm Medline small cannulated screw.

• Surgical time is likely to be considerably decreased due to cut guide and predesigned implants allowing for fewer intraoperative measurements/errors.
• A variety of proprietary porous structures are available. The senior author currently prefers a gyroid structure.
• The porous architecture allows for bony ingrowth.
• The wedge is designed larger medially to allow for correction out of varus.
• 3D-printed implants allow for intended fixation designed into the implant, which also decreases surgical time and the ideal implant position. The senior author prefers to use a 7-mm–diameter MedShape DynaMini and a 4.0-mm Medline screw for subtalar fixation through the implant, as seen in Fig. 12.3.
• To account for intraoperative flexibility, three different-sized implants are recommended.

Surgical Management With 3D-Printed Devices

• Preoperative planning: measure the degree of correction desired based on hindfoot varus alignment as well as the amount of height needed to be restored. In addition, the desired fixation should be incorporated into planning based on bone stock and the surgeon's preference.
• The implant can be filled with biologic products according to the surgeon's preference. The senior author prefers bone marrow aspirate concentrate, autograft, OsteoAmp, and Augment.
• The patient is positioned in the prone position with a thigh tourniquet and a mini c-arm.
• The posterior approach is used with Z-lengthening of the Achilles tendon to provide exposure. The Achilles tendon is repaired at the end of the case with Ethibond suture.
• The posterior capsule is released with a #15 blade scalpel to release the contracture.
• A lamina spreader is used to distract the subtalar joint. The remaining cartilage is removed using a combination of sharp osteotomes, rongeurs, and curettes.
• Any calcaneal nonunion is taken down with osteotomes and debrided to expose bleeding cancellous bone.
• The joint is then irrigated copiously and prepped by drilling holes in the subchondral bone and fishscaling with osteotomes on both sides of the joint.
• Restor3d cutting guides are then used as appropriate and fixated to the bone with multiple k-wires, as seen in Fig. 12.4. The osteotomy is made using an oscillating saw. The k-wires and cutting guide are then removed.
• The restor3d trials (Fig. 12.5) are then used to assess for final implant size and restoration of alignment and height, as seen in Fig. 12.6. The appropriate associated final implant is then chosen and filled with the biologic mix (Fig. 12.7).
• The subtalar joint is then pinned with k-wires and alignment is assessed with fluoroscopy.

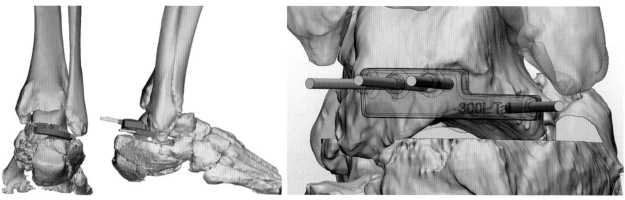

• **Fig. 12.4** Example of a proposed cutting guide showing planned provisional fixation with k-wires.

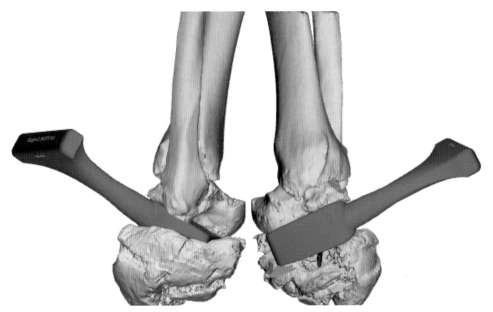

• **Fig. 12.5** Trial implant with a handle to assess for appropriate restoration of hindfoot alignment.

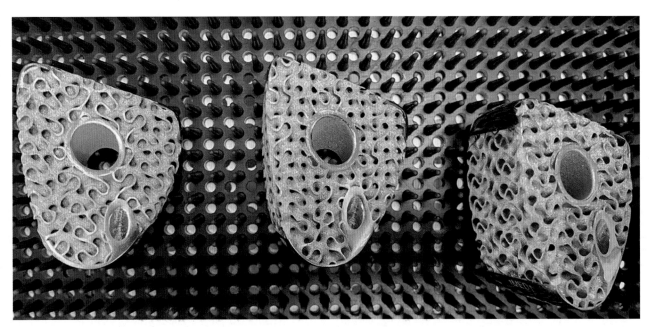

• **Fig. 12.6** Three different-sized custom subtalar wedge implants available for intraoperative use as needed for the desired correction.

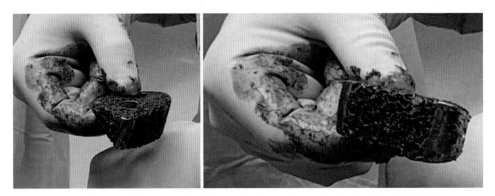

• **Fig. 12.7** A patient-specific restor3d subtalar wedge for calcaneal malunion filled with biologic slurry prior to implantation.

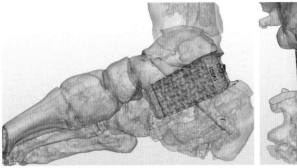
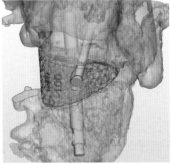

• **Fig. 12.8** The final restor3d proposed custom implant design, correction, and fixation.

- The final implant, as seen in Fig. 12.8, is then inserted and fixated using the surgeon's technique preference. The senior author uses the DynaMini as it allows for postoperative compression using nitinol technology.
- If there is residual peroneal dislocation from the original injury, this should be addressed through a separate incision. Typically, fibular groove deepening and superior peroneal retinaculum (SPR) repair with a suture anchor works well to reduce the peroneal tendons.

Postoperative Protocol

- The patient is placed in a well-padded splint in the operating room.
- The patient should be non–weight bearing for 6 weeks.
- The patient should be followed-up in clinic at 2 weeks for suture removal if appropriate and placed into a cast at neutral for another 4 weeks.
- At 6 weeks, the patient is placed into a boot and is touchdown weight bearing for another 2 weeks. At 8 weeks postoperatively the patient is allowed to advance weight bearing in the boot and then wean the boot as tolerated.
- Radiographs at the 2-week and 9-week mark consist of anteroposterior (AP) foot, AP ankle, lateral, and axial heel views.

Results/Outcomes

- The senior author has had success with this technique in a patient who sustained a fall from height and sustained a calcaneus fracture. The patient was initially seen at an outside hospital and was lost to follow-up. Upon presentation to our clinic, the calcaneus fracture had gone on to malunion/nonunion with persistent SPR injury and peroneal dislocation, and the patient experienced significant anterior ankle impingement and hindfoot varus, as seen in Fig. 12.9.
- Months after the injury the patient underwent ORIF and subtalar distraction arthrodesis with a restor3d custom implant and DynaMini for fixation. A suture anchor was used to repair the SPR after deepening the fibular groove and reducing the peroneal tendons.
- At 6 months postoperatively the patient had healed his calcaneal nonunion and subtalar arthrodesis (Fig. 12.10), was doing well clinically, and had returned to work as a laborer.
- Complications potentially include under- or overcorrection, but this is hopefully limited due to preoperative planning and custom-designed implants. Any standard complications from surgery such as arthrodesis are possible, including infection or nonunion. The patient should be adequately counseled on these prior to any surgery.

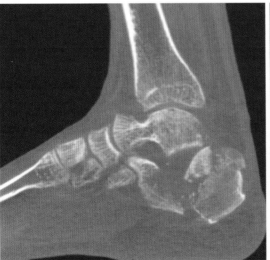
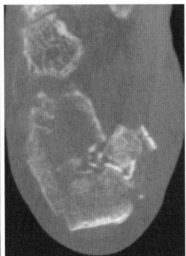
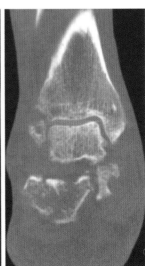

• **Fig. 12.9** A 45-year-old male sustained a fall from height, resulting in a calcaneus fracture. Lateral, axial, and coronal CT slices demonstrate a comminuted, intraarticular calcaneus fracture with a displaced articular posterior facet fragment, loss of height and length, and varus malalignment.

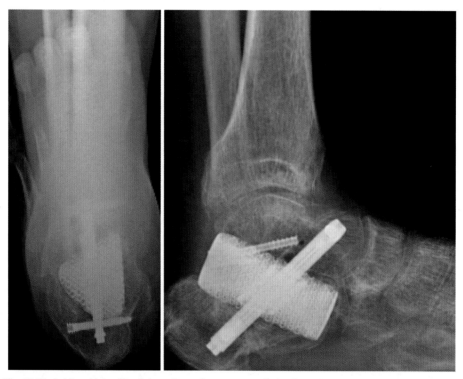

• **Fig. 12.10** Axial and lateral heel views 6 months postoperatively after subtalar distraction arthrodesis with custom 3D-printed implant. Radiographs demonstrate healed fusion site as well as improved hindfoot alignment out of varus, restoration of calcaneal height and length as well as reduced anterior ankle impingement.

TIPS AND TRICKS

Indications	Calcaneal malunion/nonunion with varus alignment and anterior ankle impingement
Goal of reconstruction	Restore heel alignment and height to improve lateral column overload and anterior ankle impingement
Imaging	A preoperative CT scan is necessary for implant planning and assessment of fracture
Labs/work up	It is important to rule out infectious process
Design	We recommend a gyroid, porous architecture with through holes for a planned fixation technique
Implantation	Prepare the joint surface for fusion using standard technique. Use cut guides and implant trials prior to final implant. Insert the final implant after packing with preferred biologic slurry
Fixation	Our fixation preference is with a DynaMini hindfoot nail, which allows for postoperative compression with nitinol technology, as well as a 4.0 mm Medline screw

PEARLS AND PITFALLS

Indications and contraindications	• Calcaneal malunion/nonunion with varus alignment and anterior ankle impingement • Subtalar arthrodesis malunion • Contraindicated in cases of active infection
Implant design	• The implant's porosity and gyroid structure should provide inherent stability and enhance bony ingrowth • Use CT and CAD images to determine the nominal implant size in all planes • The implant is designed with holes for proposed subtalar arthrodesis/implant fixation
Surgical technique	• Posterior approach, Z-lengthen the Achilles tendon • Prepare the subtalar joint • Use bone resection guides and trials to select the appropriate final implant size that will restore the hindfoot alignment and calcaneal height • Fill the prepared joint surface and final implant with biologic slurry • Insert the final implant and fixate into the bone using planned instrumentation

CAD, Computer-aided design.

References

1. Bartoníček J, Rammelt S, Naňka O. Anatomy of the subtalar joint. *Foot Ankle Clin.* 2018;23(3):315-340. doi:10.1016/j.fcl.2018.04.001.

2. Piazza SJ. Mechanics of the subtalar joint and its function during walking. *Foot Ankle Clin.* 2005;10(3):425-442. doi:10.1016/j.fcl.2005.04.001.

3. Espinosa N. The subtalar joint. *Foot Ankle Clin.* 2018;23(3):xi-xii. doi:10.1016/j.fcl.2018.05.001.

4. Sangeorzan A, Sangeorzan B. Subtalar joint biomechanics: from normal to pathologic. *Foot Ankle Clin.* 2018;23(3):341-352. doi:10.1016/j.fcl.2018.04.002.

5. Gotha HE, Zide JR. Current controversies in management of calcaneus fractures. *Orthop Clin North Am.* 2017;48(1):91-103. doi:10.1016/j.ocl.2016.08.005.

6. Myerson M, Quill GE. Late complications of fractures of the calcaneus. *J Bone Joint Surg Am.* 1993;75(3):331-341. doi:10.2106/00004623-199303000-00004.

7. Radnay CS, Clare MP, Sanders RW. Subtalar fusion after displaced intra-articular calcaneal fractures: does initial operative treatment matter? Surgical technique. *J Bone Joint Surg Am.* 2010;92(suppl 1 Part 1):32-43. doi:10.2106/JBJS.I.01267.

8. Schepers T. The subtalar distraction bone block arthrodesis following the late complications of calcaneal fractures: a systematic review. *Foot.* 2013;23(1):39-44. doi:10.1016/j.foot.2012.10.004.

9. Trnka HJ, Easley ME, Lam PW, Anderson CD, Schon LC, Myerson MS. Subtalar distraction bone block arthrodesis. *J Bone Joint Surg Br.* 2001;83(6):849-854. doi:10.1302/0301-620x.83b6.10537.

10. Jackson JB, Jacobson L, Banerjee R, Nickisch F. Distraction subtalar arthrodesis. *Foot Ankle Clin.* 2015;20(2):335-351. doi:10.1016/j.fcl.2015.02.004.

11. Espinosa N, Vacas E. Subtalar distraction arthrodesis. *Foot Ankle Clin.* 2018;23(3):485-498. doi:10.1016/j.fcl.2018.04.008.

12. Woo SH, Goh TS, Ahn TY, You JS, Bae SY, Chung HJ. Subtalar distraction arthrodesis for calcaneal malunion—comparison of structural freeze-dried versus autologous iliac bone graft. *Injury.* 2021;52(4):1048-1053. doi:10.1016/j.injury.2020.12.012.

13. Carr JB, Hansen ST, Benirschke SK. Subtalar distraction bone block fusion for late complications of os calcis fractures. *Foot Ankle.* 1988;9(2):81-86. doi:10.1177/107110078800900204.

14. Rammelt S, Grass R, Zawadski T, Biewener A, Zwipp H. Foot function after subtalar distraction bone-block arthrodesis. A prospective study. *J Bone Joint Surg Br.* 2004;86(5):659-668. doi:10.1302/0301-620X.86B5.

15. Burton DC, Olney BW, Horton GA. Late results of subtalar distraction fusion. *Foot Ankle Int.* 1998;19(4):197-202. doi:10.1177/107110079801900402.

16. Tuijthof GJ, Beimers L, Kerkhoffs GM, Dankelman J, van Dijk CN. Overview of subtalar arthrodesis techniques: options, pitfalls and solutions. *Foot Ankle Surg.* 2010;16(3):107-116. doi:10.1016/j.fas.2009.07.002.

17. Chiang CC, Tzeng YH, Lin CFJ, et al. Subtalar distraction arthrodesis using fresh-frozen allogeneic femoral head augmented with local autograft. *Foot Ankle Int.* 2013;34(4):550-556. doi:10.1177/1071100713481432.

18. Garras DN, Santangelo JR, Wang DW, Easley ME. Subtalar distraction arthrodesis using interpositional frozen structural allograft. *Foot Ankle Int.* 2008;29(6):561-567. doi:10.3113/FAI.2008.0561.

19. Persaud SJ, Catanzariti AR. Subtalar joint distraction arthrodesis utilizing a titanium truss: a case series. *J Foot Ankle Surg.* 2019;58(4):785-791. doi:10.1053/j.jfas.2018.11.022.

20. Papadelis EA, Karampinas PK, Kavroudakis E, Vlamis J, Polizois VD, Pneumaticos SG. Isolated subtalar distraction arthrodesis using porous tantalum. *Foot Ankle Int.* 2015;36(9):1084-1088. doi:10.1177/1071100715581450.

21. Niazi NS, Aljawadi A, Pillai A. Shaped titanium wedges for subtalar distraction arthrodesis: early clinical and radiological results. *Foot.* 2020;42:101647. doi:10.1016/j.foot.2019.10.002.

13

Subtalar Joint Distraction Arthrodesis Utilizing Titanium Truss Technology for Posttraumatic Calcaneal Fracture Arthritis

SHAM J. PERSAUD, ALAN CATANZARITI

Definition

- Posttraumatic subtalar joint distraction arthrodesis utilizing porous titanium wedge spacers in order to restore talar tilt and renew ankle joint range of motion as well as fuse the subtalar joint to treat pain.

Anatomy

- The subtalar joint is a complex triplanar joint consisting of the inferior surface of the talus and the superior surface of the calcaneus.[1]
- There are three articulations between the two tarsal bones that make up the joint—the anterior, middle, and posterior facets.[1]
- Normal positioning of the joint would be considered a rectus vertical position with no signs of either varus or valgus tilt. Traditional literature states the normal position would include a complete neutral position with allowable deformity to up to 5 degrees of hindfoot valgus.[1]
- Calcaneal fractures generally lead to deformity and malposition of the subtalar joint. Deformity seen with calcaneal fractures is a result of both primary and secondary fracture lines.[2]
- In general, the calcaneus is shortened and flattened with varus malalignment after severe calcaneal fractures. This is demonstrated radiographically by a decrease in Bohler's angle, an increase in Gissane's angle, and a horizontal position of the talus with a decreased talar declination angle on lateral radiographs.[2-8]
- This varus position of the subtalar joint also leads to impingement of the talar neck to the tibia with ankle

joint dorsiflexion secondary to varus position of the talus, including minimal-to-negative talar declination angle (Fig. 13.1).[3,9,10]
- Unless these deformities are corrected, they will ultimately lead to posttraumatic arthritis of the subtalar joint, anterior ankle impingement, and structural equinus.[1]

Pathogenesis

- Varus malalignment of the subtalar joint may be secondary to:
  - Genetic hindfoot varus deformity
  - Acquired hindfoot varus deformity
  - Intra-articular, depression calcaneal fractures/trauma
  - Malunion of previous subtalar joint arthrodesis.
- Genetic varus deformity is generally secondary to a group of inherited disorders that cause peroneal nerve injury. These generally fall into a category of disorders under the term Charcot-Marie-Tooth (CMT) disease. Although there are other disorders, CMT is generally the most common.
- Acquired hindfoot varus deformity develops via one of two routes. Injury of the superficial peroneal nerve or injury to the peroneal tendons. This imbalance within the foot generally leads to overpowering of the tibialis posterior tendon, which leads to hindfoot varus.
- As stated above, intraarticular depression calcaneal fractures generally lead to varus malalignment of the hindfoot.
- Primary subtalar joint arthrodesis, if not carefully evaluated, may lead to varus malunion and hindfoot deformity, leading to similar difficulties.[11]

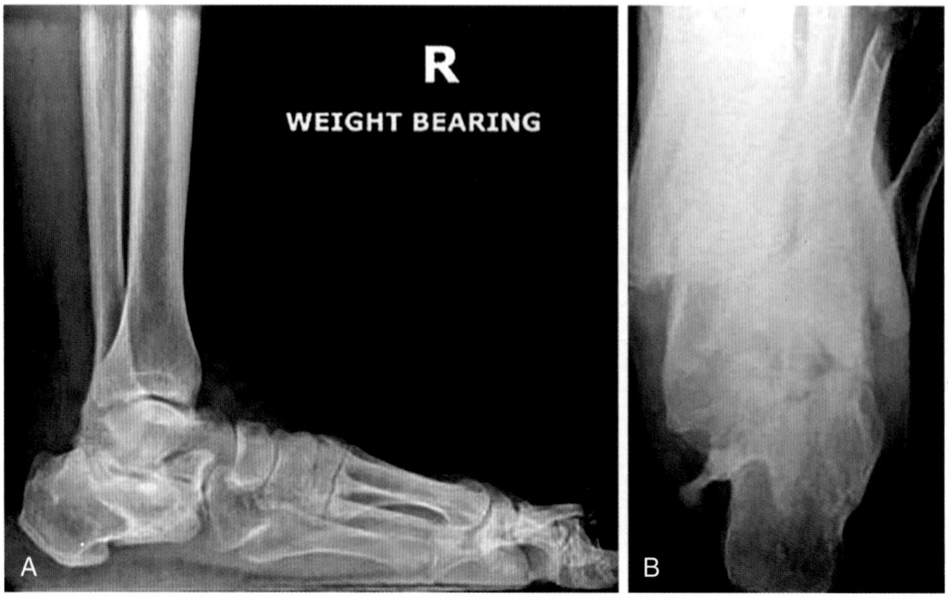

• **Fig. 13.1** Preoperative radiographs showing varus deformity secondary to intraarticular calcaneal fracture. (A) Lateral foot radiograph. (B) Calcaneal axial radiograph.

Patient History and Physical Findings

- Localized/diffuse pain throughout the subtalar joint and anterior ankle joint.
- Limited and painful range of motion of the subtalar joint.
- Pain with a hard stop with ankle dorsiflexion (structural equinus).
- Pain and weakness of the peroneal tendons.
- Lateral ankle instability with possible laxity and pain with anterior drawer and inversion stress test.
- Hindfoot varus position in a neutral stance. Deformity may be reducible or not. Generally, a Coleman block test shows a hindfoot origin of deformity.
- Difficulty with weight-bearing activities including walking.
- Neurovascular compromise with peroneal nerve testing (common and superficial peroneal nerves).[11]

Imaging and Other Diagnostic Testing

- Radiographs:
  - On lateral view, a nontraumatic patient will show a bullet hole sinus tarsi sign, increased calcaneal inclination greater than 25 degrees, an increased talar-1st metatarsal angle greater than 5 degrees, and Hibb's angle greater than 45 degrees.[11]
  - Lateral view in traumatic patients will identify the above along with a decrease in Bohler's angle (less than 30 degrees and an increase in critical angle of Gissane greater than 130 degrees).[11]
  - Most important for this procedure is whether the talus position has a decreased to negative talar declination angle less than 25 degrees and a tibiotalar angle greater than 105 degrees.[11]

- Calcaneal axial views are also recommended in order to identify the amount of varus deformity of the subtalar joint. Normal values should be neutral to no more than 5° of valgus. This will prepare the surgeon as to how much varus needs to be addressed during the joint-preparation portion of the procedure.[1]
- With standard radiographs evaluation for ankle varus should be performed and evaluation for metatarsus adductus should also be evaluated.
- Advanced imaging (MRI):
  - MRI is useful for evaluating the soft tissue injury, which can occur with varus deformity of the hindfoot or which can act as the initial injury to progress to varus deformity (Fig. 13.2).
  - Structures to evaluate carefully would include the peroneal tendons and retinaculum, the anterior talofibular ligaments, the calcaneal fibular ligament, and the posterior talofibular ligament.
  - Other structures to evaluate would be the subtalar and ankle joint for signs of degeneration, avascular necrosis, and inflammation.
  - Although fusion of the subtalar joint does limit varus and valgus rotation of the hindfoot, repair of the soft tissues should always be considered for long-term protection of the ankle joint.
- Other testing:
  - Electromyography and nerve conduction–velocity studies should be considered for patients with neurological compromise concerns.
  - Noninvasive vascular studies should be considered for patients with a poor vascular exam and patients with a smoking history.
  - Genetic testing should be considered for patients with genetically caused cavus foot concerns.

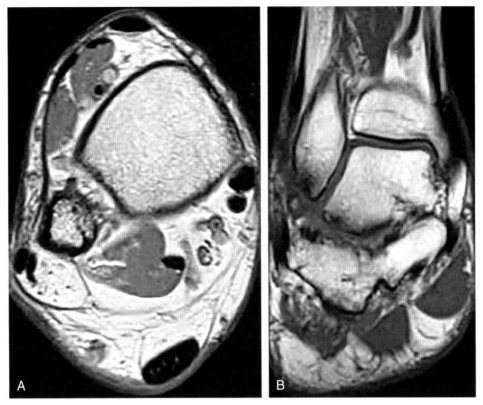

• **Fig. 13.2** Preoperative MRI showing peroneal tendon pathology with subluxation, and subtalar joint degeneration. (A) Axial T1 MRI view. (B) Coronal T1 MRI view.

• Vitamin D testing should be done to optimize patient healing before, during, and after the procedure. Patients with low vitamin D levels are generally supplemented with vitamin D 50,000 IU per week or 5000 IU per day throughout preoperative and postoperative periods.
• Cotinine/nicotine testing.

Nonoperative Management

• Ankle foot orthosis (AFO) bracing including Richie, Arizona, and custom posterior leaf AFO.
• Orthotic treatment for mild deformity with minimal ankle symptoms. May consider a University of California Berkeley Laboratories (UCBL) device for more hindfoot deformity control.
• Immobilization.
• Rest, ice, compression, elevation (RICE) therapy and nonsteroidal antiinflammatory drugs.
• Oral steroid packs or subtalar and ankle joint steroid injections.

Traditional Surgical Management: Concerns and Disadvantages

• The use of structural autografts and allograft wedges for subtalar joint distraction arthrodesis has traditionally been used for this specific procedure.

• Structural autografts from the iliac crest have been the gold standard for reestablishing talar declination in subtalar joint distraction arthrodesis.[12-18]
• Unfortunately, autografts are associated with an up to 41% risk of donor site morbidity, large hematomas in 9.6% of patients, and wound dehiscence at the donor site in 2.7% of patients.[12-18]
• Autografts have also been associated with elongated hospital stay, limited quantity and size options, and poor-quality grafts in patients with poor protoplasm.[12-18]
• In order to combat donor site complications, allografts, particularly frozen femoral head allografts, have also been discussed at length within the literature as an acceptable alternative to using autografts for subtalar joint distraction arthrodesis.
• Although allograft use does limit the donor site morbidity seen with autograft use, both have been associated with graft collapse and a relatively high nonunion rate over the long term. This is secondary to the structural graft's inability to withstand the excessive forces from axial loading.[17,18]
• Allograft use also carries the risk of disease transmission; however, the incidence of this occurring is exceptionally low.[15]
• In situ fusion has also been used as an option. Unfortunately for these patients, this generally leads to significant ankle pathology over time.[16]

Titanium Truss Design Specifications and Considerations

- An alternative to structural bone grafts is the use of structural titanium trusses. These implants inherently prevent the donor site morbidity associated with autografts, as well as the collapse and failure seen with structural bone grafts in general.
- Titanium has shown to be osteoconductive, with minimal bioactivity of concern for an allergic response.
- The porous nature of the graft also allows the surgeon to make the osteoconductive titanium also become osteogenic and osteoinductive with the addition of orthobiologics within the porous structures.
- The authors generally use a wedge-shaped truss design that allows for an increased talar declination position with fixation.
- The authors use a company with multiple truss widths and heights, which come standard along with multiple sizers in order to identify the most optimal implant for each patient.
- Although custom-designed implants can be used with the creation of holes for fixation, the authors have found an excellent construct that allows for cost savings and adequate fixation and compression at the fusion sites.
- Truss size and shape is decided with the use of joint distraction along with fluoroscopy evaluation.
- Titanium trusses, cages, and trabecular porous wedges have been discussed throughout the literature as successful means to bridge bony deficits. Reports in the orthopedic literature have shown successful use with bridging large bony defects for hip and knee arthroplasties, spinal fusions, cranioplasty plates, and pacemaker electrodes.[19-22]
- The use of titanium trusses within foot and ankle surgery is relatively new, with the earliest literature ranging from 2004 by Bouchard et al.[15] to recent studies by Coriaty et al.[23] and So et al. in 2018.[24] All of the studies have shown excellent bony ingrowth with long-term stability.[15,25-27]

Surgical Management With a Titanium Truss for Subtalar Joint Distraction Arthrodesis

- Surgical implants and instruments recommended:
  - A podiatry tray with a smooth lamina spreader. The authors recommend having a Cobb elevator and pituitary rongeur to help with joint preparation.
  - Straight and curved osteotomes and curettes for joint preparation.
  - A drill with a 2.5-mm drill bit for joint subchondral drilling.
  - A bone marrow aspiration (BMA) and bone harvester kit. The authors recommend either demineralized bone matrix (DBM) or allograft/autograft through a bone mill if available.
  - 4.5-mm to 7.0-mm cannular short thread compression screws of choice.
  - A wedge truss set.
- Positioning: lateral decubitus position with a thigh tourniquet and adequate padding and protection for the patient.
- Anesthesia: general anesthesia.
- Approach: a curvilinear incision is made along the posterior medial aspect of the fibula extending distally toward the distal tip of the lateral malleolus of the right lower extremity.
- Technique:
  - Dissection is carried down to the level of the calcaneus and subtalar joint. Any spurring noted within the local area and synovitis was removed with a combination of instruments.
  - With the use of fluoroscopy, the subtalar joint is identified and the joint is mobilized.
  - Once mobilized, a lamina spreader is used to distract the joint for cartilage removal and preparation. All articular cartilage is removed from the subtalar joint with the use of osteotomes and curettes.
  - After removal of the articular cartilage, the joint is further prepared using both subchondral drilling and fishscaling techniques until a healthy cancellous substrate is developed.
  - The subtalar joint is then posteriorly distracted using a smooth lamina spreader under lateral fluoroscopy (Fig. 13.3).
  - The joint is distracted until all deformity is accounted for, including reduction of calcaneal inclination angle, talar declination angle, and Bohler's and Gissane's angles.

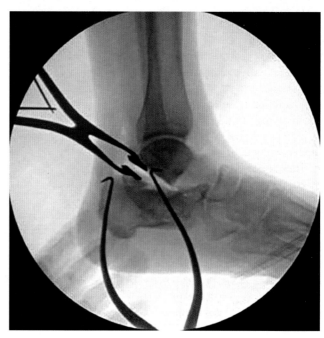

• **Fig. 13.3** Distraction of the subtalar joint to normal angles.

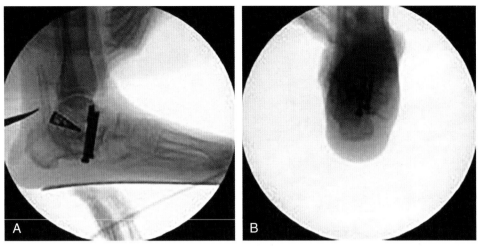

• **Fig. 13.4** Insertion of a truss with fixation. (A) Lateral and (B) axial views.

- Trial sizers for the titanium truss are then inserted into the subtalar joint until the most optimal size is identified. Although each patient is different, the authors have found that a 12-mm medium-sized truss is generally the optimal size for reduction of deformity.
- Once a size is chosen, the truss is opened and augmented by packing the porous trust with bone marrow aspirate, bone graft, and/or orthobiologic of choice.
- Once optimized per the surgeon's preference, the truss is then inserted into the posterior facet of the subtalar joint. Adequate positioning is confirmed via fluoroscopy using multiple views.
- Once adequate positioning is confirmed, the subtalar joint is then fixed using two partially threaded cannulated compression screws per the surgeon's choice. Both screws are delivered anterior to the truss, extending into the neck and body of the talus (Fig. 13.4).
- Other adjunctive procedures may include but are not limited to peroneal tendon repair, ankle arthrotomy with synovectomy/ankle arthroscopy, and lateral ankle ligament repair.

Postoperative Protocol

- The patient is generally placed in a posterior splint with a Jackson-Pratt (JP) drain if needed. The patient is generally kept for 23 hours observation in order to monitor drain output, undergo physical therapy assessment, and control pain.
- If drain output is minimal and the patient's pain is managed well, the patient is then transferred into a short leg cast upon discharge and sent home with non–weight-bearing status with the use of an assistive device.
- The patient remains non-weight bearing and in a short leg cast for 8 to 12 weeks pending radiographic incorporation of the truss within the subtalar joint. This is confirmed

with a CT scan prior to progression to assisted weight bearing.
- The patient is then transferred into a controlled angle motion (CAM) walking boot for progression to full weight bearing. This generally requires the patient to be in the CAM boot for 2 to 4 weeks.
- The patient is transferred to full weight bearing with an ankle-stabilizing orthosis (ASO) brace in regular shoe gear. The patient may remain in the brace until they feel comfortable to walk without it. Usually this takes another 4 weeks.
- Physical therapy is used as needed.

Results/Outcomes

- The authors have been successful in addressing posttraumatic subtalar joint arthritis following calcaneal fracture with subtalar joint distraction arthrodesis using the titanium truss technique.
- This technique has been successful in all patients to date. The authors believe that a combination of pre- and postoperative patient optimization along with joint preparation and fusion position has led us to their success.
- The most difficult portion of the procedure is the surgical approach. The posterior approach to the subtalar joint can be difficult at times, especially when identifying it from the ankle joint. It is highly recommended that fluoroscopy be used as a tool to aid in finding the subtalar joint from this posterolateral approach.
- The authors also recommend confirmation of bony ingrowth with the use of a CT scan as it is difficult to truly assess ingrowth based on radiographs. A CT scan at 12 weeks generally shows successful union (Fig. 13.5).
- Our results have shown a biomechanical reduction in deformity with improved patient pain and function (Tables 13.1 and 13.2).

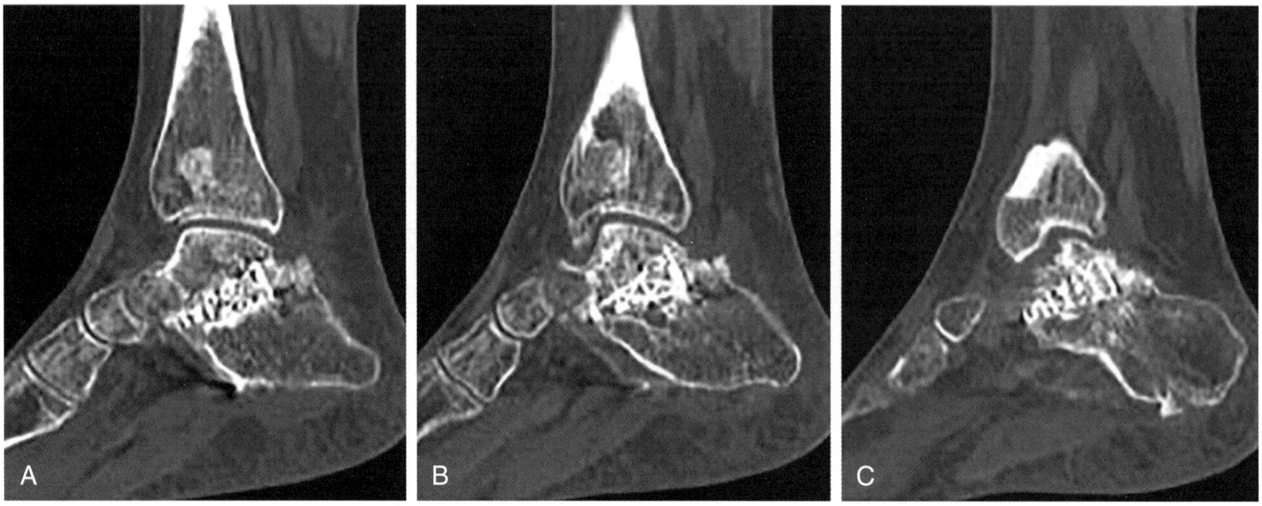

• **Fig. 13.5** Postoperative CT scan revealing the incorporation of bony ingrowth into the titanium truss (A–C) lateral to medial.

TABLE 13.1	Comparison of Preoperative and Postoperative Sagittal Plane Angles in Patient 1	
Angle Measured	Preoperative Angle (Degrees)	Postoperative Angle (Degrees)
Calcaneal inclination angle	13.6	17.5
Talar declination angle lateral	6.5	15.7
Talocalcaneal angle	18.4	33.5
Angle of Gissane	136.4	123.9
Bohler's angle	12.4	29.3

TABLE 13.2	Comparison of Preoperative and Postoperative Sagittal Plane Angles in Patient 2	
Angle Measured	Preoperative Angle (Degrees)	Postoperative Angle (Degrees)
Calcaneal inclination angle	26.12	26.57
Talar declination angle lateral	8.45	18.67
Talocalcaneal angle	29.97	46.31
Angle of Gissane	138.74	130.47
Bohler's angle	27.5	35.38

PEARLS AND PITFALLS

Indications and contraindications	• Posttraumatic or primary STJ arthritis with varus deformity, especially lack of talar declination • Contraindicated in cases of active infection • Use prudence in patients with a history of deep infection
Implant design	• Titanium appears to be the ideal material • Implant shape and porosity should provide inherent stability and enhance bony ingrowth • Use fluoroscopy and trial sizes to determine the optimum implant size • Screw holes for direct fixation are not necessary as anterior STJ fixation has been shown to work well • Positioning and deformity reduction is the key to success
Surgical technique	• Ensure all of the cartilage and subchondral plate is removed • A Cobb elevator and pituitary rongeur are great tools for identifying, mobilizing, and prepping the STJ • Use joint preparation to help reduce any frontal plane deformity noted • The ideal implant size yields physiologic tension of the adjacent soft tissues, inherent stability, and provides normal talocalcaneal angles

STJ, Subtalar joint.

Previously Published Results

- Persaud SJ, Catanzariti AR. Subtalar joint distraction arthrodesis utilizing a titanium truss: a case series. *J. Foot Ankle Surg.* 2019; 58(4): 785-791.
  - Two patient case series for subtalar joint distraction arthrodesis using trusses.
  - Minimum 1 year follow-up.
  - Both patients had successful unions with deformity correction.
  - All patients had CT confirmation of union at 12 weeks.

Possible Complications

- Nonunion
- Malunion
- Infection
- Hardware failure
- Ankle joint deformity or arthritis
- Loss of limb

TIPS AND TRICKS

Indications	Varus hindfoot alignment with STJ arthritis
	Anterior ankle pain/impingement
	Pain
Goal of reconstruction	Restore length and alignment
	Pain relief
	Improve function
Imaging	Preoperative MRI is necessary for implant planning and assessment of soft tissue injury
Labs/work up	Important to rule out a neurologic cause if not traumatic
	Vitamin D
	Vascular status
	Nicotine/cotinine
	Optimize the patient for optimal results
Design	The authors recommend a wedge-shaped implant with a minimal need for customization. Can truly dial in correction with intraoperative sizing and achieve great fixation with anterior screw placement
Implantation	The authors recommend using a 12 medium implant for most cases; however, each patient is unique. The authors optimize the implant with the addition of BMA, orthobiologics, and bone graft
Fixation	The authors recommend two screws anterior to the truss in order to provide compression with rotational stability

BMA, Bone marrow aspiration; *STJ*, subtalar joint.

References

1. Hentges MJ, Gesheff MG, Lamm BM. Realignment subtalar joint arthrodesis. *J Foot Ankle Surg.* 2016;55(1):16-21.
2. Bohler L. Diagnosis, pathology, and treatment of fractures of the os calcis. *J Bone Joint Surg Am.* 1931;13:75-89.
3. Jackson JB III, Jacobson L, Banerjee R, Nickisch F. Distraction subtalar arthrodesis. *Foot Ankle Clin.* 2015;20:335-351.
4. Gissane W. Discussion on "fractures of the os calcis." Proceedings of the British Orthopedic Association. *J Bone Joint Surg.* 1947; 29:254-255.
5. Rammelt S, Grass R, Zawadski T, Biewener A, Zwipp H. Foot function after subtalar distraction bone-block arthrodesis. A prospective study. *J Bone Joint Surg Br.* 2004;86:659-668.
6. Toussaint RJ, Lin D, Ehrlichman LK, Ellington JK, Strasser N, Kwon JY. Peroneal tendon displacement accompanying intra-articular calcaneal fractures. *J Bone Joint Surg Am.* 2014;96:310-315.
7. Isbister JF. Calcaneo-fibular abutment following crush fracture of the calcaneus. *J Bone Joint Surg Br.* 1974;56:274-278.
8. Rosenberg ZS, Feldman F, Singson RD, Price GJ. Peroneal tendon injury associated with calcaneal fractures: CT findings. *AJR Am J Roentgenol.* 1987;149:125-129.
9. Kitaoka HB, Schaap EJ, Chao EY, An KN. Displaced intra-articular fractures of the calcaneus treated non-operatively. Clinical results and analysis of motion and ground-reaction and temporal forces. *J Bone Joint Surg Am.* 1994;76:1531-1540.
10. Romash MM. Reconstructive osteotomy of the calcaneus with subtalar arthrodesis for malunited calcaneal fractures. *Clin Orthop Relat Res.* 1993;(290):157-167.
11. Maynou C, Szymanski C, Thiounn A. The adult cavus foot. *EFORT Open Rev.* 2017;2(5):221-229.
12. Papadelis EA, Karampinas PK, Kavroudakis E, Vlamis J, Polizois VD, Pneumaticos SG. Isolated subtalar distraction arthrodesis using porous tantalum: a pilot study. *Foot Ankle Int.* 2015;36: 1084-1088.
13. Sasso RC, LeHuec JC, Shaffrey C, Spine Interbody Research Group. Iliac crest bone graft donor site pain after anterior lumbar interbody fusion: a prospective patient satisfaction outcome assessment. *J Spinal Disord Tech.* 2005;18(suppl):S77-S81.
14. Niedhart C, Pingsmann A, Jürgens C, Marr A, Blatt R, Niethard FU. [Complications after harvesting of autologous bone from the ventral and dorsal iliac crest—a prospective, controlled study]. *Z Orthop Ihre Grenzgeb.* 2003;141:481-486.
15. Bouchard M, Barker LG, Claridge RJ. Technique tip: tantalum: a structural bone graft option for foot and ankle surgery. *Foot Ankle Int.* 2004;25:39-42.
16. Flemister AS Jr, Infante AF, Sanders RW, Walling AK. Subtalar arthrodesis for complications of intra-articular calcaneal fractures. *Foot Ankle Int.* 2000;21:392-399.
17. Egol KA. Bone grafting: sourcing, timing, strategies and alternatives. *J Orthop Trauma.* 2015;29:12.
18. Panchbhavi VK. Synthetic bone grafting in foot and ankle surgery. *Foot Ankle Clin.* 2010;15:559-576.
19. Flecher X, Paprosky W, Grillo JC, Aubaniac JM, Argenson JN. Do tantalum components provide adequate primary fixation in all acetabular revisions? *Orthop Traumatol Surg Res.* 2010;96: 235-241.
20. Kim WY, Greidanus NV, Duncan CP, Masri BA, Garbuz DS. Porous tantalum uncemented acetabular shells in revision total hip replacement: two to four year clinical and radiographic results. *Hip Int.* 2008;18:17-22.

21. Levine BR, Sporer S, Poggie RA, Della Valle CJ, Jacobs JJ. Experimental and clinical performance of porous tantalum in orthopedic surgery. *Biomaterials*. 2006;27:4671-4681.

22. Meneghini RM, Lewallen DG, Hanssen AD. Use of porous tantalum metaphyseal cones for severe tibial bone loss during revision total knee replacement. *J Bone Joint Surg Am*. 2008;90: 78-84.

23. Coriaty N, Pettibone K, Todd N, Rush S, Carter R, Zdenek C. Titanium scaffolding: an innovative modality for salvage of failed first ray procedures. *J Foot Ankle Surg*. 2018;57(3):593-599.

24. So E, Mandas VH, Hlad L. Large osseous defect reconstruction using a custom three dimensional printed titanium truss implant. *J Foot Ankle Surg*. 2018;57:196-204.

25. Mulhern JL, Protzman NM, White AM, Brigido SA. Salvage of failed total ankle replacement using a custom titanium truss. *J Foot Ankle Surg*. 2016;55:868-873.

26. Hamid KS, Parekh SG, Adams SB. Salvage of severe foot and ankle trauma with a 3D printed scaffold. *Foot Ankle Int*. 2016;37:433-439.

27. Sagherian BH, Claridge RJ. Porous tantalum as a structural graft in foot and ankle surgery. *Foot Ankle Int*. 2012;33:179-189.

14

Treatment of Navicular Avascular Necrosis in the Sensate Patient

PETER D. HIGHLANDER, AMAR R. GULATI, LANCE JOHNSON

Definition

- Utilizing patient-specific custom 3D-printed metallic navicular cages for the treatment of chronic navicular pathology in sensate patients without Charcot neuroarthropathy.

Anatomy and Biomechanics

- The navicular is an irregular-shaped tarsal bone which has a concave surface that articulates with the talus and a convex surface that articulates with the cuneiforms.
- There are ligamentous and capsular attachments on all four sides of the navicular, while there is a solitary tendon attachment. The posterior tibial tendon attaches to the navicular tuberosity and acts as a dynamic stabilizer of the rearfoot during pronation while providing supination during push-off or propulsion.[1-3]
- The navicular is a vital part of the medial column, which also includes the 1st metatarsal, medial cuneiform, and the talus. These bones and corresponding articulations are important for maintaining foot structure and function.[4] It is essential for the medial column to operate as a rigid lever for normal biomechanical function during propulsion.
- The alignment of the medial column radiographically is assessed on:
  - Lateral projections via Meary's angle, which may be defined as normal where the axis between the midline of the talus and 1st metatarsal is 0 degrees. Abnormal values may be considered when the axis is >4 degrees.[5] Increased angles downward may be described as medial column sag, which infers inability of the medial column to act as a rigid lever during propulsion.
  - Anteroposterior (AP) projections via talar-navicular coverage, which compares the articular surface of the talar head and that of the proximal navicular. An axis

of >7 degrees is considered abnormal and consistent with transverse plane deformity that occurs in pes planus.[5]
- Vascular supply to the navicular primarily comes from the dorsalis pedis artery, which supplies dorsal arterial supply via three to five terminal perforators, and the medial plantar artery, which provides plantar vascularization. Abundant vascular supply from these two networks is supplied predominantly to the medial and lateral superficial of the navicular. The navicular however lacks substantial vascular supply to the deep and central portions. This anatomic discrepancy leads to higher risk of stress fracture and avascular necrosis (AVN) within the central navicular.[6]
- Nervous innervation is provided from the medial plantar and deep peroneal nerves.[7]

Pathogenesis

- An array of etiologies exists for navicular pathology which include AVN, acute fractures, and stress fractures, all of which have a poor prognosis.[8]
- Köhler disease, a rare idiopathic AVN of the navicular, most commonly occurs in children aged 4 to 7 years. The poor blood supply to the central third of the talus paired with the increasing weight of the child is thought to increase the chance of Köhler disease. Fortunately, the process is self-limiting and surgical intervention is rarely necessary.[9]
- Mueller-Weiss syndrome is also a spontaneous, idiopathic form of navicular AVN; however, it occurs in adults most commonly between the fifth and seventh decade of life. Theories regarding the development of Mueller-Weiss syndrome include congenital etiologies and chronic microtrauma secondary to poor biomechanics, which lead to overload of the lateral third of the

navicular which tends to be less ossified.[10] Radiographically, the lateral collapse of the navicular appears as a comma-shaped navicular.[11]

- Navicular stress fractures compromise 10% to 35% of all stress fractures and are most commonly seen in young, active individuals.[12-14]
- Regardless of etiology, AVN is secondary to disruption of the vascular supply to the navicular.
- The progression of AVN, regardless of etiology, can be monitored radiographically. Ficat and Arlet classified femoral head AVN,[15] and later Mont et al.[16] modified the classification for the talus. Despite no classification specific for navicular AVN, descriptions are often similar to other bones.
- Medial column shortening, transverse forefoot deformity, and loss of arch height may be observed in late-stage navicular AVN due to progressive collapse of the navicular.[17-19]

Patient History and Physical Exam Findings

- Navicular pathology is associated with pain and swelling due to a localized inflammatory process.
- Dysfunction and pain are worse with activity.
- Vague midfoot pain, often with normal subtalar and ankle range of motion, is observed.
- Navicular fractures may occur secondary to a known acute injury, whereas chronic overuse with high functional demands often presents with navicular stress fractures.
- Deformity of the forefoot, midfoot, and hindfoot occurs in late-stage navicular AVN (Fig. 14.1).

Imaging and Other Diagnostic Testing

- There are four types of navicular fractures: cortical avulsion, tuberosity avulsion, body, and stress fractures. Sangeorzan et al.[20] classified acute navicular fractures based on orientation of the fracture line, adjacent joint involvement, and the presence of foot deformity.
- Stress fractures most often occur in the central third of the navicular body. If a high index of suspicion for navicular stress fracture exists despite unremarkable initial X-rays, then consideration is given to MRI or CT evaluation.
- Navicular AVN progression (Fig. 14.2):
  - Initially plain radiographs may appear normal but alterations are visible on MRI, thus MRI remains the most reliable diagnostic test for stage 1 AVN.
  - Osteosclerotic and cystic changes without navicular collapse are observed at stage 2. Often contralateral views can be helpful to determine if early collapse is present.
  - Subchondral lucency may be indicative of subchondral collapse, which is characteristic of stage 3 AVN. During this stage the adjacent joints are spared and subtle deformity may be present.

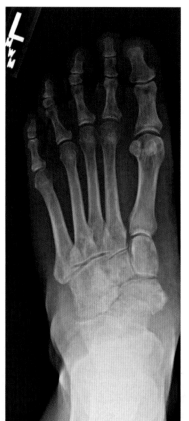
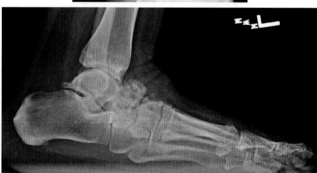

• **Fig. 14.1** Anteroposterior (AP) and lateral radiographs of a patient with late-stage avascular necrosis with resultant deformity in the transverse and sagittal planes.

- Stage 4 characteristically displays collapse, deformity of the forefoot with or without hindfoot involvement, and adjacent joint degeneration.
- For surgical planning purposes, the authors recommend CT and MRI evaluation to determine the extent of AVN.
- If there is a possibility of infection, further work-up may include laboratory assessment, including inflammatory markers and bone biopsy.
- If a previous procedure resulted in a nonunion, then further work-up should be considered and possible systemic causes such as osteoporosis and endocrine etiologies may need to be assessed. The patient should be optimized appropriately. This may include smoking cessation and nutritional optimization.

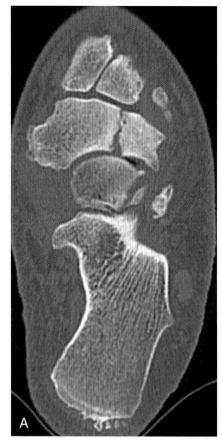

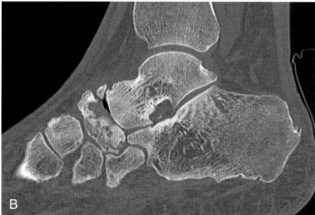

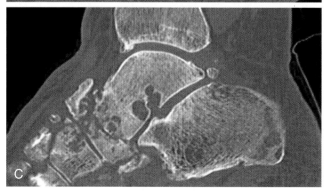

• **Fig. 14.2** The progression of navicular avascular necrosis on CT images. (A) Osteosclerotic changes without collapse is indicative of stage 2. (B) Subchondral lucency and early collapse is noted in stage 3. (C) Significant collapse with adjacent joint changes is evident in stage 4. Stage 1 may appear normal on radiographs and CT.

- Noninvasive vascular studies are recommended for primary and revision cases. Pending results, the patient may benefit from further endovascular optimization.

Nonoperative Management

- Nondisplaced acute or stress fractures are often initially treated nonsurgically; however, considerable debate remains due to a high risk of nonunion, refracture, and AVN.[8]
- Nonoperative management may be successful in early-stage AVN. This may involve immobilization with a period of non-weight bearing followed by protective weight bearing with noninvasive bone stimulation and/or extracorporeal shockwave therapy.[21]
- Close follow-up with serial imaging is recommended.
- In the authors' experience, nonoperative management tends to be less successful with symptomatic late-stage AVN, especially in younger and physically active patients.
- Only low-level evidence exists for operative and nonoperative management of AVN in the foot and ankle.[21]

Traditional Surgical Management

- When nonoperative treatment fails to improve symptoms or there is continued progression of AVN, operative treatment may be considered.
- Operative intervention for nondisplaced fractures has been shown to lower rates of delayed union, nonunion, and AVN; however, potential risks and complications are possible.[20,22]
- Core decompression may be considered for early-stage (without collapse) navicular AVN; however, poor efficacy due to the tenuous blood supply may exist.[23]
- Vascularized bone grafting for several donor sites has been described with some success; however, this may be limited to early-stage AVN if preservation of joint function is desired. If arthritis is present, fusion should be strongly considered.[24-26]
- When fusion is indicated, necrotic bone must be thoroughly debrided, which may be approximated on CT and MRI. In the authors' experience this leads to a considerable osseous deficit, in which case in situ fusion (talar-cuneiform) is a poor option, as this would lead to considerable deformity.
- Prior to the advent of 3D printing, the authors would employ bridge plating with bone grafting to the medial column to preserve length. Often the osseous deficit being grafted is >2 to 3 cm, therefore the concern for nonunion is high and these cases remain at high risk for failure and need for multiple surgeries.

3D-Printed Implant Considerations

- In the United States, titanium (Ti) alloys and cobalt chromium (CoCr) are currently the ideal biocompatible materials for 3D printing. Typically, CoCr is used when the implant articulates with native cartilage or polyethylene components used in joint replacement. Ti has a higher coefficient of friction, therefore making it inferior to CoCr for articular components.[27-29]

- When osseous integration into the implant is desired such as during an arthrodesis procedure, Ti tends to be used more often. Research continues to explain osseous integration abilities of CoCr compared to Ti.[27-29]

- A major limitation in the use of CoCr implants is the lack of complementary fixation methods and mixing different types of metals is to be avoided. That is, screws, plates, and intramedullary fixation is not available in CoCr. On the contrary, Ti fixation is widely available, therefore if supplemental fixation is necessary then Ti 3D-printed implants are preferred.

- If corrective osteotomies are planned, the surgeon may consider using a patient-specific cut guide to improve accuracy and reduce surgical time.

- Basic implant design considerations:
  - If osseous integration is desired, the authors recommend porous Ti implants to preserve the length and alignment of the medial column while promoting biologic stability through the bony ingrowth into the implant.
  - Ti implants with a rough-surface finish provide additional advantages. The rough surface increases friction at the bone-implant interface, thus making the implant more stable.

- Ideal porosity has yet to be determined. Ultimately, the porosity should provide a network of structural strength and permit the packing and retention of the bone graft or biologics of choice (Fig. 14.3).

- The implant should be smooth and polished to decrease friction where the implant is to articulate with native, adjacent joint cartilage. Although CoCr would be preferable at the articulation, there is no CoCr off-the-shelf fixation available. This may represent an area of future advancement (Fig. 14.4).

- The implant shape is patient specific and should replicate the osseous deficit created after aggressive bone debridement.

- Sizing options should mimic the minimum and maximum amount of bone to be excised. In the authors' experience, for navicular AVN the implant will vary based on proximal to distal length alone. In other words, the medial-to-lateral width remains constant while the implant length may vary based on osseous resection and resultant deficit as well as adjunctive procedures. Medial column length, in absolute measurement as well as compared to lateral column length, may be determined based on contralateral CT scans preoperatively (Fig. 14.5).

- The authors recommend requesting a minimum of three sizes to ensure ideal fit and alignment restoration.

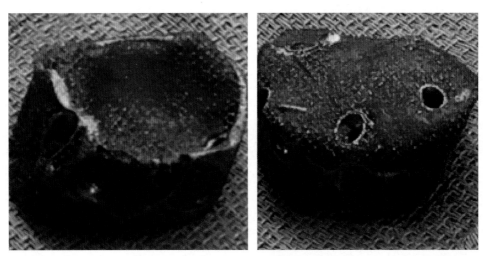

• **Fig. 14.3** 3D-printed titanium implant designed for medial column fusion which is packed with bone graft and biologics. The porosity allows for bone graft retention and osseous integration. This implant was designed to be fixated with multiple 3.5-mm screws.

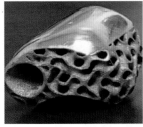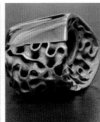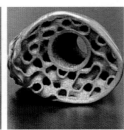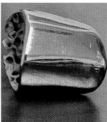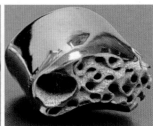

• **Fig. 14.4** 3D-printed titanium navicular implant with porous areas with surface roughness in locations of desired osseous integration, while smooth areas are close in proximity to soft tissues that could be affected by the implant. This implant has a 9-mm hole to accommodate a midfoot beam.

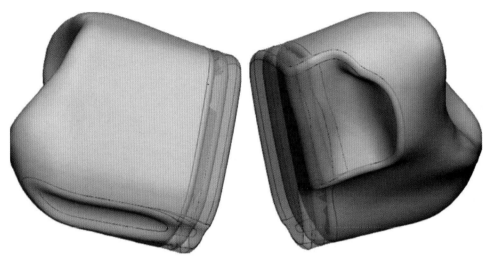

• **Fig. 14.5** Computer-aided design images depicting three sizes of a navicular implant. This implant's width (medial to lateral) remains constant while it varies in length (anterior to posterior). (Reprinted with permission from restor3d, Inc, Durham, NC.)

- Further implant specifications may be dependent on the osseous involvement and adjacent joint arthritis. In the authors' experience, the need for 3D-printed navicular implants most often presents in one of three patterns. The basic implant design and procedure selection is often dictated on the pattern of pathology (Table 14.1).
- Pattern 1: An osseous deficit limited to the navicular without degeneration to the talar head with or without cuneiform degeneration:
  - This situation may be seen in Ficat/Mont stage 2 or 3 navicular AVN.
  - Implant design features include a smooth, concave surface of the proximal navicular, which articulates with the talar head and porous distal surface to promote osseous integration from the cuneiforms.
  - Fixation may include holes within the implant body as well as flanges to allow passage of screws into the cuneiforms. Osseous integration serves to stabilize the implant but is inherently limited to one surface, therefore the soft tissues are vital to implant stability.
  - Attachment of the posterior tibial tendon to the implant is vital for function. Adams and Danilkowicz[8] recommended a tunnel within the implant from the medial aspect to the dorsal aspect of the implant to allow passage of the posterior tibial tendon, which can be anchored to the cuneiforms. Additional eyelets can be incorporated into the implant to allow attachment of adjacent ligaments and capsular tissue. The footprint of the ligaments may be roughened to promote soft tissue ingrowth and scar formation.
- Pattern 2: An osseous deficit limited to the navicular with degeneration of the talar head and cuneiforms:
  - This situation may be seen with stage 4 navicular AVN, nonunion of navicular fracture, nonunion of previous talonavicular joint (TNJ) fusion, or osteomyelitis limited to the navicular.

- The navicular implant is designed to recreate medial column length and alignment. Unlike Pattern 1 implants, soft tissue attachments are much less important given the much larger surface area available for osseous integration.
- Porosity for osseous integration should be designed on all surfaces except where scar contracture and vital soft tissues are adjacent to the implant.
- Obtaining adequate fixation in the talus can be challenging but is paramount to providing stability of the overall construct. The surgeon should consider intramedullary beams or external fixation for Pattern 2 implants.
- From the authors' experience, spanning the entire medial column from talus to 1st metatarsal is preferable, even in sensate patients. Attempts to preserve the first tarsometatarsal joint have led to inadequate fixation, hardware breakage, and the need for revision.
- Pattern 3: Osseous deficit involving multiple bones including the navicular with adjacent joint arthritis:
  - This situation may be seen subsequent to severe rearfoot/ankle trauma, nonunion of previous fusions, AVN, and osteomyelitis involving multiple rearfoot/ankle bones.
  - Pattern 3 cases may require vastly more bone debridement and excision, which may be staged especially if the pathology is secondary to chronic infection.
  - The implant size and shape should reflect the deficient created. These implants tend to span a much larger area. Fixation should therefore be robust.
  - Similar to Pattern 1 and 2 implant designs, abundant porosity should exist at areas of osseous integration, and smooth surfaces should exist where articulating with native cartilage or areas of concern for undesirable soft tissue ingrowth and contracture.

TABLE 14.1   **Indications for Navicular Implants Commonly Present in Three Different Patterns, Which May Aid in Implant Design and Procedure Selection**

Pattern	Findings	Procedure Selection	Implant Example
1	Osseous deficit limited to the navicular without degeneration to the talar head with or without cuneiform degeneration. May be consistent with mid-stage AVN (Ficat 2 or 3)	TNJ-sparing navicular replacement[8]	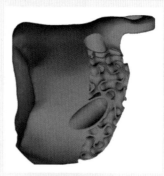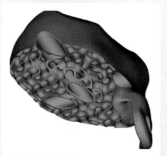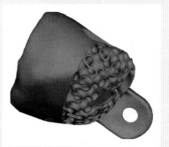
2	Osseous deficit limited to the navicular with degeneration of the talar head and cuneiforms. May be consistent with late-stage AVN	Medial column fusion with a 3D-printed porous navicular implant	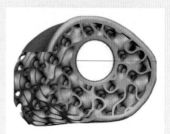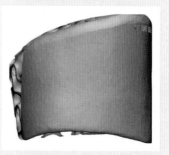

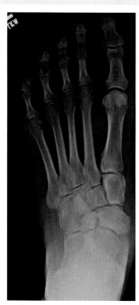

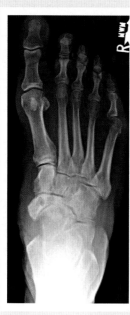

TABLE 14.1	Indications for Navicular Implants Commonly Present in Three Different Patterns, Which May Aid in Implant Design and Procedure Selection—cont'd		
Pattern	Findings	Procedure Selection	Implant Example
3	Osseous deficit of the navicular and other hindfoot bones. May be consistent following high-energy trauma or infection	Hindfoot fusion with large 3D-printed porous implant with possible selective adjacent joint sparing	

AVN, Avascular necrosis; *TNJ*, talonavicular joint.
CAD images depicting implant examples reprinted with permission from restor3d, Inc, Durham, NC.

- Fixation methods are surgeon and pathology dependent:
  - The authors recommend using a 3D-printed cage-type implant to accommodate the osseous deficit, which may have holes for screw fixation. Screw fixation from the implant to the adjacent bone provides compression at the bone-implant interface and enhanced stability of the implant; however, it decreases the surface area available for osseous integration into the implant. Screw trajectory is determined in the preoperative planning stage and additional guides may be created to ensure the desired placement is achieved.

- Solid screws may provide higher fatigue strength compared to cannulated screws. Using a cannulated technique is recommended when using solid screws to confirm the trajectory fluoroscopically and compared to preoperative computer-aided design (CAD) images.
- The authors typically use a combination of 3.0, 3.5, and 4.0 mm screws.
- Additional supplemental fixation is recommended. Off-the-shelf traditional Ti internal fixation such as spanning locking plates, intramedullary beams, and external fixation may be considered.

Surgical Management With 3D-Printed Devices

- The authors recommend general anesthesia with regional nerve block for this procedure.
- The patient is placed supine with an ipsilateral hip bump and thigh tourniquet.
- Treatment of navicular AVN without TNJ arthritis (Pattern 1) with TNJ sparing navicular replacement[8]:
  - A dorsomedial approach is recommended to allow access to the posterior tibial tendon. If visualization of the lateral navicular is difficult, then a dorsal lateral/sinus tarsi incision should be considered.
  - Once the navicular is exposed, it is sharply released of soft tissue attachments including the posterior tibial tendon, which is tagged.
  - The authors recommend using a patient-specific cutting guide and sagittal saw to remove the cuneiform bases, which aids in implant fit and determining the fixation trajectory (Fig. 14.6).
  - After the osteotomy of the cuneiforms is performed, the guide is removed and the navicular and cuneiform bases are removed using osteotomes and rongeurs. The surgeon is to take caution to avoid damaging the talar head cartilage as well as preserving vital ligaments, which may

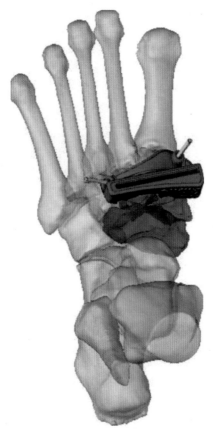

• **Fig. 14.6** Computer-aided design image depicting a patient-specific cutting guide pinned with 2.0-mm wires. The bone in red represents bone to be excised. The guide accommodates a sagittal saw, allowing precise osseous resection which promotes ideal fit and implant placement. (Reprinted with permission from restor3d, Inc, Durham, NC.)

be tagged with suture. The intercuneiform joints are prepared for fusion using standard technique. Copious irrigation is used to ensure all debris is removed.

- Trial navicular implants are used to determine the ideal size. An ideal-sized implant will maintain length and alignment of the medial column with physiologic tension of the adjacent soft tissues. Avoid overstuffing the joint, as this will lead to increased friction and wear on the talar head. Range of motion (ROM) and stability are assessed on the table as well as under fluoroscopy. If available, trials impregnated with barium sulfate render the trial radiopaque, making radiographic evaluation easier.
- After size is determined and the trial is removed, copious irrigation is performed while the final implant is packed with bone graft and/or biologics of choice. The final implant is placed and the placement location confirmed on fluoroscopy may then be pinned in place temporarily.
- The implant is then fixated with nonlocking screws per the preoperative plan. It may be advantageous to avoid fully seating any screw until all are in place to avoid migration of the implant, which may occur as the screw compresses the bone-implant interface.
- Ligaments, particularly the spring ligament, which were previously tagged are reapproximated with nonabsorbable suture. Ensure no impingement occurs with ROM after the ligaments are attached.
- The posterior tibial tendon may be reattached using different methods per the surgeon's preference:
  - A tendon allograft may be utilized to provide sufficient length to the attachment site on the dorsal cuneiforms. The allograft is interwoven and sewn to the distal end of the posterior tibial tendon. The suture is passed through the tunnel within the implant, tensioned, and attached to the cuneiform with tenodesis and/or suture anchors while holding the foot slightly supinated.[8]
  - Alternatively, the tendon may be reattached directly to the medial aspect of the medial cuneiform. A tendon allograft is typically necessary to provide sufficient length. To enhance fixation strength the surgeon may consider sewing the tendon and passing the suture through eyelets in the navicular implant.
  - If there is sufficient tendon length, then the tendon may be whip stitched and passed through a tunnel in the navicular implant. The suture is secured on the dorsal aspect of the navicular implant (Fig. 14.7).
- Closure per the surgeon's protocol is performed and the foot is splinted in supination.
- Treatment of navicular AVN with TNJ arthritis (Pattern 2), treated with a porous 3D-printed navicular implant and medial column fusion:
  - The medial column may be approached dorsomedially or dorsally:

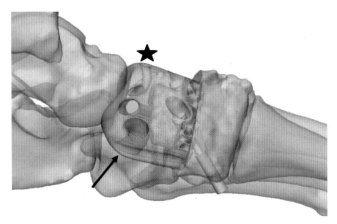

• **Fig. 14.7** Computer-aided design image depicting an option for reattachment of the posterior tibial tendon. The tendon is whip stitched and passed into the tunnel at plantar medial aspect of the implant *(arrow)*. The sutures are passed through the tunnel dorsal laterally and secured on the dorsal implant surface *(star)*. (Reprinted with permission from restor3d, Inc, Durham, NC.)

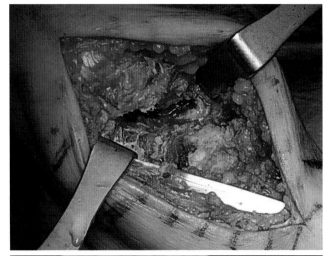

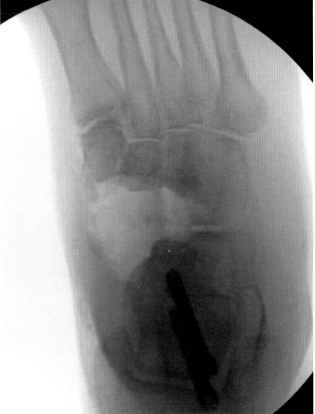

• **Fig. 14.8** Intraoperative photograph and radiograph taken after a naviculectomy has been performed. To ensure all nonviable bone has been excised, the surgeon may consider deflating the tourniquet to ensure normal perfusion to all remaining osseous structures. In this case there was poor bone quality noted in the medial talar head, which required excision as well.

- A dorsomedial approach may allow plantar plating and screw fixation, which may enhance stability. However, a dorsomedial approach may limit access to the lateral aspects of the talar head, navicular, and lateral cuneiform. Further, it is difficult to fixate the lateral aspect of the navicular implant, therefore the surgeon should consider a 2nd incision over the sinus tarsi.
- A dorsal approach between the tibialis anterior and extensor hallucis longus tendon provides great visualization and access to the entire navicular, talar head, and cuneiform bases. It can be more difficult to release the posterior tibial tendon from a dorsal approach.
- All necrotic and devitalized bone is excised. In the authors' experience, the central third is profoundly affected in AVN and often extends medially and laterally depending on chronicity (Fig. 14.8).
- Joint surfaces are prepared for fusion using standard technique.
- Radiopaque trials are placed in the navicular space. the ideal size is demonstrated by physiologic tension of the adjacent soft tissues as well as anatomic length and alignment of the medial column (Fig. 14.9).
- The trial is removed and the surgical site is irrigated continuously while the final navicular implant is packed with the bone graft and biologics of choice (see Fig. 14.3).
- Final implantation:
  - Plate and screw fixation: the implant is temporarily fixated and the position confirmed. Screws through the implant are placed to compress the bone-implant interface. When tightening the screws closely, watch for changes in the implant alignment, which may occur due to asymmetric compression caused by overtightening the screws. A medial column plate is used to span the implant and adjacent bones, which may include the 1st metatarsal (Fig. 14.10).
  - Beam fixation: a guide pin is placed through the trial and into the talus using an integrated drill guide. The guide is removed and reaming performed over the wire and through the trial. The beam length is determined and all trials/wires are removed. The navicular implant is placed followed

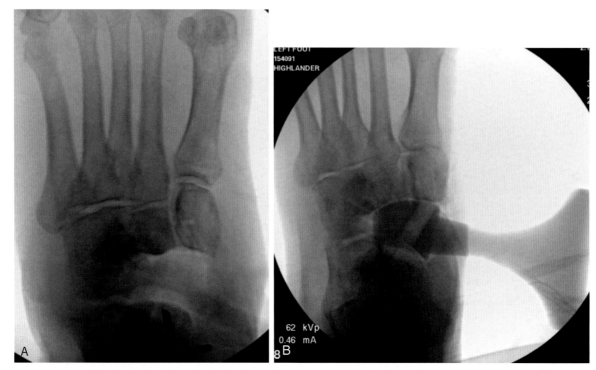

• **Fig. 14.9** Intraoperative radiographs of two different cases comparing sizing assessment with (A) radiolucent and (B) radiopaque trial implants. The radiopaque trials, if available, are preferable to evaluate fit and placement compared with the adjacent bones.

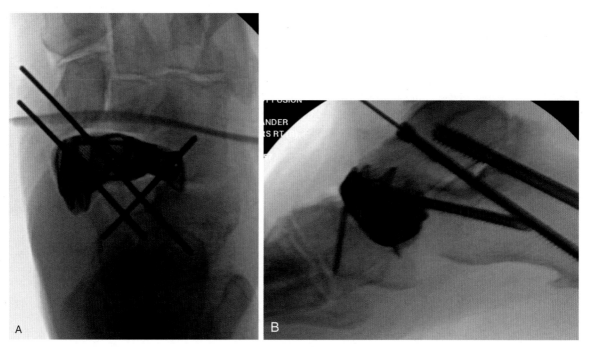

• **Fig. 14.10** Navicular implant with plate and screw fixation for medial column fusion. (A) The implant is pinned in place and alignment assessed. All screws through the implant are then inserted and tightened. (B) The surgeon should observe compression of the implant-bone interface while ensuring the implant position is not altered.

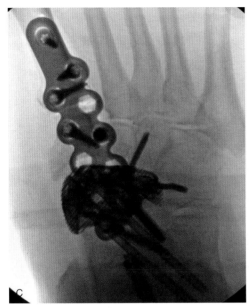
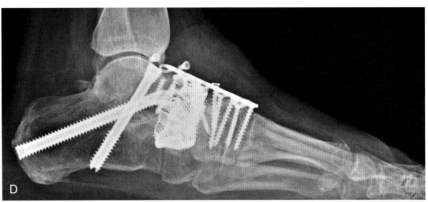

• **Fig. 14.10, cont'd** (C) A medial column plate is then placed for additional stability. (D) In the authors' experience there is a higher rate of hardware failure when the first tarsometatarsal joint is spared.

by the beam. The beam is compressed and fixated accordingly.

- In the authors' experience, medial column stability appears to be paramount for achieving good outcomes.
  - When using plates and screws, preserving the first tarsometatarsal joint has been associated with hardware failure and the need for additional surgery (Fig. 14.10D).
  - Medial column beaming is an alternative option or it may be used with plates and screws. In sensate patients, placing a beam from the 1st metatarsal phalangeal joint may lead to chronic issues, therefore consider a starting point from the medial cuneiform or 1st metatarsal base. Patient-specific targeting guides are recommended to ensure proper placement within the medial column as well as through the implant (Fig. 14.11).
  - External fixation may also be considered for supplemental fixation to improve stability. However, risks do exist, which include patient intolerance, need for surgical removal, cost, and pin site infections.
- Closure per the surgeon's protocol is performed and a short-leg splint is applied with the foot and ankle held in a neutral position.
- Treatment of large osseous deficits due to pathology affecting the navicular, talus, and navicular (Pattern 3), with staged hindfoot fusion with preservation of the navicular cuneiform joints (Fig. 14.12):
  - This approach may be limited due to the soft tissue envelope and prior incisions, because often patients with an osseous deficit involving multiple bones have had multiple surgeries and/or suffered high-energy trauma.
    - An anterior approach between the tibialis anterior and extensor hallucis longus allows access to the tibia, talus, and navicular.

- A dual anteromedial and anterolateral approach may also be considered.
- All necrotic bone is excised in a stepwise fashion. Bones requiring excision may be determined by:
  - Bone biopsy.
  - MRI and CT scan may aide in determining the extent of osseous involvement.
- The talar head and neck are removed first.
- Once the talar head and neck are excised, there is ample room to release all soft tissue attachments to the navicular, which makes removal more efficient. When removing the navicular, care is taken to avoid damage to the cartilage on the proximal cuneiforms.
- Removal of the talar body may be more difficult if the tibiotalar joint is severely arthritic or autofused. In these situations a tibial resection is may be considered. A patient-specific cut guide for the distal tibia was used to ensure potential optimized bone is resected as well as contoured to mirror that of the implant design
- Removal of the distal tibia and talar body can be performed simultaneously:
  - In situations of previous infection, it is recommended that the procedure be staged to ensure clean margins and adequate excision and debridement.
  - We recommend using antibiotic-impregnated nonbiodegradable cement such as poly(methyl methacrylate) (PMMA) as a temporary spacer until cultures return (Fig. 14.12B,C).
- Once it is clear that only healthy bone remains, the antibiotic cement is removed and the calcaneal facets are prepared for fusion:
  - The authors prefer to use an acetabular reamer for preparation of the calcaneus, which increases the

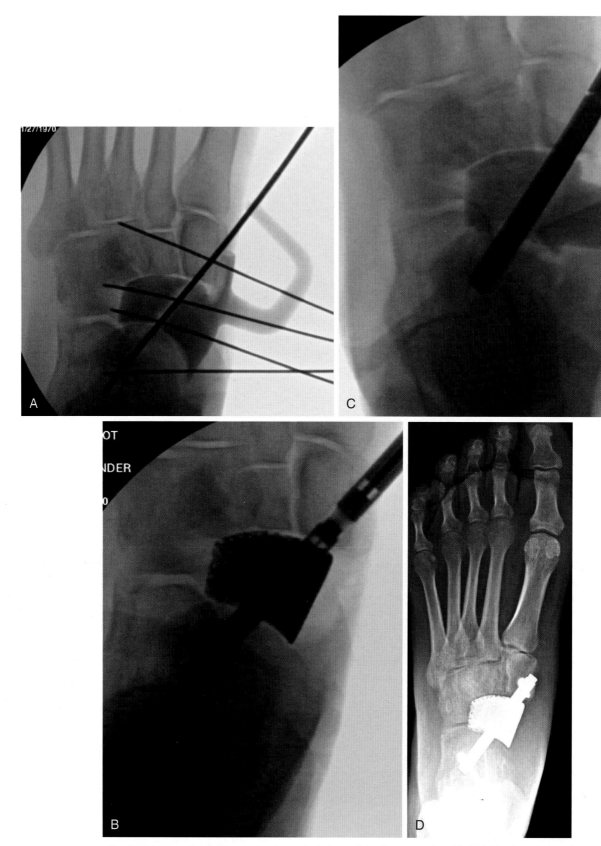

• **Fig. 14.11** Alternative fixation methods may include medial column beaming. (A) A trial implant designed with a drill guide is temporarily fixated after the ideal implant size is determined. A guidewire is placed through the implant, then temporary fixation and the drill guide component are removed. Reaming proceeds over the guidewire and through the trial implant. (B) The guidewire is removed and the beam length determined. (C and D) The beam is then placed through the implant, compressed, and fixated accordingly.

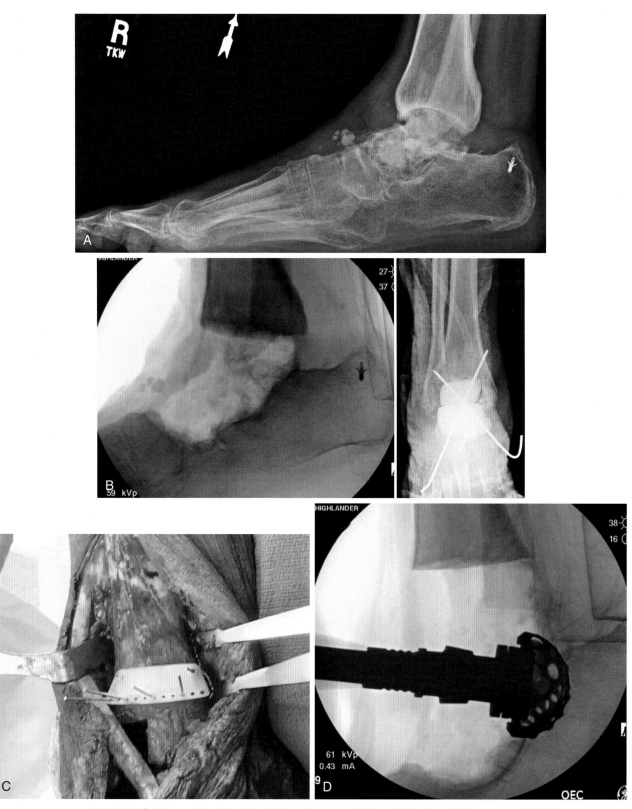

• **Fig. 14.12** A 47-year-old male with a history of an open talar neck fracture which was complicated by infection. (A) After the injury the patient had been unable to ambulate due to pain for nearly 2 years. A staged reconstruction was initiated. Stage I involved identifying infection location via bone biopsies which confirmed chronic infection of the navicular and talus. (B) Stage II required multiple surgeries to ensure all infected and potentially contaminated bone was excised. Excision of the navicular, talus, and the tibial plafond was required. (C–G) Stage III, or final reconstruction, involved arthrodesis of the ankle and subtalar joint with arthroplasty of the navicular-cuneiform joints with a 3D-printed implant. (C) The distal tibia resection was finalized using a patient-specific cut guide to optimize implant fit. (D) The calcaneal facets were prepared with an acetabular reamer.

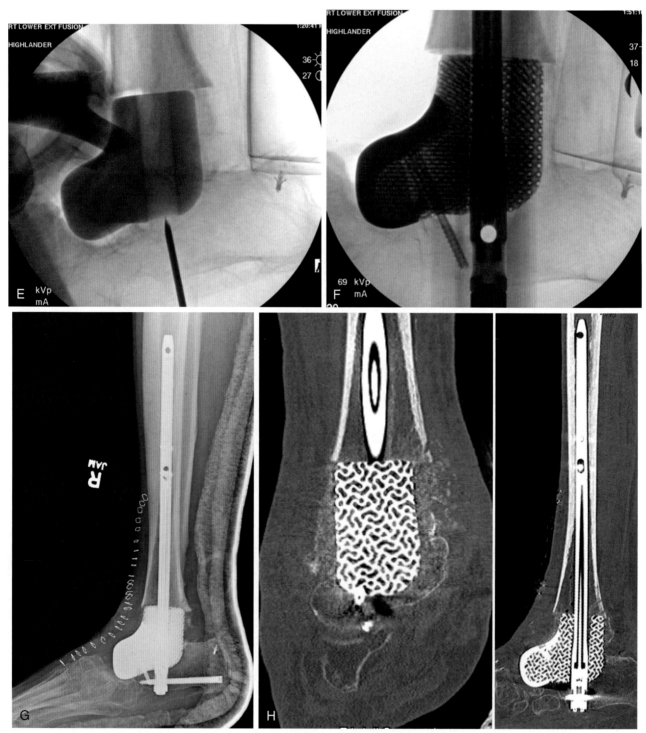

• **Fig. 14.12, cont'd** (E) The ideally sized trial is placed, a guide wire is placed, and reaming proceeds for intramedullary nail fixation. (F) The final implant is placed and fixated to prevent rotation. (G) The intramedullary nail is fixated and compressed accordingly to complete the construct. (H) A 3-month follow-up CT scan demonstrates a stable, osseous integration at the bone-implant interface and overgrowth surrounding the implant. At 1 year follow-up, the patient showed significant improvement in quality of life, pain, and function.

surface area of the bone-implant interface compared to in situ fusion using curettage (Fig. 14.12D).

- The contour and size of the inferior aspect of the implant is designed based on the desired acetabular reamer size.
- If the cuneiform cartilage is largely free of degenerative changes, the authors recommend consideration toward preserving navicular cuneiform motion:
  - The distal aspect of the implant is smooth and polished, and should mirror the morphology of the proximal cuneiforms.
  - A pantalar fusion is essentially the result of this technique. Preserving navicular cuneiform articulation allows the foot to adapt to the sagittal plane rigidity provided by the ankle and TNJ fusions.[30]
  - Biomechanical studies have suggested that plantarflexion of the medial column is primarily provided at the medial navicular cuneiform joint during propulsion,[31] therefore preserving this articulation promotes more normal function.
- Radiopaque trials are used to determine the ideal size of the implant:
  - Close evaluation for fit and contact of the bone-implant interface, length and alignment of the limb, and physiologic tension of the adjacent soft tissues.
  - If the adjacent soft tissues are overly tensed, then the implant may be inherently more stable due to the compressive forces exerted at the bone-implant interface. However, overly tensed/stretched soft tissues may result in neurovascular compromise and/or deformity.
  - If the adjacent soft tissues are relaxed (do not reach physiologic tension), the implant is undersized and is inherently less stable.
  - Once the size is determined, reaming for the intramedullary nail is performed with the trial maintained in its preferred position (Fig. 14.12E).
  - While reaming the tibial canal for nail insertion, the reamings are collected and separated into liquid and solid components utilizing the Hensler Bone Press (Hensler Surgical Technologies, Willmington, NC).
- The surgical site is irrigated continuously while the porous aspect of the final implant is packed with solid bone graft obtained during reaming. Additional allograft and biologics may be used if desired. The success of this technique as well as the implant design relies on osseous integration at the calcaneus-implant and tibial-implant interfaces.
- The final implant is placed and the intramedullary nail is placed through the implant under fluoroscopic guidance:
  - Prior to fixating the nail, transverse plane alignment is evaluated on the AP foot view. Once alignment is ideal, a screw is placed from the dorsal aspect of the implant into the calcaneus. The screw should be retightened once all components of the

intramedullary nail are completed, including external compression if provided by the surgeon's preferred nail.
  - The authors prefer longer intramedullary nails to allow stability and rigidity.
  - For optimal stability of the distal nail, it is strongly recommended that the surgeon utilizes an intramedullary nail that provides two points of fixation in the calcaneus, preferably 90 degrees to one another.
- The nail is fixated and compressed accordingly (Fig. 14.12F).
- Closure per the surgeon's protocol is performed and a short-leg splint is applied with the foot and ankle held in a neutral position (Fig. 14.12G).
- Ancillary procedures may include:
  - Gastrocnemius recession.
  - Bone graft harvest.
  - Corrective osteotomies of the hindfoot and/or forefoot if deformity is present.
  - The authors recommend strong consideration for contaminant subtalar joint fusion with medial column fusion. Fusion of the subtalar joint decreases talar excursion and enhances the stability of the talar-implant interface.[32,33]

Postoperative Protocol

- The authors recommend a similar postoperative protocol regardless of pathology pattern or ancillary procedures.
- An immediate postoperative CT scan should be considered to serve as a comparison to follow-up CT scans.
- Non-weight bearing for 6 to 8 weeks.
- Splint removed and incision should be evaluated 5 to 10 days postoperatively.
- A cast is applied and maintained for 2 to 3 weeks or until the incisions have healed.
- At 3 to 4 weeks postoperatively:
  - Transition to a controlled ankle motion (CAM) boot but remain non-weight bearing.
  - Begin active ROM exercise without resistance.
- At 6 to 8 weeks, if the pain is controlled and radiographs are stable, the patient may begin partial protected weight bearing in a CAM boot.
- Physical therapy may begin at 8 weeks postoperatively but is limited to non–weight-bearing exercise.
- A follow-up CT scan is obtained at 12 weeks (Fig. 14.12H).
  - If bony consolidation, close bone-implant interface (absence of periprosthetic lucency), and maintenance of hardware placement and limb alignment are observed, the patient may:
    - Begin weight bearing as tolerated in a CAM boot.
    - Progress physical therapy to weight-bearing exercise.
    - Transition to a lace-up ankle brace and supportive shoes as tolerated.
  - If periprosthetic lucency exists, then a noninvasive bone stimulator is initiated and the patient is to remain in a CAM boot with partial weight bearing.

- The authors obtain additional follow-up CT scans at 6 months, 12 months, and then yearly, while follow-up X-rays are evaluated every 6 to 8 weeks from 3 to 6 months postoperatively. X-rays are then obtained every 6 months unless needed otherwise.

Results/Outcomes

- There is limited research on the surgical treatment of navicular AVN and most publications are case studies or small case series.[34-37]
- Adams and Danilkowicz[8] were the first to publish a single case study of navicular AVN-treated 3D-printed TNJ-sparing navicular replacement. At 4 years' follow-up, the patient improved in all subjective and objective measures, and CT scan demonstrated osseous integration.
- Navicular AVN with adjacent joint arthritis has traditionally been treated similarly to talar AVN with arthritis: fusion with structural allograft to restore length and alignment.[34-37] Steele et al.[38] demonstrated improved outcomes and fusion rates when performing fusion for talar AVN using a 3D-printed porous implant compared to traditional methods. It appears that the osteoconductive and structural properties of porous titanium spacers may be a reason for improved results; however, research comparing 3D-printed implants and traditional methods for navicular AVN has yet to be published.
- In the senior author's (P.D.H.) experience, increased complications occur when performing medial column fusion with a 3D-printed navicular implant:
  - A high rate of hardware failure with plate and screw fixation alone.
  - A higher revision rate when the first tarsometatarsal joint is not incorporated into the arthrodesis.
- For substantial osseous deficits compromising multiple bones, large fusions paired with structural allografts have higher failure rates with increasing size of the deficit. It appears this limitation may not be as apparent with 3D-printed porous implants, which may lessen the need for amputation.
- More research is needed on the treatment of navicular AVN. Anecdotally, there appears to be a benefit to both the patient and surgeon when treating navicular AVN with 3D-printed patient-specific implants. Nonetheless, these cases are rare and when encountered surgeons should consider traditional reconstruction methods versus that of 3D printing on a case-by-case basis.

PEARLS AND PITFALLS

Indications & Contraindications	• Avascular Necrosis of the Navicular
	• Acute fractures of the Navicular
	• Stress fracture of the Navicular
	• Nonunion of the navicular
	• Contraindicated in cases of active infection
	• Use prudence in patients with a history of deep infection
Implant Design	• Titanium appears to be ideal material for fusion/osseous integration
	• Porous structure is recommended for titanium implants/osseous integration
	• Cobalt chrome and smooth surfaces are ideal for contact with cartilaginous surfaces
	• Patient specific cut guides may be used in conjunction for increased accuracy and efficiency
	• Implant shape is patient specific
Surgical Technique	• Dorsal approach provides better visualization but may result in more difficulty releasing posterior tibial tendon
	• Remove all non-viable bone
	• Use instrumentation that replicates the shape & size of the implant to promote optimal bone-implant contact
	• Minimum of three sizes to ensure ideal fit and alignment restoration.
	• Size of implant and fixation method is patient specific. Consideration for fixation targeting guides can be considered.
	• Spanning fusions across the medial column or subtalar joint can also be considered.

TIPS AND TRICKS

Procedure Selection	• Joint involvement will aide in determination to preserve the talar head or to fuse the talus to the navicular implant • The major limitation to preserving the talar head is reliably attaching the posterior tibial tendon to the implant. Failure to do so will result in postoperative deformity and asymmetric wear of the talar head. • Fixation to the cuneiforms can be problematic therefore strongly consider spanning fixation across the 1st tarsometatarsal joint.
Goals of Reconstruction	• Improve function & relieve pain • Restore medial column length & alignment
Imaging	• MRI is most sensitive for diagnosis of avascular necrosis • CT is best for assessing collapse, osseous deficit and joint involvement • CT is required for preoperative planning & should be compared to contralateral scans
Labs/Work-up	• Labs should aide in determination of existing infection or metabolic deficiencies required for bone healing • Bone biopsy should be considered
Implant Design	• If the implant is to articulate with adjacent native cartilage materials with a low coefficient of friction should be considered to decrease cartilage wear. • When fusion is desired implant surface roughness will increase friction at the bone-implant interface enhancing stability. • Implant porosity should allow packing & maintenance of bone graft & biologics of choice
Implantation	• Using a pin distractor to recreate physiologic tension of adjacent soft tissues will help determine ideal implant size. • Radiopaque trials are preferred. • Ensure the implant position is ideal prior to any fixation
Fixation	• Disposable guides will ensure temporary fixation is centered within the implant screw holes. • Sequentially tighten screws to prevent implant migration. • Achieving stability along the medial column with a navicular implant can be challenging & often underestimated. If stability is not adequate hardware failure is inevitable. • Strongly consider incorporating the 1st tarsometatarsal joint into the fusion construct. • Medial column plates & intramedullary nails are often preferable for fixation.

References

1. Guelfi M, Pantalone A, Mirapeix RM, et al. Anatomy, pathophysiology and classification of posterior tibial tendon dysfunction. *Eur Rev Med Pharmacol Sci.* 2017;21(1):13-19.
2. Smith CF. Anatomy, function, and pathophysiology of the posterior tibial tendon. *Clin Podiatr Med Surg.* 1999;16(3):399-406.
3. Kaye RA, Jahss MH. Tibialis posterior: a review of anatomy and biomechanics in relation to support of the medial longitudinal arch. *Foot Ankle.* 1991;11(4):244-247.
4. Roling BA, Christensen JC, Johnson CH. Biomechanics of the first ray. Part IV: the effect of selected medial column arthrodeses. A three-dimensional kinematic analysis in a cadaver model. *J Foot Ankle Surg.* 2002;41(5):278-285.
5. Flores DV, Mejía Gómez C, Fernández Hernando M, Davis MA, Pathria MN. Adult acquired flatfoot deformity: anatomy, biomechanics, staging, and imaging findings. *RadioGraphics.* 2019;39(5): 1437-1460.
6. Song D, Yang X, Wu Z, et al. Anatomic basis and clinical application of the distally based medialis pedis flaps. *Surg Radiol Anat.* 2016;38(2):213-221.
7. Shi GG, Williams MA, Whalen JL, Wilke BK, Kraus JC. An anatomic and clinical study of the innervation of the dorsal midfoot capsule. *Foot Ankle Int.* 2019;40(10):1209-1213.
8. Adams SB, Danilkowicz RM. Talonavicular joint-sparing 3D printed navicular replacement for osteonecrosis of the navicular. *Foot Ankle Int.* 2021;42(9):1197-1204.
9. Chan JY, Young JL. Köhler disease: avascular necrosis in the child. *Foot Ankle Clin.* 2019;24(1):83-88.
10. Perisano C, Greco T, Vitiello R, et al. Mueller-Weiss disease: review of the literature. *J Biol Regul Homeost Agents.* 2018;32 (6 suppl 1):157-162.

11. Samim M, Moukaddam HA, Smitaman E. Imaging of Mueller-Weiss syndrome: a review of clinical presentations and imaging spectrum. *AJR Am J Roentgenol.* 2016;207(2):W8-W18.

12. Brukner P, Bradshaw C, Khan KM, et al. Stress fractures: a review of 180 cases. *Clin J Sport Med.* 1996;6:85.

13. Bennell KL, Malcolm SA, Thomas SA, et al. The incidence and distribution of stress fractures in competitive track and field athletes. A twelve-month prospective study. *Am J Sports Med.* 1996; 24:211.

14. Jones MH, Amendola AS. Navicular stress fractures. *Clin Sports Med.* 2006;25:151.

15. Ficat RP, Arlet J. Necrosis of the femoral head. In: Hungerford DS, ed. *Ischemia and Necrosis of Bone.* Baltimore, MD: Williams & Wilkins; 1980:171-182.

16. Mont MA, Schon LC, Hungerford MW, Hundeford DS. Avascular necrosis of the talus treated by core decompression. *J Bone Joint Surg.* 1996;78:827-830.

17. Ahmed AA, Kandil MI, Tabl EA, Elgazzar AS. Müller-Weiss disease: a topical review. *Foot Ankle Int.* 2019;40(12):1447-1457.

18. Maceira E, Rochera R. Müller-Weiss disease: clinical and biomechanical features. *Foot Ankle Clin.* 2004;9(1):105-125.

19. Welck MJ, Kaplan J, Myerson MS. Müller-Weiss syndrome: radiological features and the role of weightbearing computed tomography scan. *Foot Ankle Spec.* 2016;9(3):245-251.

20. Sangeorzan BJ, Benirschke SK, Mosca V, Mayo KA, Hansen ST. Displaced intra-articular fractures of the tarsal navicular. *J Bone Joint Surg Am.* 1989;71(10):1504-1510.

21. Dhillon MS, Rana B, Panda I, Patel S, Kumar P. Management options in avascular necrosis of the talus. *Indian J Orthop.* 2018; 52(3):284-296.

22. Coulibaly MO, Jones CB, Sietsema DL, Schildhauer TA. Results and complications of operative and non-operative navicular fracture treatment. *Injury.* 2015;46(8):1669-1677.

23. Chang SM, Chen PY, Tsai MS, Shee BW. Light bulb procedure for the treatment of tarsal navicular osteonecrosis after failed percutaneous decompression: a case report. *J Foot Ankle Surg.* 2019;58(1):187-191.

24. Fishman FG, Adams SB, Easley ME, Nunley JA II. Vascularized pedicle bone grafting for nonunions of the tarsal navicular. *Foot Ankle Int.* 2012;33(9):734-739.

25. Gilbert BJ, Horst F, Nunley JA. Potential donor rotational bone grafts using vascular territories in the foot and ankle. *J Bone Joint Surg Am.* 2004;86(9):1857-1873.

26. Levinson H, Miller KJ, Adams SB Jr, Parekh SG. Treatment of spontaneous osteonecrosis of the tarsal navicular with a free medial femoral condyle vascularized bone graft: a new approach to managing a difficult problem. *Foot Ankle Spec.* 2014;7(4): 332-337.

27. Poh CK, Shi Z, Tan XW, et al. Cobalt chromium alloy with immobilized BMP peptide for enhanced bone growth. *J Orthop Res.* 2011;29(9):1424-1430.

28. Marti A. Cobalt-based alloys used in bone surgery. *Injury.* 2000;31(suppl 4):18-21.

29. Mavrogenis AF, Papagelopoulos PJ, Babis GC. Osseointegration of cobalt-chrome alloy implants. *J Long Term Eff Med Implants.* 2011;21(4):349-358.

30. Sealey RJ, Myerson MS, Molloy A, Gamba C, Jeng C, Kalesan B. Sagittal plane motion of the hindfoot following ankle arthrodesis: a prospective analysis. *Foot Ankle Int.* 2009;30(3):187-196.

31. Phillips RD, Law EA, Ward ED. Functional motion of the medial column joints of the foot during propulsion. *J Am Podiatr Med Assoc.* 1996;86(10):474-486.

32. Zhang K, Chen Y, Qiang M, Hao Y. Effects of five hindfoot arthrodeses on foot and ankle motion: measurements in cadaver specimens. *Sci Rep.* 2016;6:35493.

33. Astion DJ, Deland JT, Otis JC, Kenneally S. Motion of the hindfoot after simulated arthrodesis. *J Bone Joint Surg Am.* 1997;79(2):241-246.

34. Greenhagen RM, Crim BE, Shinabarger AB, Burns PR. Bilateral osteonecrosis of the navicular and medial cuneiform in a patient with systemic lupus erythematosus: a case report. *Foot Ankle Spec.* 2012;5(3):180-184.

35. Kitaura Y, Nishimura A, Nakazora S, et al. Spontaneous osteonecrosis of the tarsal navicular: a report of two cases. *Case Rep Orthop.* 2019;2019:5952435.

36. Zapolsky IJ, Gajewski CR, Webb M, Wapner KL, Levin LS. A case report of bilateral navicular osteonecrosis successfully treated with medial femoral condyle vascularized autografts: a case report. *JBJS Case Connect.* 2020;10(3):e2000010.

37. Cao HH, Tang KL, Xu JZ. Peri-navicular arthrodesis for the stage III Müller-Weiss disease. *Foot Ankle Int.* 2012;33(6):475-478.

38. Steele JR, Kadakia RJ, Cunningham DJ, Dekker TJ, Kildow BJ, Adams SB. Comparison of 3D printed spherical implants versus femoral head allografts for tibiotalocalcaneal arthrodesis. *J Foot Ankle Surg.* 2020;59(6):1167-1170.

15

Midfoot Fusion With a Custom 3D-Printed Cage for Charcot Deformity

DANIEL J. TORINO, BENJAMIN R. WAGNER, GERARD J. CUSH Jr.

Definition

- Currently, diabetes mellitus (DM) is the most common predisposing medical condition for the development of Charcot arthropathy.
- The midfoot is most commonly affected in Charcot arthropathy and historically was treated with total contact casting in the acute phase with a later transition to accommodative bracing after resolution of symptoms. Prior studies have shown that bracing does not always correlate with a good patient outcome.[1-3]
- Progressive bony deformity and resorption that may accompany Charcot arthropathy have led to advocating for surgical intervention. Recent literature has demonstrated successful operative corrections of midfoot deformity with improved quality of life for patients.[4]
- Sammarco[5] has described super construct concepts, which focus on four main factors:
  - Extending the fusion beyond the zone of injury to the unaffected joints to improve fixation.
  - Performing bony rection as needed to allow adequate deformity reduction without placing undue tension on the soft tissue envelop.
  - Using the strongest device that can be tolerated by the soft tissue envelope.
  - Application of the device in a position that maximizes mechanical function.
- Intramedullary beaming fixation is a more recently described technique which allows for decreased soft tissue dissection, simultaneous compression across multiple arthrodesis sites, minimally invasive insertion, and the ability to span across the zone of injury.[6] The primary goal of surgery is an ulcer-free plantigrade foot.

Diagnosis

- Specific conditions for which such fusion is commonly indicated include:
  - Inflammatory arthropathies
  - Congenital deformity
  - Neuropathic arthritis secondary to DM or inherited/acquired polyneuropathies
  - Failed total ankle arthroplasty
  - Severe pes planovalgus deformity
  - Fracture malunion and nonunion
  - Bone loss and collapse secondary to trauma, tumor, osteonecrosis, Charcot arthropathy, or infection.
- Patient factors that have been shown to affect outcomes of midfoot and hindfoot fusion include medical comorbidities such as DM, previous ulcerations, peripheral vascular disease, renal disease, immunosuppression, chronic steroid use, rheumatologic disease, malnutrition, and smoking.
- In addition, a history of surgical intervention, particularly with postoperative complications (e.g., deep infection, problems with wound healing) may affect postoperative outcomes.

Anatomy

- The midfoot includes the navicular, cuboid, and cuneiform bones and their articulations with the proximal metatarsal bones.
- The heads of the first and fifth metatarsal bones and the calcaneus constitute a tripod necessary for foot stability.
- The key joints in the foot for maintenance of mobility are the hindfoot joints, including the tibiotalar, subtalar, and talonavicular articulations. The lateral and fourth and fifth tarsometatarsal (TMT) joints that are important for normal foot function are more mobile than other TMT joints. The remaining hindfoot and midfoot joints, including the calcaneocuboid and the first, second, and third TMT joints, do not require a full range of motion to maintain function of the foot.
- The transverse tarsal joint (Chopart joint) is composed of the talonavicular and calcaneocuboid joints and acts in concert with the subtalar joint to control foot flexibility during gait.

- The talonavicular joint is supported by the spring ligament complex, which has two separate components: the superior medial calcaneonavicular ligament and the inferior calcaneonavicular ligament.
- The calcaneocuboid joint is saddle shaped. It is supported plantarly by the inferior calcaneocuboid ligaments (superficial and deep) and superiorly by the lateral limb of the bifurcate ligament.

Biomechanics

- TMT joints
  - Little motion occurs through the intercuneiform and naviculocuneiform (NC) joints.
  - The fourth and fifth TMT joints are the most mobile, with a range of motion from 5 to 17 degrees. The second TMT is the least mobile, with 1 degree of motion.
  - Dorsiflexion of the metatarsal-phalangeal (MTP) joints during propulsion tightens the plantar fascia through a windlass effect, raising the longitudinal arch and inverting the heel.

Pathogenesis

- Midfoot arthritis in the sensate foot
  - The first, second, and third TMT joints of the midfoot may be viewed as nonessential joints, and if fused in anatomic alignment, physiologic foot function is generally anticipated.
  - The etiology of midfoot arthritis can be primary, inflammatory, or posttraumatic (Fig. 15.1).
  - Primary osteoarthritis of the midfoot is the most common type of midfoot arthritis.

- Untreated TMT joint (Lisfranc) fracture-dislocation typically leads to loss of the longitudinal arch and forefoot abduction.
- The pathogenesis of Charcot arthropathy (also termed Charcot foot or Charcot neuroarthropathy [CN]) has been explained using two major theories:
  - The neurotraumatic theory attributes bone destruction to the loss of pain sensation and proprioception, combined with repetitive and mechanical trauma to the foot.
  - The neurovascular theory suggests that joint destruction is secondary to an autonomic stimulated vascular reflex causing hyperemia and periarticular osteopenia with contributory trauma.
- There is a growing body of evidence that dysregulation of inflammatory and bone metabolism pathways, with upregulation of receptor activator of nuclear factor K-B ligand (RANK-L), lead to osteoclast over-activation and bone resorption.[4,6,7]
- Clinically, midfoot osteoarthropathy manifests as a noninfectious, osteolytic process that may ultimately result in profound deformity and instability from bone and joint collapse.[8] Deformity with neuropathy may lead to ulceration and potentially to a limb-threatening condition.
- In 1966, orthopedic surgeon Sidney N. Eichenholtz (1909–2000) published a monograph entitled "Charcot Joints" in which the clinical, radiographic, and pathologic data of 68 consecutive patients were used to define three stages of Charcot arthropathy based on the natural history of the condition.[9] The three stages he described were (1) development, (2) coalescence, and (3) reconstruction and reconstitution.

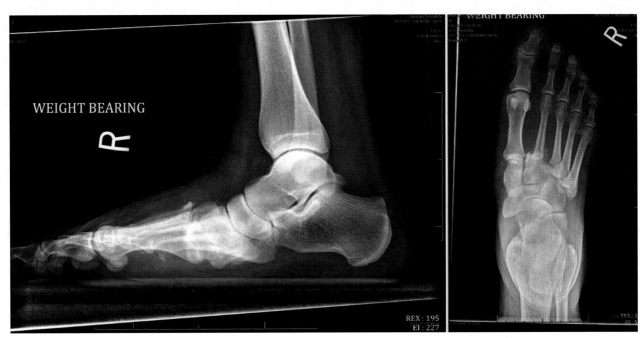

• **Fig. 15.1** Pes planovalgus foot alignment secondary to posttraumatic midfoot arthritis.

TABLE 15.1 Charcot Neuroarthropathy Staging Based on Eichenholtz and Shibata et al.[9,11]

Stage	Characteristic
0: Acute inflammatory phase	Foot is swollen, erythematous, warm, hyperemic; radiographs reveal periarticular soft tissue swelling and varying degrees of osteopenia
1: Developmental or fragmentation	Periarticular fracture and joint subluxation with risk of instability and deformity
2: Coalescence stage; subacute	Resorption of bone debris and soft tissue homeostasis
3: Consolidation or reparative stage; chronic	Restabilization of the foot with fibrous or bony arthrodesis of the involved joints

- Clinical signs (such as swelling, warmth, and erythema) regularly precede the radiographic findings seen with Eichenholtz stage I arthropathy.[10] As such, in 1990 Shibata et al. added a fourth stage, Charcot foot stage 0, to the conventional Eichenholtz classification[11] (Table 15.1).

Patient History and Physical Exam Findings

- Patients reports midfoot/arch pain with weight bearing, particularly with push-off during gait. Pain is elicited with palpation or stress. Bone prominences of the midfoot may be present.
- Examination of the patient should begin with assessment of the skin and pedal pulses. If there is any question about the vascular status of the limb in which surgery is being considered, further workup is warranted and may include vascular studies or consultation with a vascular surgeon. A neurologic evaluation should include sensation testing with a 5.07-gauge monofilament and an evaluation of the muscular strength in all planes of the leg that is to be treated.
- Assessment of the alignment of the foot and ankle begins with an evaluation of the standing alignment and during gait. Loss of the longitudinal arch (often associated with forefoot abduction) is frequently seen on weight bearing and with radiographic alignment. Midfoot arthritis is the second most common cause of longitudinal arch loss behind posterior tibial tendon dysfunction.
- Special attention should be paid to the alignment in both the sagittal and coronal planes. An equinus posture (i.e., fixed ankle plantar flexion) is important to detect, along with any varus or valgus positioning of the hindfoot. Attention should then be turned to the forefoot. To assess the need for forefoot correction, the hindfoot can be held in the corrected position while the clinician assesses the position of the forefoot in the coronal plane relative to the long axis of the tibia while the patient is seated.
- When evaluating the patient with Charcot arthropathy of the midfoot, the location and severity of the deformity must be determined radiographically and clinically to decide which treatment will most likely lead to a good result.

Imaging and Other Diagnostic Testing

- Weight-bearing radiographs of the ankle and foot are mandatory in the evaluation for deformity and alignment. Findings may include:
  - A nonlinear talus-first metatarsal relationship with the apex of the deformity at the midfoot.
  - Loss of longitudinal arch and forefoot abduction.
  - Evidence of arthrosis, bone loss, shortening, or existing implants from prior surgeries (particularly broken screws).
  - Bilateral weight-bearing anteroposterior (AP) view of both feet and ankles give an excellent indication of the degree of actual or functional shortening caused by bone loss or malalignment.
- Radiographic parameters examined include the lateral talo-first metatarsal angle (Meary's angle), AP talo-first metatarsal angle, calcaneal pitch, and cuboid height—weight bearing preoperative and final postoperative data are collected for comparison.
- In addition to plain radiography, a CT scan may be indicated in patients with substantial disruption of the normal bone architecture of the foot and ankle, and it is also useful in revision arthrodesis for determining the status of a previous fusion.

Nonoperative Management

- Nonsurgical treatment of arthritis of the ankle and foot include nonsteroidal antiinflammatories (systemic or topical), activity modification, corticosteroid injections, shoe modifications, and bracing treatment (ankle foot orthosis [AFO]). Most cases of acute Charcot arthropathy can be treated effectively with pressure-relieving methods such as total contact casting or a Charcot restraint orthotic walker (CROW).
- Longitudinal arch supports with rigid inserts.
- Typical advanced midfoot deformities require accommodative (not corrective) orthotics with recess to relieve pressure from prominences.
- Shoe modifications (rocker soles).
- Fixed ankle bracing treatment in combination with shoe modifications (rocker soles) may further unload the midfoot during gait.
- Early-stage Charcot arthropathy, where the arch is low and the foot is at risk, can often be managed with orthotics or accommodative shoes. Later stages, when the arch has collapsed, requires aggressive nonsurgical treatment such at total contact casting, and surgery may be required.

Traditional Surgical Management

- Prior studies have shown that bracing does not always correlate with a good patient outcome.[1-3] Progressive bony deformity and resorption that may accompany CN have led to advocating for surgical intervention.
- Late-stage CN, where the arch is below the plane of the calcaneus and the metatarsal heads, has a poor prognosis and a high risk of chronic ulcers and osteomyelitis. These patients likely require surgery.[12]
- The primary goal of surgery is an ulcer-free plantigrade foot.
- Surgical treatment consists of either an ostectomy or correction of the deformity and fusion. An ostectomy is indicated in patients who have continuous breakdown resulting from a bony prominence that prevents casting or bracing, as well as in patients who have sustained a fracture that has fragmented and consolidated into a stable deformity and now has symptomatic bony prominences. One caveat is that in completing the ostectomy you may destabilize the joint, as the resected, prominent bone may have been contributing to stability. An ostectomy is also indicated in patients who have recurrent ulcers owing to bony prominences, to allow the ulcers to heal before definitive correction and fusion.[13]
- Operative intervention may be indicated to realign the midfoot, which is typically achieved in conjunction with internal plate/screw or circular external (thin-wire) fixation.
- In general, fusion should involve the joints that are most obviously affected. In more mild deformities a more limited fusion may suffice. In severe cases, a first through fifth tarso-metatarsal (TMT) fusion is required. Additionally, fixation without fusion of the NC, talonavicular, and calcaneocuboid joints may also be beneficial to gain stability in better bone stock.
- "Beaming," which refers to a technique that utilizes intramedullary large-bolt fixation, has been described (Fig. 15.2). Utilizing medial and lateral column beams across the midfoot may allow surgeons to decrease the amount of hardware required to achieve stability, provide improved compression, and do so with both less soft tissue stripping and a lower chance of hardware exposure in the event of wound breakdown.[14]
- Subtalar and or hindfoot arthrodesis is often included as part of a Charcot midfoot reconstruction to restore calcaneal pitch and reduce the lateral talo-first metatarsal angle.
- Manchanda et al. demonstrated an 80% reduction in the odds of a complication when a subtalar arthrodesis was included in midfoot CN reconstruction in their retrospective review of complication rates for intramedullary beaming of midfoot Charcot reconstruction with and without subtalar arthrodesis.[15]
- Schon and Marks[12] described a comprehensive approach to Charcot of the midfoot. Depending on the location and magnitude of the deformity and the presence of infection, a combination of axial interfragmentary screws and plantar plates or external fixation was used for fixation of the deformity. The approach emphasized osteotomy and fusion of the entire midfoot from medial to lateral to achieve realignment and stability, if necessary.

Surgical Management With 3D-Printed Devices

- Physiologic foot function for ambulation, in particular during propulsion, can be reestablished with successful realignment and arthrodesis of the first, second and third TMT and/or NC joints. The fourth and fifth TMT joints are not fused to preserve the accommodation function of the foot.
- Internal fixation of the midfoot articulations has evolved to include screws, staples, and plates specifically indicated for midfoot arthrodesis.
- A tendon-Achilles lengthening is performed first, if necessary, through a triple-stab incision, step-cut fashion.
- A lateral incision over the sinus tarsi is made and carried sharply down through the subcutaneous tissue. Electrocautery was used for hemostasis. The subtalar joint is

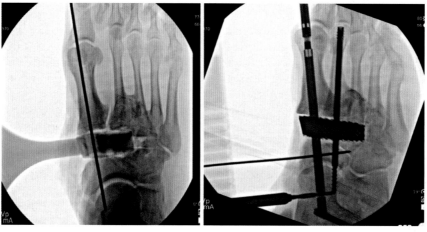

• **Fig. 15.2** Intraoperative midfoot reconstruction with a 3D-printed cage and beaming technique.

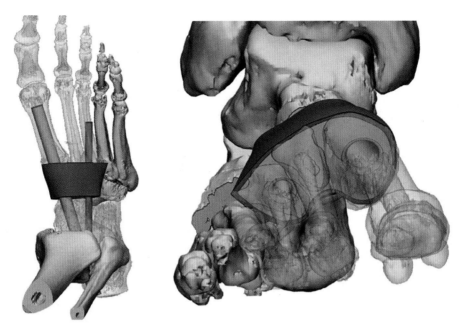

• **Fig. 15.3** Fixation trajectory for intramedullary fixation through the 3D-printed cage provides stability and compression at the bone-implant interfaces. (Reprinted with permission from restor3d, Inc Durham, NC.)

debrided of the articular cartilage with a combination of curettes, chisel, and double-action rongeur in preparation for fusion. A guidewire is placed under fluoroscopic imaging from the plantar aspect of the calcaneus traversing the subtalar joint. Alignment is confirmed and a 7.0 cannulated screw is placed across the joint to complete the subtalar fusion.

• A medial incision is then made across the midfoot and carried down sharply through the subcutaneous tissue. Electrocautery is used for hemostasis. Wedge resection is performed of the tarsal metatarsal articulation and cuneiforms to correct midfoot adductus/abduction, to correct cavus or rocker at the midfoot, and to correct varus/valgus at the hindfoot or ankle. The remaining joint surfaces are prepared for fusion and the 3D wedge guide is placed into the fusion bed. A guidewire is then placed from the metatarsal head, up the metatarsal shaft, through the guide for the 3D cage into the talar head. The talo-first metatarsal deformity correction is confirmed on orthogonal fluoroscopic views. At this point, if there is an abduction deformity a medial-based closing wedge osteotomy is performed, and for a rocker deformity with abduction a plantar-medial closing wedge osteotomy is performed.

• Sequential guidewires are then placed up the second metatarsal through the cage. Bone marrow aspiration is harvested from the proximal tibia via stable incision and added to Trinity as well as local autograft bone to augment the fusion site and cage itself. The cage is appropriately fitted within the talonavicular articulation and between the first metatarsal and navicular. Then for impaction, a mini DynaNail (Medshape Inc, Atlanta, GA) across the medial column is performed with subsequent placement of the screw beam up the second metatarsal, securing both

proximally and distally and then releasing the nitinol tension to get additional compression (Fig. 15.3). An additional independent screw is placed from the dorsal aspect to get additional compression across the talonavicular articulation. Upon completion of the case, alignment on multiple fluoroscopic views of the indwelling hardware with compression across the joints is confirmed. The surgical sites are irrigated copiously with saline and closed in standard layered fashion. A sterile dressing is applied and the patient is transferred to the recovery room in a stable condition after splint placement.

Implant Design and Specifications

• Materials: all implants were fabricated via laser powder bed fusion (L-PBF) of medical-grade titanium alloy (Ti6Al4V ELI) (Fig. 15.4).

• Polished versus rough surfaces: after printing, the implants undergo multiple postprocessing steps before being delivered for surgery. The first of these steps is known as hot isostatic pressing (HIP; "hipping"), a process during which the parts are subjected to both high temperature and pressure to relieve the implants of residual thermal stresses and close any internal voids. Next, the parts undergo microblasting, during which titanium powder is blown at the implant surface under high pressure to remove any partially adhered particles of powder. Finally, the parts are subjected to a chemical passivation process, which results in a thin surface oxide layer that improves the corrosion resistance of the implants.

• Shape: the implants are designed as spheres. This geometry was selected after proving to offer significant intraoperative flexibility in terms of repositioning.

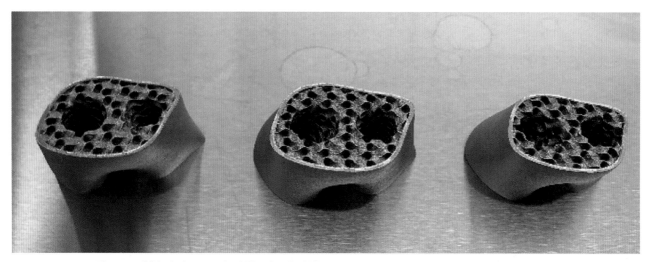

• **Fig. 15.4** Clinical photograph of 3D-printed midfoot cages in three sizes depicting polished and rough surfaces.

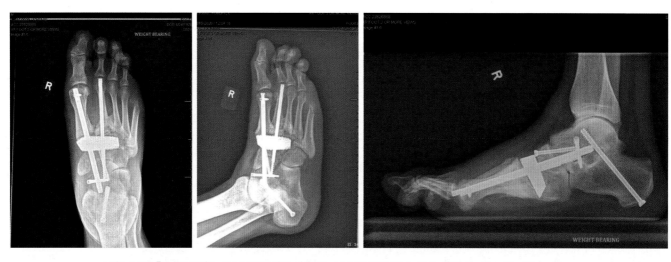

• **Fig. 15.5** Postoperative anteroposterior, oblique, and lateral views of a midfoot reconstruction with a 3D-printed cage and beaming technique.

- Sizing: the surgeon's preference is nominal ±5% to 10%.
- Any other special features: some spherical cage designs were utilized while the remaining cases employed spherical implants with a flattened lateral side to aid in soft tissue closure.
- Corresponding off-the-shelf fixation and how that may influence overall design: the implants were all designed for use with a tibiotalocalcaneal (TTC) fusion nail that is offered in 10- and 12-mm diameter options. All cages were designed with 14-mm cannulations such that they would be able to accommodate either nail size and allow for intraoperative flexibility.

Postoperative Protocol

- Non–weight bearing for a minimum of 6 weeks.
- A soft tissue evaluation and removal of sutures is performed at 2 weeks postoperatively.

- The operative limb is maintained in a short-leg splint versus a cast for 6 weeks for swelling management.
- At the 6-week postoperative visit, three-view ankle X-rays are obtained and the patient is transitioned to a controlled ankle motion (CAM) boot but is to remain non–weight bearing for an additional 6 weeks.
- At 3 months, three-view X-rays of the ankle are obtained and the patient is provided with a physical therapy script for gradual return to full weight bearing, from 10% to 100% and weaning of the CAM boot. Additionally, orthotics is consulted for a molded ankle foot orthosis (MAFO) brace with a normal shoe wear for additional support if needed (Fig. 15.5).

Results/Outcomes

- Early results of select cases are promising. The goals of achieving a stable plantigrade foot that is shoe-able can be quite difficult in any situation. The use of midfoot cages as load sharing along with beaming has made this more achievable in the authors' practice. The struggles with the soft tissue envelope continue, but the boney architecture appears to be more maintainable when using 3D patient–specific technology.

- Complications associated with Charcot midfoot reconstruction include infection, ulceration, recurrence of deformity, nonunion, problems with patient compliance, hardware failure, hardware prominence, and amputation, which may occur using traditional reconstruction methods as well as with 3D printing:
  - Postoperative infection has been reported in up to 10%.[16-18]
  - Nonunion rates range from 0% to 50%.[16-18]
  - Hardware fracture has been reported to range from 0% to 32%, with a higher occurrence in intramedullary screw fixation.[16-18]
  - Hardware prominence can lead to another surgery and had been reported to rage from 0% to 19%.[16-18]
  - Wound complication rates range from 0% to 29%.[16-18]
  - Amputation in the setting of uncontrollable infection has been reported to range from 0% to 10%.[16-18]

Approach/ exposure	Be prepared to make multiple incisions to allow for implant placement but keep in mind soft tissue closure
Soft tissue protection	Consider adding solid and polished portions to the implant in certain areas (dorsal, plantar, lateral, medial) to protect soft tissues
Advanced imaging	Carry out a CT scan as soon as possible close to surgery to avoid anatomic or worsening pathologic changes. The contralateral limb should also be scanned in cases where there is significant hardware, deformity, or defect in the side of interest

PEARLS AND PITFALLS

a. Select cases of symptomatic fourth and fifth tarsometatarsal (TMT) joints arthritis diagnosed using selective corticosteroid joint injections may be treated with interposition arthroplasty, which maintains the lateral column and accommodates gait.

b. TMT joints are 2 to 3 cm deep; full joint preparation must extend to the plantar surface to optimize physiologic alignment and fusion.

c. Care must be taken not to malposition the second and third TMT joints during fusion. Excessive plantar flexion will cause metatarsalgia of the involved ray, and excessive dorsiflexion will cause transfer metatarsalgia of the adjacent rays.

d. Severe deformity may warrant a biplanar midfoot osteotomy in conjunction with arthrodesis, particularly in nonbraceable Charcot midfoot deformity.

e. Given the high prevalence of midfoot arthritis following Lisfranc injury, primary arthrodesis maybe be considered, especially in the setting of associated metatarsal base fractures. Surgical management of arthritis of the midfoot may warrant simultaneous Achilles tendon lengthening and hindfoot realignment.

TIPS AND TRICKS

| Implant options | Always ensure that you have small/undersized (not providing full correction) implant options |
| Fixation options | Consider adding additional fixation options into the implant design if one is not able to be utilized due to alignment issues/soft tissue constraints |

References

1. Pakarinen TK, Laine HJ, Maenpaa H, Mattila P, Lahtela J. Long-term outcome and quality of life in patients with Charcot foot. *Foot Ankle Surg.* 2009;15:187-191.
2. Kroin E, Schiff AP, Pinzur MS, Davis ES, Chaharbakhshi E, DiSilvio FA Jr. Functional impairment of patients undergoing surgical correction for Charcot foot arthropathy. *Foot Ankle Int.* 2017;38:705-709.
3. Raspovic KR, Wukich DK. Self-reported quality of life in patients with diabetes: a comparison of patients with and without Charcot neuroarthropathy. *Foot Ankle Int.* 2014;35:195-200.
4. Hingsammer AM, Bauer D, Renner N, Borbas P, Boeni T, Berli M. Correlation of systemic inflammatory markers with radiographic stages of Charcot osteoarthropathy. *Foot Ankle Int.* 2016;37(9):924-928.
5. Sammarco VJ. Superconstructs in the treatment of Charcot foot deformity: plantar plating, locked plating and axial screw fixation. *Foot Ankle Clin.* 2009;14:393-407.
6. Sinacore DR, Bohnert KL, Smith KE, et al. Persistent inflammation with pedal osteolysis 1 year after Charcot neuropathic osteoarthropathy. *J Diabetes Complications.* 2017;31(6):1014-1020.
7. Zhao H-M, Diao J-Y, Liang X-J, Zhang F, Hao D-J. Pathogenesis and potential relative risk factors of diabetic neuropathic osteoarthropathy. *J Orthop Surg Res.* 2017;12(1):142.
8. Pinzur MS. Current concepts review: Charcot arthropathy of the foot and ankle. *Foot Ankle Int.* 2007;28(8):952-959.
9. Eichenholtz SN. *Charcot Joints.* IL, USA: Springfield; 1966.
10. Classen JN, Rolley RT, Carneiro R, Martire JR. Management of foot conditions of the diabetic patient. *Am Surg.* 1976;42:81-88.
11. Shibata T, Tada K, Hashizume C. The results of arthrodesis of the ankle for leprotic neuroarthropathy. *J Bone Joint Surg Am.* 1990;72:749-756.
12. Schon LC, Marks RM. The management of neuroarthropathic fracture dislocations in the diabetic patient. *Orthop Clin North Am.* 1995;26:375-392.
13. Kroin E, Chaharbakhshi EO, Schiff A, Pinzur MS. Improvement in quality of life following operative correction of midtarsal Charcot foot deformity. *Foot Ankle Int.* 2018;39:808-811.

14. Jones CP. Beaming for Charcot foot reconstruction. *Foot Ankle Int.* 2015;36(7):853-859. doi:10.1177/1071100715588637.

15. Manchanda K, Wallace SB, Ahn J, et al. Charcot midfoot reconstruction: does subtalar arthrodesis or medial column fixation improve outcomes? *J Foot Ankle Surg.* 2020;59(6):1219-1223. doi:10.1053/j.jfas.2020.07.001.

16. Ford SE, Cohen BE, Davis WH, Jones CP. Clinical outcomes and complications of midfoot Charcot reconstruction with intramedullary beaming. *Foot Ankle Int.* 2019;40(1):18-23. doi:10.1177/1071100718799966.

17. Lieberman JR. *AAOS Comprehensive Orthopaedic Review.* Rosemont, IL: American Academy of Orthopaedic Surgeons; 2020.

18. Ha J, Hester T, Foley R, et al. Charcot foot reconstruction outcomes: a systematic review. *J Clin Orthop Trauma.* 2020;11(3): 357-368. doi:10.1016/j.jcot.2020.03.025.

16

A 3D-Printed Solution for Evans Calcaneal Osteotomy Nonunion

ERIC SO, LEE M. HLAD

Definition

- A custom/patient-specific 3D-printed porous metallic spacer for revision of Evans calcaneal osteotomy nonunion.

Anatomy and Pathogenesis

- With Evans calcaneal osteotomy the foot follows the displacement of the calcaneocuboid joint, suggesting that the long plantar ligament acts as a pivot, the talonavicular joint as the axis of rotation, and the spring ligament as a hinge.
- This 3D movement allows the peroneus longus tendon to recover its plantarflexory effect on the first metatarsal. These changes and the recovery of the windlass mechanism of the plantar fascia increase the bowstring effect, which restores the longitudinal arch and increases the stability of the osteotomy.[1]
- The rich vascularization of the calcaneus and press-fit nature of the graft allows for a relatively low rate of nonunion.
- In a systematic review of 73 feet with a mean age of 22 years and an average follow-up of 3.6 years, Prissel and Roukis found that the incidence of nonunion in unfixated Evans osteotomies was 1.4%.[2] Other studies have shown similar incidences, as Haeseker et al. reported a nonunion rate of 5.3%.[3]
- Other complications of the Evans calcaneal osteotomy include[1,4]:
  - Dorsal displacement of the anterior calcaneal tuberosity
  - Lateral column pain
  - Loss of calcaneal lengthening
  - Overcorrection
  - Undercorrection.
- Structures at risk[5]:
  - The sural nerve
  - Peroneal tendons
  - Anterior and middle facets of the subtalar joint.

Patient History and Physical Exam Findings

- Assess for location of pain.
- Assess the function of the posterior tibial tendon.
- Assess for undercorrected or recurrent forefoot varus, hindfoot valgus, medial ankle instability, subfibular impingement, or forefoot abduction.
- Assess the range of motion to the subtalar, talonavicular, and ankle joints.
- Assess for contractures to the gastrocsoleus and peroneal tendons.
- Obtain prior operative records to understand the size of graft used and type of hardware implanted.

Imaging

- Radiographs: nonunion may be represented by[6]:
  - lack of callus and/or trabeculation along osteotomy site (Fig. 16.1)
  - bony sclerosis
  - loss of correction of the hindfoot joints
  - subluxation/dislocation of the capital fragment
  - hardware failure.
- CT is useful in assessing for the presence of nonunion, implant loosening, and overall alignment of the hindfoot:
  - CT is helpful in surgical planning and procedure selection.
  - Currently, CT is the imaging modality of choice if 3D printing technology is being utilized.[7]

Nonoperative Management

- Shoe modification: a wide, rigid toe box
- Orthotics/shoe modifications
- Immobilization
- Rest, ice, compression, and elevation (RICE) therapy and nonsteroidal antiinflammatory drugs
- Bone stimulator for the treatment of aseptic nonunion.

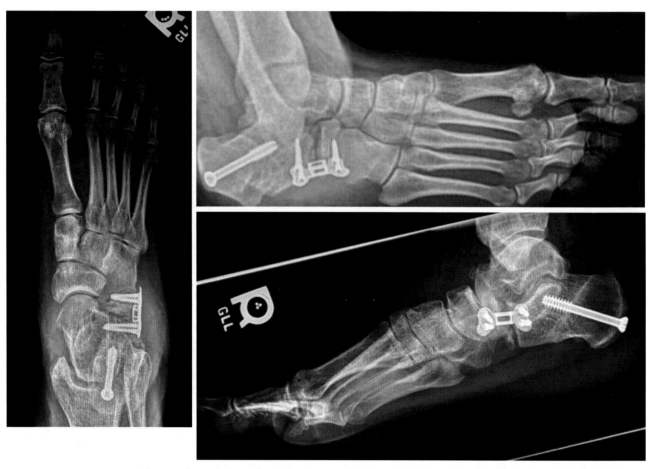

• **Fig. 16.1** Preoperative radiographs of a nonunion of an Evans calcaneal osteotomy.

Traditional Surgical Management

- Revision:
  - Results in retained motion through the talonavicular and subtalar joints.
  - Must consider the size of the prior graft.
  - Must consider local anatomic constraints such as the calcaneocuboid joint.
  - Autograft may be obtained from the iliac crest; however, donor site morbidity is a significant concern.
  - Cancellous autograft from the distal or proximal tibia.
  - Allograft and other biologics may be considered.
- Revision with calcaneocuboid joint arthrodesis:
  - Due to the location of the Evans calcaneal osteotomy, a revision may require inclusion of the calcaneocuboid joint for adequate bone stock and fixation purchase.
  - This results in limited range of motion through the talonavicular and subtalar joints by 48% and 30%, respectively.[8]
- Triple arthrodesis:
  - Allows for correction of any residual hindfoot deformity, particularly if there is degenerative arthritic disease or if the deformity has become rigid.

- Allows a stable, plantigrade hindfoot during weight bearing.
- Sacrifices motion through the hindfoot.
- May be performed in combination with revision of the osteotomy.
- Ancillary procedures:
  - Consider the need to perform a gastrocnemius recession, Cotton osteotomy, posterior tibial tendon debridement and repair, FDL tendon transfer, peroneal brevis lengthening, or spring or deltoid ligament reconstruction to address any residual deformity.

3D-Printed Implant and Instrumentation Considerations

- Titanium has been shown to have osteoconductive properties and is biologically inert, therefore titanium is the material of choice[9,10]:
  - Pore size has been described in the literature from 300 to 1000 μm.[11]
  - Truss configurations provide the greatest strength with the least mass. These allow for a mechanically robust construct that resists the load-bearing forces of the foot and ankle. The truss configuration acts as

a lattice for bone grafting and other orthobiologic material.[12]

- The 3D configuration of the implant must be designed to allow it to be successfully implanted through the planned surgical exposure, cognizant of the constraints imposed by the local anatomy and previous implants.[12]
- The length of the implant is case specific and based on the proposed resection level. The length of osseous deficit after resection of nonviable bone and preparation for fusion determines the nominal length. Custom cutting guides may be created and used to ensure the resection is accurate.
- Degree of porosity: the percentage of porosity is inversely proportional to implant strength. This should be considered during implant design.
  - A rectangular/trapezoidal-shaped implant is recommended (Fig. 16.2), which promotes a larger surface area for fusion and enhanced interposition of the implant to bone.
  - Inherent stability is provided by the rough texture, which enhances friction at the bone-implant interface, thereby resisting torsional forces.
  - The porous surface is in direct contact with the adjacent bone and areas of smooth/polished surfaces to prevent soft tissue ingrowth and contracture.
- Diameter, width, length, and height are patient specific and based on the size at the proposed resection level (Fig. 16.3).
  - The implant can be designed with screw holes to allow direct implant to bone fixation; however, the more screws used, the less surface area available for bone ingrowth and fusion.
- A preoperative CT is obtained to guide surgical planning.
  - Images as scanned are used to gain an appreciation for the amount of bone resection required (Fig. 16.4).

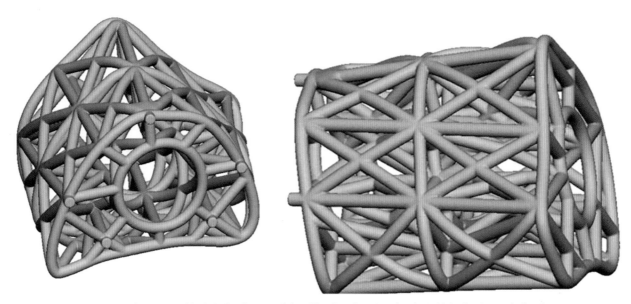

• **Fig. 16.2** Computer-aided design image of the 3D-printed custom implant. Note the truss design to serve as a lattice for osseous incorporation through the implant. (Reprinted with permission from 4WEDB Medical, Frisco, TX.)

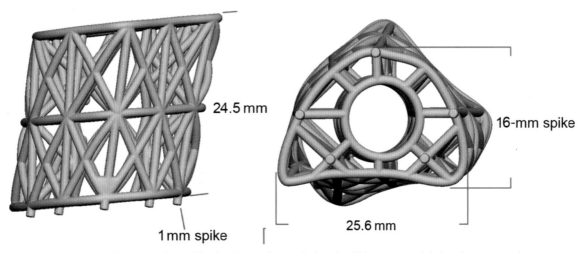

24.5 mm

1 mm spike

16-mm spike

25.6 mm

• **Fig. 16.3** The dimensions of the implant and screw holes should be measured during the preoperative planning stage. (Reprinted with permission from 4WEDB Medical, Frisco, TX.)

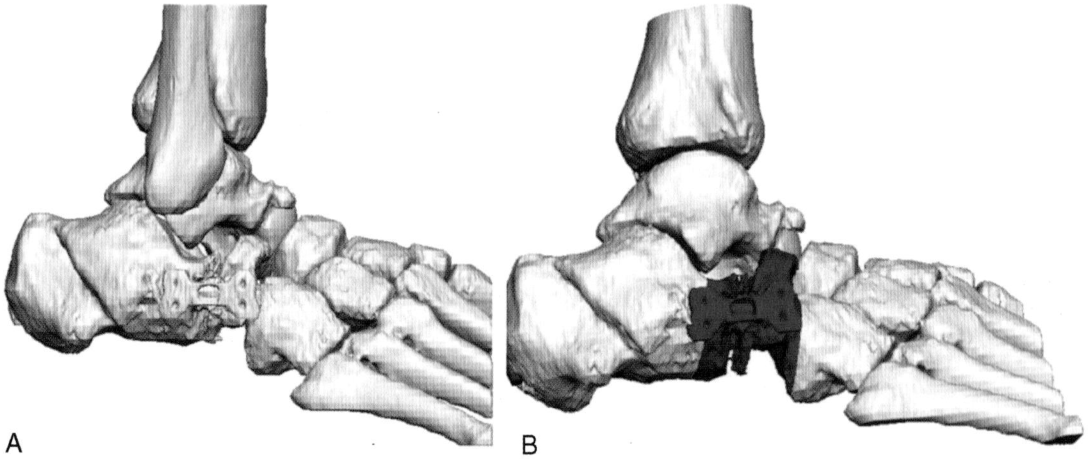

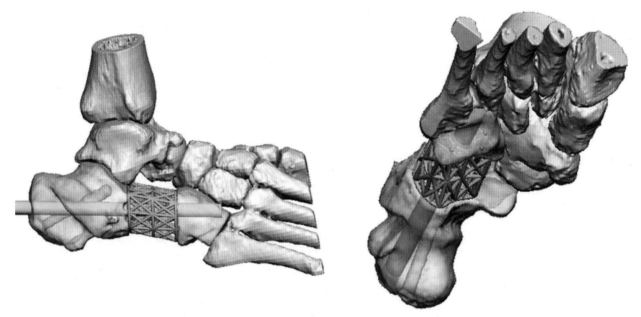

A   B

• **Fig. 16.4** Preoperative computer-aided design image depicting the nonunion of the first tarsometatarsal joint with the presence of (A) hardware and (B) the planned osseous resection *(red)*. (Reprinted with permission from 4WEDB Medical, Frisco, TX.)

• **Fig. 16.5** Preoperative computer-aided design images demonstrating the accurate trajectory for the intramedullary fixation. (Reprinted with permission from 4WEDB Medical, Frisco, TX.)

- Consider the trajectory of screw placement. Important considerations are local anatomy, anticipated surgical exposure, and internal fixation options. Fixation can include retrograde nails, plates, or screws, or a combination thereof. Compression should be achieved across the implant. Fixation should provide stability and compression but also not provide a source of prominence or soft tissue impingement.
- In the case of a revision of Evans nonunion, primary fixation should compose of intramedullary fixation through the implant. A 7.0-mm diameter screw

should be considered. Longitudinal fixation will resist shear and bending forces. Secondary fixation may compose of spanning fixation from the calcaneus to the cuboid to resist torsional forces; however soft tissue constraints (i.e., peroneal tendons) should be taken into consideration (Fig. 16.5).
- If intramedullary fixation is planned, an outrigger trajectory guide should be manufactured to allow precise and accurate placement of intramedullary fixation (Fig. 16.6). The guide should be able to accommodate the guide pin used for the cannulated screw fixation.

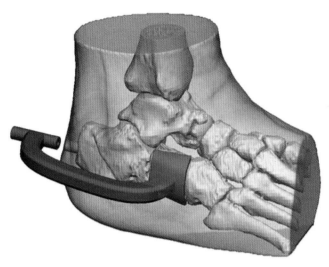

• **Fig. 16.6** Preoperative computer-aided design images depicting the outrigger trajectory guide. (Reprinted with permission from 4WEDB Medical, Frisco, TX.)

Surgical Management With 3D-Printed Devices

- Off-the-shelf items required:
  - A sagittal saw to resect the bone at the appropriate level.
  - A 2.0-mm solid core drill bit to fenestrate either bone ends to promote osseous ingrowth.
  - Biologics, bone allograft and/or autograft harvester per the surgeon's preferences to promote osteoconduction, osteoinduction and osteogenesis.
  - A distractor.
- Positioning: supine with an ipsilateral bump.
- Anesthesia: general with regional blockade.
- Approach: lateral; however, consider placement of preexisting incisions or previous surgical wounds.
- Technique:
  - Expose the osteotomy and nonunion site. Remove any preexisting hardware.
  - Obtain adequate visualization of the nonunion site and calcaneocuboid joint. The peroneal tendons and sural nerve should be retracted throughout the procedure.
  - A Reamer-Irrigator-Aspirator (DePuy Synthes, Warsaw, IN) from the femur may be considered to obtain autogenous graft that may be packed within the porous structure of the 3D-printed implant. This may be augmented with allogeneic orthobiologics.
  - Use a sagittal saw to perform bone resection at the preplanned level. Excise nonviable bone. Ensure the presence of healthy, viable bone in the calcaneus and cuboid.
  - At this time a trial is inserted into the defect, which should be press fitted into the defect. Use the trial to ensure that the implant-bone interface is perfectly matched. If a perfect fit is not obtained, make certain that all debris and interposing soft tissue is removed.

Now remove the trial and pack the implant with the desired biologics. Insert the implant into the defect.
- Next, utilize the outrigger guide to place the guide pin from the posterior aspect of the calcaneus through the implant and into the cuboid. Utilize fluoroscopy to judge the placement of the implant and alignment of the hindfoot. At this point, a cannulated drill is used to drill through the calcaneus, implant, and cuboid. An appropriate-length 7.0-mm screw is inserted from posterior to anterior. It is the surgeon's discretion to use a large cannulated screw or to exchange the cannulated wire for a solid core screw. The screw should obtain purchase, compression, and stability into the cuboid.
- Test the stability and position directly and under fluoroscopy.
- Perform the aforementioned ancillary procedure as needed.
- Closure and bandaging per the surgeon's protocol.

Postoperative Protocol

- Non–weight bearing in a splint for 1 to 2 week(s).
- Non–weight bearing in a short-leg cast for 2 to 6 weeks.
- Non–weight bearing in a controlled ankle motion (CAM) boot for 6 to 12 weeks.
- Weight bearing as tolerated in a CAM boot for 12 to 24 weeks.
- Weight bearing as tolerated in a stiff-soled shoe from 24 to 52 weeks.
- CT scan obtained at 12 months postoperatively.

Results/Outcomes

- Lack of pain, clinical stability, and radiographic consolidation should be achieved prior to transitioning to weight bearing (Fig. 16.7).
- A 12-month postoperative CT scan shows adequate bony ingrowth surrounding the implant, and no signs of hardware failure or stress shielding (Fig. 16.8).
- Ensure any infection is eradicated prior to utilizing this technique. Follow proper infectious disease guidelines and surgical principles to clear infection prior to implantation and final reconstruction of the bone defect.
- Possible complications:
  - Infection
  - Nonunion/malunion
  - Hardware failure
  - Deep venous thrombosis
  - Wound complication
  - Deformity
  - Stress fracture of the fifth metatarsal.
- Previously published results:
  - So E, Mandas V, Hlad L. Large osseous defect reconstruction using a custom three-dimensional printed titanium truss implant. *J Foot Ankle Surg.* 2018; 57(1): 196-204.

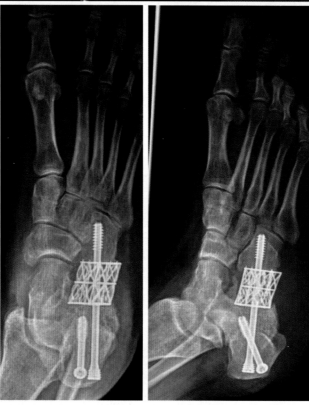

• **Fig. 16.7** Postoperative radiographs demonstrating appropriate alignment of the hindfoot and midfoot, osseous consolidation, and stable hardware.

PEARLS AND PITFALLS

Indications and contraindications	• Osseous deficits of the anterior process of the calcaneus after Evans osteotomy nonunion • Contraindicated in patients with sensory neuropathy, active infection, and peripheral arterial disease • Active infection must be cleared prior to insertion of the implant
Implant design	• Titanium appears to be the ideal material • Implant shape and porosity should provide inherent stability and enhance bony ingrowth • Use CT and CAD images to determine implant size, shape after bony resection • Screw holes for direct fixation should be easy to access • Consider local anatomy with regards to internal fixation options • Consider intramedullary fixation along the long axis of the implant
Surgical technique	• Ensure all compromised and nonviable bone is removed • Use instrumentation that replicates the shape and size of the implant to promote optimal bone-implant contact • An ideal implant size yields physiologic tension of the adjacent soft tissues and inherent stability, and restores the length relationship of the hindfoot without compromising neurovascular structures • Utilize outrigger trajectory guides to ensure accurate placement of internal fixation through the implant • Utilize autogenous bone grafting when possible and supplement with allograft orthobiologics as needed

CAD, Computer-aided design.

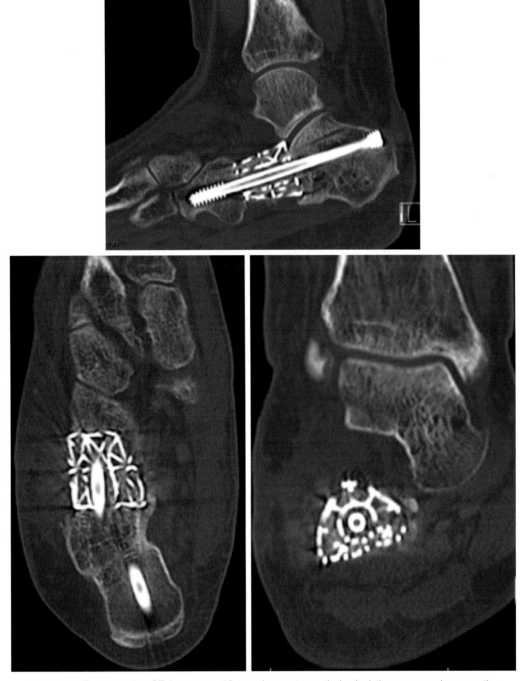

• **Fig. 16.8** Postoperative CT images at 12 months postoperatively depicting osseous incorporation through the implant and union across the calcaneocuboid joint.

References

1. Jara M. Evans osteotomy complications. *Foot Ankle Clin.* 2017; (22):573-585.
2. Prissel M, Roukis T. Incidence of nonunion of the unfixated, isolated Evans calcaneal osteotomy: a systematic review. *J Foot Ankle Surg.* 2012;51(3):323-325.
3. Haeseker G, Mureau M, Faber F. Lateral column lengthening for acquired adult flatfoot deformity caused by posterior tibial tendon dysfunction stage II: a retrospective comparison of calcaneus osteotomy with calcaneocuboid distraction arthrodesis. *J Foot Ankle Surg.* 2010;49(4):380-384.
4. Thomas R, Wells B, Garrison R, et al. Preliminary results comparing two methods of lateral column lengthening. *Foot Ankle Int.* 2001;22(2):107-119.
5. Bussewitz B, DeVries J, Hyer C. Evans osteotomy and risk to subtalar joint articular facets and sustentaculum tali: a cadaver study. *J Foot Ankle Surg.* 2013;52(5):594-597.
6. Agarwal A. Principles of nonunions. In: *Nonunions.* Boston, MA: Springer; 2018:1-43.
7. Dekker TJ, Steele JR, Federer AE, Hamid KS, Adams SB Jr. Use of patient-specific 3D-printed titanium implants for complex foot and ankle limb salvage, deformity correction, and arthrodesis procedures. *Foot Ankle Int.* 2018;39(8):916-921.

8. Deland J, Otis J, Lee K, et al. Lateral column lengthening with calcaneocuboid fusion: range of motion in the triple joint complex. *Foot Ankle Int.* 1995;16(11):729-733.

9. Takemoto M, Fujibayashi S, Neo M, Suzuki J, Kokubo T, Nakamura T. Mechanical properties and osteoconductivity of porous bioactive titanium. *Biomaterials.* 2005;26(30):6014-6023.

10. de Wild M, Schumacher R, Mayer K, et al. Bone regeneration by the osteoconductivity of porous titanium implants manufactured by selective laser melting: a histological and micro computed tomography study in the rabbit. *Tissue Eng Part A.* 2013;19(23):2645-2654.

11. Taniguchi N, Fubiyashi S, Takemoto M, et al. Effect of pore size on bone ingrowth into porous titanium implants fabricated by additive manufacturing: an in vivo experiment. *Mater Sci Eng C Mater Biol Appl.* 2016;59:690-701.

12. So E, Mandas V, Hlad L. Large osseous defect reconstruction using a custom three-dimensional printed titanium truss implant. *J Foot Ankle Surg.* 2018;57(1):196-204.

17

3D-Printed Total Cuboid Replacement for Lateral Column Pathology

PAUL R. LEATHAM, PETER D. HIGHLANDER

Definition

- Excision of the cuboid in total, which is then replaced with a metallic, patient-specific 3D-printed implant.

Indications

- Posttraumatic arthritis located at the cuboid and associated articulations.[1-4]
- A shortened lateral column, typically from prior trauma, with compression cuboid fractures.[1-4]
- Avascular necrosis of the cuboid.[1-4]

Anatomy

- The cuboid has a pyramid morphology with a medial base and apex laterally.[5] The cuboid is unique as it articulates with the metatarsals as well as directly with the calcaneus[6] (Figs. 17.1 and 17.2).
- Multiple articulations with different osseous surfaces are present, including distal, proximal, and medial. There is significant ligamentous attachment including long and short plantar ligaments.[7,8]
- The peroneal groove is located anterolaterally and the peroneal longus courses around towards its insertion at the plantar 1st metatarsal base.[9]
- The cuboid is a biomechanical anchor and allows for adaptive accommodation provided from the lateral column.[9,10]

Pathogenesis

- Loss of length to the lateral column can affect the foot's shock absorption and mobile adaptation, which can increase stress to adjacent joints[11,12] (Figs. 17.3 to 17.5).
- Valgus stress causes compression of the cuboid.[13]
- Direct crush injuries to the cuboid have been described after motor vehicle accidents, horseback riding, and direct loading of heavy weight.[14,15]

- Cuboid fracture, or posttraumatic arthritis, is commonly indicative of a complex midfoot injury including involvement of the navicular, cuneiforms, and/or the Lisfranc joint complex.[5,16,17]
- Disturbance in lateral column length can lead to forefoot abduction, lateral subluxation of the tarsometatarsal joints, and pes planus.[18-21]
- Compensatory biomechanics from altered native anatomy can cause a variety of foot deformities and include posttraumatic arthritis.[17,22-25] In the same manner, tendinopathy may result in secondary altered biomechanics of the peroneal groove.[9]

Patient History and Physical Exam Findings

- Patients complain of pain along the plantar and dorsal aspect of the lateral column, to the 4th or 5th metatarsal articulations, as well as articulation with the calcaneus.[26]
- Pain may be exacerbated with propulsion in gait, with the increased demand causing stress along the lateral column.
- A previous history of trauma to the midfoot is common among patients with complaints of lateral column pain.
- Corticosteroid injections with/without fluoroscopic guidance can provide temporary relief; however, they do not eliminate symptoms.

Imaging and Other Diagnostic Testing

- Radiographs often demonstrate osteophyte formation, which represent arthritic changes to the cuboid's articulations.
- A contralateral radiograph can be useful to compare lengths of the lateral column.
- Advanced imaging, including CT scan, can assist in further analysis of arthritic changes, cyst formation, and changes in osseous morphology.

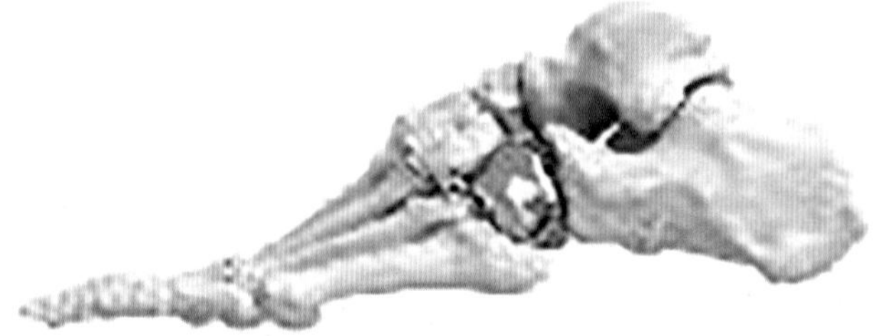

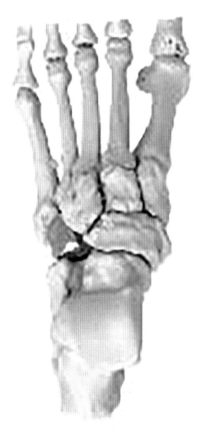

• **Fig. 17.1** Lateral view of a total cuboid replacement model. (Reprinted with permission from Paragon 28, Inc, Englewood, CO)

• **Fig. 17.2** Anteroposterior view of a total cuboid replacement model. (Reprinted with permission from Paragon 28, Inc, Englewood, CO)

Nonoperative Management

- Conservative treatment is warranted prior to consideration for surgical intervention, although oftentimes relief is minimal when posttraumatic arthritic changes are significant and advanced[27]:
  - Rest, ice, compression, and elevation (RICE)
  - Activity modification
  - Shoe modification
  - Bracing
  - Custom ankle foot orthoses (i.e., Arizona)
  - Athletic ankle-stabilizing orthoses
  - Shoe inserts (over the counter vs. custom)
  - Oral or topical nonsteroidal antiinflammatories.

Traditional Surgical Management

- Corrective osteotomy (i.e., opening wedge cuboid osteotomy).
- Lateral column lengthening ± calcaneal cuboid arthrodesis.[28]
- Calcaneocuboid arthrodesis may affect adjacent joints and decrease the mean range of motion to the talonavicular joint (TNJ) by 33% and the subtalar joint by 8%.[6,29]
- Fourth and 5th tarsometatarsal arthrodesis.[30]
- Interpositional arthroplasty.[31]
- Traditional surgical management often includes arthrodesis but elimination of motion in the highly mobile lateral column can be problematic. If the majority of the pathology is isolated to the cuboid and articulation to the 4th or 5th metatarsal, interpositional arthroplasty has traditionally provided relief. In the author's opinion and experience, patients do well after an interpositional arthroplasty for about a year and then often symptoms begin to return. Opening wedge osteotomy or calcaneal lateral lengthening osteotomy could increase articulation pressures, resulting in increasing arthritic symptoms. In addition, osteotomies and/or arthrodesis include risks of high nonunion rates. Replacing the cuboid with a patient-specific implant restores the native length of the lateral column as well as allows motion at both the tarsometatarsal and calcaneocuboid joints. Preservation of motion provides more opportunity for decreased stress adjacent to the joint in comparison to arthrodesis.[6,30]

3D-Printed Implant Design Specification and Considerations

- A 3D-printed implant for cuboid pathology allows specific and precise determination of the degree of lateral column shortening.
- Obtain a CT scan of the contralateral foot to create an inverted variant for nominal anatomy of the affected cuboid.
- The implant material can vary depending on the surgeon's preference. The implant seen throughout this chapter is made from titanium alloy (Ti6Al4V). Cobalt chromium (CoCr) is also readily available a common implant printing material.
- The implant is anchored into the lateral aspect of the lateral cuneiform via porous pegs.
- Additional fixation can be designed into the implant, including hole clearances for screw fixation. The design is patient specific to facilitate additional adjunctive procedures (Fig. 17.6).
- The medial surface of the implant is designed for osseous integration via a porous scaffold for increased stability (see Fig. 17.6).

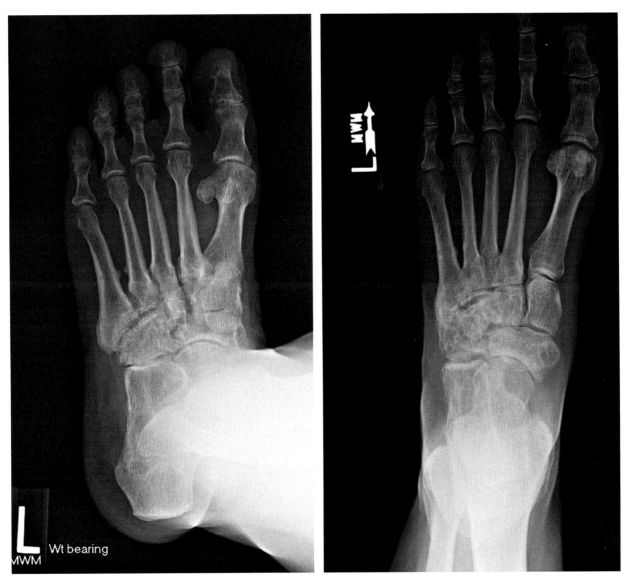

• **Fig. 17.3** Medial oblique and anteroposterior view of preoperative radiographs demonstrating a shortened lateral column and associated posttraumatic degenerative changes from a previous midfoot and cuboid injury.

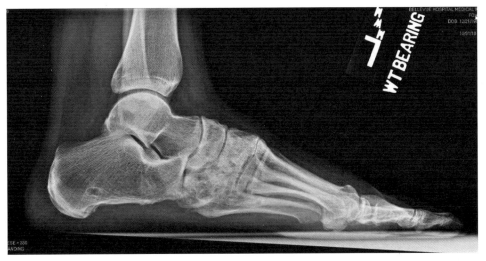

• **Fig. 17.4** Lateral view of preoperative radiographs demonstrating posttraumatic degenerative changes from a previous midfoot and cuboid injury.

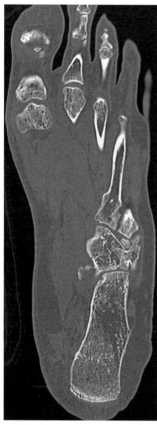

• **Fig. 17.5** Coronal CT scan of the foot demonstrating a compressed cuboid with multiple osseous cystic formations.

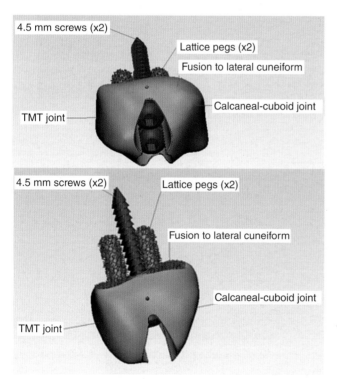

• **Fig. 17.6** Computer-aided design image of projected cuboid implants demonstrating lattice pegs and hole clearance with 4.5-mm screws for additional fixation. *TMT,* tarsometatarsal joint (Reprinted with permission from Paragon 28, Inc, Englewood, CO)

- The pore size is designed to facilitate osseous integration, and there is a range available to choose from for pore size.
- We prefer medium-sized pores, which are easily packed with bone graft and biologics but also enhance graft retention.
- The remaining surfaces, including the proximal and distal articulations, utilize a highly polished surface.
- The peroneal groove is designed with a polished surface. Eyelets (loop holes) for soft tissue attachment can be accommodated in the implant design (Figs. 17.7 and 17.8).
- Trial guides, with corresponding drill holes for pegs (Fig. 17.9). Although not pictured, radioopaque trial guides provide the benefit of easy visualization prior to implantation.
- Trial guides ±5% to 10% from nominal. In the authors' experience, the majority of final implants are nominal in size.
- Harvested bone autograft morselized and packed into the porous surface. Utilization of the Hensler Bone press condylar technique allows for easy handling and packing into the porous aspect of the implant.

Surgical Management With 3D-Printed Devices

- The surgeon's preference is general anesthesia with a preoperative regional nerve block.
- The surgical approach is best achieved through the supine position with a hip bump.
- Incision planning should be well planned in accordance with adjunctive procedures planned to be performed. However, direct visualization of the cuboid is vital to the procedure. An incision is made from the distal tip of the lateral malleolus extending to the dorsal aspect of the base of 5th metatarsal. An additional incision in-between the 2nd and 3rd tarsometatarsal joints allows for excellent exposure for adjunctive procedures as well and additional increased visualization of the lateral aspect of the lateral cuneiform.
- We recommend the use of a bone saw with osteotomes for excision of native cuboid. A bone rongeur can assist with the removal of smaller osseous fragments to ensure removal of the entire cuboid. Careful attention is needed to appropriately retract and protect the surrounding soft tissues, including the peroneal longus and brevis tendons.
- Sizing trial guides can be manufactured from a polymer, with barium sulfate allowing precise visualization on intraoperative fluoroscopy.
- Caution is required in order to select an appropriately sized implant, finding the correct balance between stability but also allowing range of motion. If an implant is selected that is too small, may create additional motion

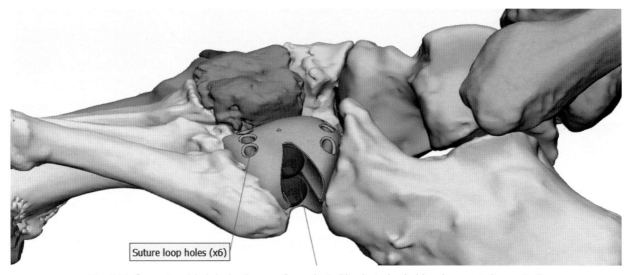

Suture loop holes (x6)

• **Fig. 17.7** Computer-aided design image of a projected implanted cuboid replacement demonstrating designed suture loop holes for soft tissue if desired. (Reprinted with permission from Paragon 28, Inc, Englewood, CO)

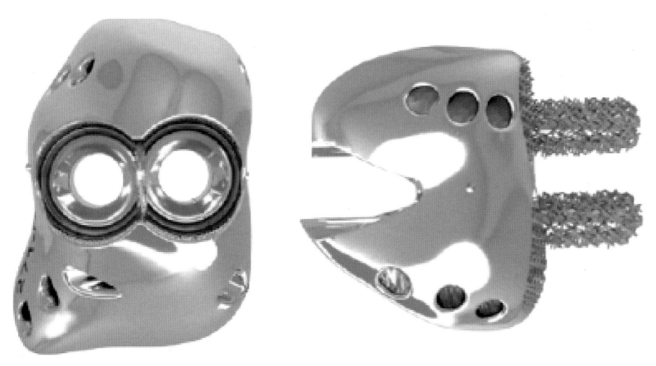

• **Fig. 17.8** Computer-aided design image of polished articular surfaces, porous pegs, soft tissue eyelets, and screw hole clearances. (Reprinted with permission from Paragon 28, Inc, Englewood, CO)

of the implant that may contribute to failure. On the other hand, if an implant is too large, this may affect the range of motion to the proximal and distal articulations of the cuboid.

• Drill holes for pegs are performed through the trial guide once the size has been selected.

• Trabecular lattice, including the pegs, is packed with morselized bone autograft. The implant is carefully tamped into position with the insertion of pegs into previously drilled peg holes (see Fig. 17.9).

• If additional screw fixation is desired, drill holes now can be drilled through the implant (Fig. 17.10).

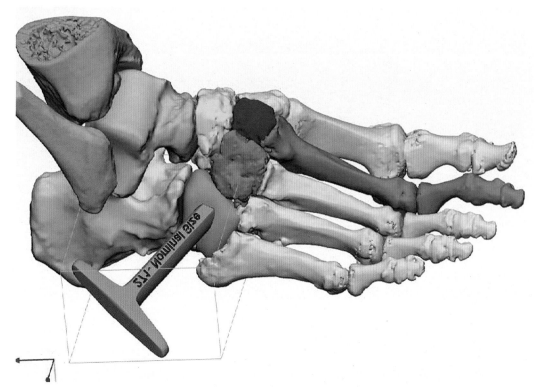

• **Fig. 17.9** Computer-aided design image demonstrating a trial implant with an easy-to-position handle. (Reprinted with permission from Paragon 28, Inc, Englewood, CO)

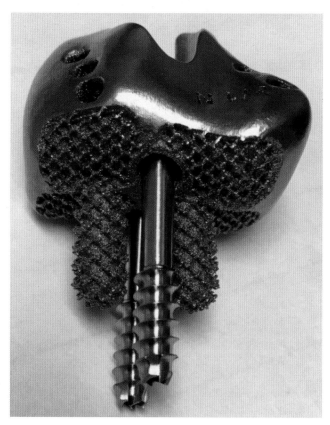

• **Fig. 17.10** Image of a 3D-printed cuboid demonstrating porous pegs, a trabecular lattice, and additional screw fixation through the implant. (Reprinted with permission from Paragon 28, Inc, Englewood, CO)

- Common adjunctive procedures are variable based on the patient's presentation, such as adjacent tarsometatarsal arthrodesis, intercuneiform arthrodesis, use of harvested autograft, and/or bone marrow aspirate concentrate.
- There is a fine balance to be achieved between implant stability/fixation and the opportunity for ingrowth of bone into the trabecular lattice of the implant. The morphology of adjacent bones, in particular the lateral cuneiform, also needs to be taken into account. If multiple points of fixation into the lateral cuneiform are needed, this may affect its viability. If there is not enough bone stock within the lateral cuneiform, there could be the potential for bone resorption after the insertion of multiple points of fixation.

Postoperative Protocol

- Initially the patient is placed into a well-padded posterior splint, non–weight bearing (NWB).
- The patient is placed into a short-leg cast at 1-week follow-up and then transitioned to a controlled ankle motion (CAM) boot at week 3, with NWB maintained.
- Protective weight bearing can begin with the use of a CAM boot 8 weeks postoperatively.
- At 12 weeks follow-up the patient can transition to normal shoe gear with the assistance of an ankle-stabilizing orthosis (ASO) brace, but with no higher impact/demand activities.

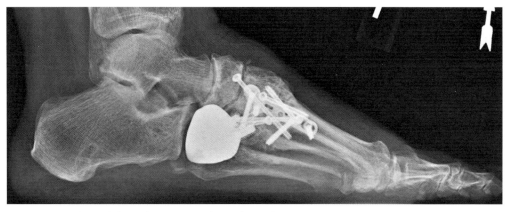

• **Fig. 17.12** Lateral view of a postoperative radiograph at 1-year follow-up demonstrating maintained cuboid height with an appropriate articulating position with the calcaneus.

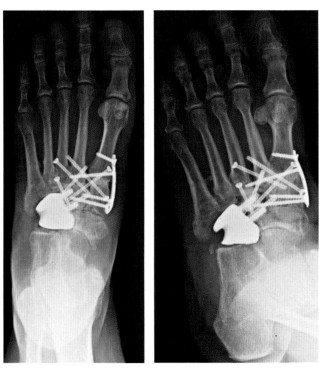

• **Fig. 17.11** One-year postoperative follow-up radiographs demonstrating stable fixation of a cuboid implant into the midfoot with the length of the lateral column maintained.

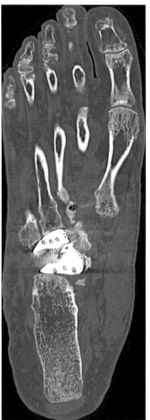

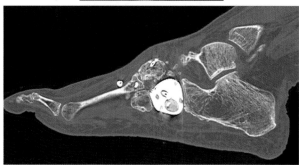

• **Fig. 17.13** Coronal and sagittal views of a postoperative CT scan at 1 year showing evidence of osseous integration to the medial face of the cuboid implant, as well as maintained anatomic position and restored lateral column length.

- At 6 months the patient can begin to transition to higher demand activities (i.e., a longer period of standing/prolonged walking).
- X-rays should be obtained at every postoperative visit, with the exception of the first postoperative visit (Figs. 17.11 and 17.12).
- CT scans should be obtained immediately postoperatively and at 3, 6, and 12 months after operation. These are used to evaluate for bony ingrowth and incorporation of the implant (Fig. 17.13).

Summary (Table 17.1)

TABLE 17.1	Recommendation Summary for 3D-Printed Total Cuboid Replacement for Lateral Column Pathology
Indications	Prior cuboid trauma with a residual shortened lateral column Pain Avascular necrosis of the cuboid
Goal of reconstruction	Restore length, alignment, and rotation Pain relief Improve function and associated articulations
Imaging	A preoperative CT scan is necessary for implant planning and assessment of bone quality A contralateral CT scan is necessary for native morphologic implant planning
Labs/work up	It is important to rule out metabolic and infectious causes of nonunion or implant arthroplasty failure
Design	The implant material should contain characteristics for osseous integration into its surface and be compatible with native cartilage articulation. Additional clearances in the implant for screw fixation are recommended. Eyelets for potential soft tissue augmentation are easy to accommodate and can provide additional stability
Implantation	The authors recommend using Hintermann retractors to maintain the opening of the lateral column while completing implantation
Fixation	The authors recommend direct fixation consisting of both pegs and additional screws. The pegs provide a trabecular lattice for osseous integration

PEARLS AND PITFALLS

Implant design	• Multiple metals are available as the implant material, most commonly used are titanium alloy (Ti6Al4V) or cobalt chromium (CoCr) • The shape and porosity if the implant should provide inherent stability and enhance bony ingrowth • Use CT and CAD images to determine the nominal implant size in all planes • Screw holes for direct fixation should be easy to access and allow clearance • Direct fixation is achieved with pegs, which provide trabecular lattice or porosity for osseous integration • Eyelets can be incorporated for potential eyelet augmentation
Surgical technique	• Ensure all compromised bone is removed • Use instrumentation that replicates the shape and size of the implant to promote optimal bone-implant contact • Drill direct fixation for screws and pegs through trial implants • The ideal implant size yields physiologic tension of the adjacent soft tissues, inherent stability, and restores the length of the lateral column without compromising neurovascular structures

CAD, Computer-aided design.

References

1. Blumberg K, Patterson RJ. Fractures of the cuboid bone in toddlers. *Pediatr Radiol.* 1999;29(7):563.
2. Blumberg K, Patterson RJ. The toddler's cuboid fracture. *Radiology.* 1991;179(1):93-94.
3. Beaman DN, Roeser WM, Holmes JR, Saltzman CL. Cuboid stress fractures: a report of two cases. *Foot Ankle.* 1993;14(9):525-528.
4. Greaney RB, Gerber FH, Laughlin RL, et al. Distribution and natural history of stress fractures in U.S. Marine recruits. *Radiology.* 1983;146(2):339-346.
5. Borrelli J Jr, De S, VanPelt M. Fracture of the cuboid. *J Am Acad Orthop Surg.* 2012;20(7):472-477.
6. Astion DJ, Deland JT, Otis JC, Kenneally S. Motion of the hind foot after simulated arthrodesis. *J Bone Joint Surg Am.* 1997;79(2):241-246.
7. Sarrafian S. Osteology. *Anatomy of the Foot and Ankle.* Hagerstown: 2nd ed. Lippincott; 1993:65-70.
8. Huang CK, Kitaoka HB, An KN, Chao EY. Biomechanical evaluation of longitudinal arch stability. *Foot Ankle.* 1993;14(6):353-357.
9. Engelmann E, Rammelt S, Schepers T. Fractures of the cuboid bone. *JBJS Rev.* 2020;8(4):173.
10. Clements JR, Dijour F, Leong W. Surgical management navicular and cuboid fractures. *Clin Podiatr Med Surg.* 2018;35(2):145-159.
11. Hansen S. *Functional Reconstruction of the Foot and Ankle.* Hagerstown: Lippincott; 2000.
12. Rammelt S, Zwipp H, Hansen S. Posttraumatic reconstruction of the foot and ankle. In: *Skeletal Trauma.* Philadelphia PA: Elsevier Saunders; 2019:2641-2690.
13. Enns P, Pavlidis T, Stahl JP, Horas U, Schnettler R. Sonographic detection of an isolated cuboid bone fracture not visualized on plain radiographs. *J Clin Ultrasound.* 2004;32(3):154-157.
14. Angoules AG, Angoules NA, Georgoudis M, Kapetanakis S. Update on diagnosis and management of cuboid fractures. *World J Orthop.* 2019;10(2):71-80.

15. Chen JB. Cuboid stress fracture. A case report. *J Am Podiatr Med Assoc.* 1993;83(3):153-155.

16. Court-Brown CM, Zinna S, Ekrol I. Classification and epidemiology of mid-foot fractures. *The Foot.* 2006;16(3):138-141.

17. Main BJ, Jowett RL. Injuries of the midtarsal joint. *J Bone Joint Surg Br.* 1975;57(1):89-97.

18. Rammelt S, Zwipp H, Schneiders W, Heineck J. Anatomical reconstruction of malunited Chopart joint injuries. *Eur J Trauma Emerg Surg.* 2010;36(3):196-205.

19. Schneiders W, Rammelt S. Joint-sparing corrections of malunited Chopart joint injuries. *Foot Ankle Clin.* 2016;21(1):147-160.

20. Brunet JA, Wiley JJ. The late results of tarsometatarsal joint injuries. *J Bone Joint Surg Br.* 1987;69(3):437-440.

21. Thordarson D, Tornetta P, Einhorn T. Anatomy and biomechanics of the foot and ankle. In: *Orthopaedic Surgery Essentials: The Foot and Ankle.* Hagerstown: Lippincott; 2004:18-23.

22. Kotter A, Wieberneit J, Braun W, Ruter A. [The Chopart dislocation. A frequently underestimated injury and its sequelae. A clinical study]. *Unfallchirurg.* 1997;100(9):737-741. German.

23. Rammelt S, Zwipp H, Hansen S. Posttraumatic reconstruction of the foot and ankle. In: *Skeletal Trauma.* Philadelphia PA: Elsevier Saunders; 2019:2641-2690.

24. Sangeorzan BJ, Swiontkowski MF. Displaced fractures of the cuboid. *J Bone Joint Surg Br.* 1990;72(3):376-378.

25. Rammelt S, Schneiders W, Schikore H, Holch M, Heineck J, Zwipp H. Primary open reduction and fixation compared with delayed corrective arthrodesis in the treatment of tarsometatarsal (Lisfranc) fracture dislocation. *J Bone Joint Surg Br.* 2008;90(11):1499-1506.

26. Dewar FP, Evans DC. Occult fracture subluxation of the midtarsal joint. *J Bone Joint Surg Br.* 1968;50(2):386-388.

27. Weber M, Locher S. Reconstruction of the cuboid in compression fractures: short to midterm results in 12 patients. *Foot Ankle Int.* 2002;23(11):1008-1013.

28. Rammelt S, Schepers T. Chopart injuries: when to fix and when to fuse? *Foot Ankle Clin.* 2017;22(1):163-180.

29. Barmada M, Shapiro HS, Boc SF. Calcaneocuboid arthrodesis. *Clin Podiatr Med Surg.* 2012;29(1):77-89.

30. Koenis MJ, Louwerens JW. Simple resection arthroplasty for treatment of 4th and 5th tarsometatarsal joint problems. A technical tip and a small case series. *Foot Ankle Surg.* 2015;21(1):70-72.

31. Shawen SB, Anderson RB, Cohen BE, Hammit MD, Davis WH. Spherical ceramic interpositional arthroplasty for basal fourth and fifth metatarsal arthritis. *Foot Ankle Int.* 2007;28(8):896-901.

18

A 3D-Printed Solution for Revision Lapidus Bunionectomy

ERIC SO, LEE M. HLAD

Definition

- Custom/patient-specific 3D-printed metallic porous spacer for revision of first tarsometatarsal (TMT) joint arthrodesis nonunion.

Anatomy and Pathogenesis

- The first TMT joint is a trapezoid-shaped joint with a complex anatomic configuration.[1]
- It is well constrained by soft tissue structures but allows a certain amount of rotational and sagittal plane movement.
- The dorsalis pedis artery and deep peroneal nerve are encountered in the interval between the extensor hallucis longus and the extensor hallucis brevis.
- The dorsoplantar extent of the first TMT joint is approximately 30 mm.
- The medial cuneiform is approximately 1.5 cm wide.
- The neurovascular bundle traverses from dorsal to plantar within the first intermetatarsal 18 mm distal to the second TMT joint.[2]
- The nonunion rate has been reported to range from 4% to 12%.[3-5]
- Transfer metatarsalgia, hardware pain, and infection may also occur after Lapidus bunionectomy.

Patient History and Physical Exam Findings

- Clinical nonunion is defined as a painful, swollen arthrodesis site 6 months postoperatively.[6]
- Assess for location of pain.
- Degree of recurrent deformity.
- Consider overall foot alignment.

Imaging and Other Diagnostic Testing

- Radiographs:
  - Nonunion may be represented by a lack of callus and/or trabeculation along the osteotomy or fusion site (Fig. 18.1), bony sclerosis, change in alignment, subluxation/dislocation of the capital fragment, and hardware failure.[7]
- Evidence of osteomyelitis: osteopenia, radiolucency, lytic changes/cortical erosion, trabecular destruction, bone necrosis, brodie abscess, sclerosis, and periosteal reaction.[8]
- CT scan:
  - CT is often more helpful in staging avascular necrosis (AVN) as well as deciphering between fusion and nonunion, and implant loosening.
  - CT is often more helpful in surgical planning and procedure selection.
  - Currently, CT is the imaging modality of choice if 3D printing technology is being utilized.[9]

Nonoperative Management

- Shoe modification: a wide, rigid toe box
- Orthotics and/or metatarsal pads
- Immobilization
- Rest, ice, compression, elevation (RICE) therapy and nonsteroidal antiinflammatory drugs (NSAIDs)
- A bone stimulator for the treatment of aseptic nonunion.

Traditional Surgical Management

- In situ fusion:
  - This results in acute shortening and consequential biomechanics.
- First TMT joint fusion with bone block:
  - Graft incorporation and fusion on both sides of the graft is required. This may increase the time to union and nonunion rate. An autograft may be used in most cases, but depending on the size of the bone defect, allograft may be considered.
  - Autograft or allograft may be used in a staged manner using the Masquelet technique.

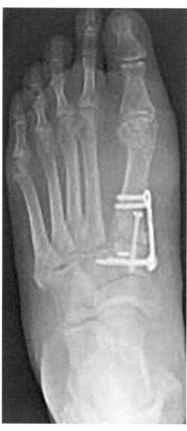

• **Fig. 18.1** Preoperative anteroposterior X-ray demonstrating a non-union of the first tarsometatarsal joint.

- Distraction osteogenesis:
  - This requires an extended time with an external fixator, which is associated with pin site infection and poor patient satisfaction. Bone regenerate formation may be compromised in patients with comorbidities such as tobacco use or diabetes.
- Amputation:
  - Partial foot amputation may be considered in situations in which there is severe infection, trauma, or failure of multiple revisions.

3D-Printed Implant and Instrumentation Considerations

- Titanium has been shown to have osteoconductive properties and is biologically inert, therefore titanium is the material of choice[10,11]:
  - Pore size has been described in the literature from 300 to 1000 μm.[12]
  - Truss configurations provide the greatest strength with the least mass. These allow for a mechanically robust construct that resists the load-bearing forces of the foot and ankle. The truss configuration acts as a lattice for bone grafting and other orthobiologic material.[13]
  - The 3D configuration of the implant must be designed to allow it to be successfully implanted through the planned surgical exposure, cognizant of the constraints imposed by the local anatomy and previous implants.[13]
  - The length of the implant is case specific and based on the proposed resection level. The length of osseous deficit after resection of nonviable bone and preparation for fusion determines the nominal length. Custom cutting guides may be created and used to ensure the resection is accurate.
- Degree of porosity: the percentage of porosity is inversely proportional to implant strength. This should be considered during implant design:
  - A rectangular/oblong-shaped implant is recommended (Fig. 18.2), which promotes a larger surface area of fusion and enhanced interposition of the implant to bone.
  - Inherent stability is provided by the rough texture, which assists in resisting torsional forces.
  - The porous surface is in direct contact with the adjacent bone and areas of smooth/polished surfaces to prevent soft tissue ingrowth and contracture.
- Diameter, width, length, and height are patient specific and are based on the size at the proposed resection level (Fig. 18.3):
  - The implant can be designed with screw holes to allow direct implant-to-bone fixation; however, the

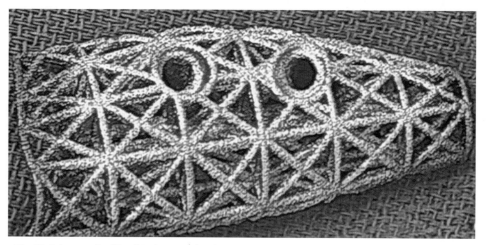

• **Fig. 18.2** Image of a 3D-printed custom implant. Note the porous design to promote osseous ingrowth as well as the truss design to serve as a lattice for osseous incorporation through the implant.

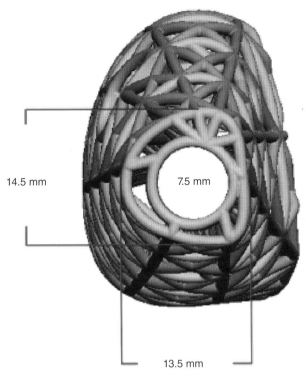

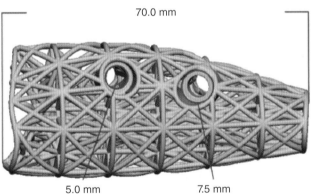

14.5 mm

7.5 mm

13.5 mm

70.0 mm

5.0 mm   7.5 mm

• **Fig. 18.3** Preoperative computer-aided design images demonstrating the dimensions of the implant and screw holes that should be measured during the preoperative planning stage. (Reprinted with permission from 4WEB Medical, Frisco, TX.)

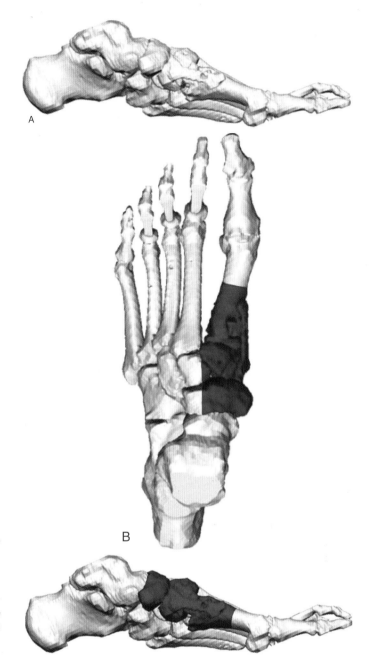

A

B

• **Fig. 18.4** Preoperative computer-aided design image depicting nonunion of the first tarsometatarsal joint with the presence of (A) hardware and (B) the planned resection *(red)*. (Reprinted with permission from 4WEB Medical, Frisco, TX.)

more screws used, the less surface area is available for bone ingrowth and fusion.

- A preoperative CT scan is obtained to guide surgical planning:
  - Images as scanned are used to gain an appreciation for the amount of bone resection required (Fig. 18.4).
  - Consider the trajectory of the screw placement. Important considerations are local anatomy, anticipated surgical exposure, and internal fixation options. Fixation can include retrograde nails, plates, or screws, or a combination thereof. Compression should be achieved across the implant. Fixation should provide stability and compression but also not provide a source of prominence or soft tissue impingement.
  - In the case of a revision Lapidus, primary fixation should comprise of intramedullary fixation through the

implant. A 6.5-mm–diameter screw should be considered. Secondary fixation should comprise of transverse fixation into the second metatarsal and cuneiforms. This provides additional stability in the sagittal and transverse planes (Fig. 18.5).[14] Transverse fixation should be 3.5-mm or 4.0-mm–diameter screws.

- If intramedullary fixation is planned, a trajectory guide should be manufactured to allow precise and accurate placement of intramedullary fixation (Fig. 18.6). The guide should be able to accommodate the guide pin used for the cannulated screw fixation.

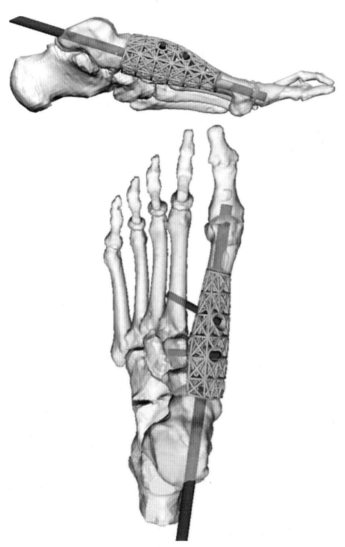

• **Fig. 18.5** Preoperative computer-aided design images demonstrating the position of the implant with planned fixation. (Reprinted with permission from 4WEB Medical, Frisco, TX.)

Surgical Management With 3D-Printed Devices

- Off-the-shelf items required:
  - A sagittal saw to resect the bone at the appropriate level.
  - A 2.0-mm solid core drill bit to fenestrate either bone ends to promote osseous ingrowth.
  - Biologics, bone allograft and/or autograft harvester per the surgeon's preferences to promote osteoconduction, osteoinduction and osteogenesis.
- Positioning:
  - Supine with an ipsilateral bump.
- Anesthesia:
  - General with regional blockade.
- Approach:
  - A dorsomedial approach, however, consider the placement of preexisting incisions or previous surgical wounds.

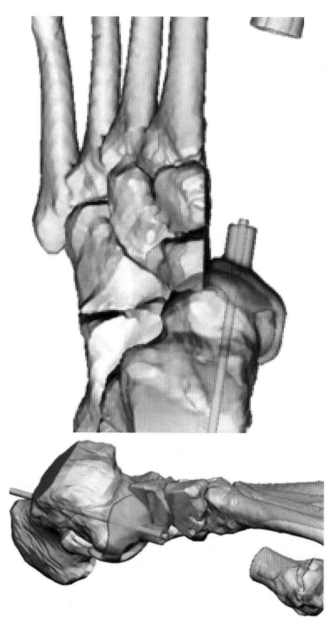

• **Fig. 18.6** Preoperative computer-aided design images demonstrating the pin guide used to obtain an accurate trajectory for the intramedullary fixation. (Reprinted with permission from 4WEB Medical, Frisco, TX.)

- Technique:
  - Expose the arthrodesis site. Remove any preexisting hardware.
  - Obtain adequate visualization of the first metatarsal, second metatarsal base, cuneiforms, and navicular.
  - A Reamer-Irrigator-Aspirator (DePuy Synthes, Warsaw, IN) from the femur may be considered to obtain autogenous graft that may be packed within the porous structure of the 3D-printed implant. This may be augmented with allogeneic orthobiologics.
  - Use a sagittal saw to perform bone resection at the preplanned level. Ensure that healthy, viable bone is present.

- Prior to insertion of the implant, predrill a fixation from the talus by placing the manufacturer's drill guide on the talus. Retrograde the provided guide pin from the anterior aspect of the talus to the posterior aspect of the talus. It is critical to obtain fluoroscopic imaging to confirm proper positioning of the guide pin and trajectory of the anticipated screw. The guide pin is exited through the posterior aspect of the ankle. Care must be taken to avoid injury to the surrounding articular surfaces. A counter incision is made at the exit point of the guide pin, typically lateral to the Achilles tendon. Care must be taken to avoid injury to the sural nerve. Blunt dissection is performed to allow passage of the cannulated drill. With the trajectory and placement of the guide pin secured, the talar head is prepared for arthrodesis using standard technique.

- At this time, a trial is inserted into the defect. The trial should be press-fitted into the defect. Ensure the implant-bone interface is perfectly matched by using the trial provisionally. If a perfect fit is not obtained, make certain that all debris and interposing soft tissue is removed. Now remove the trial and pack the implant with desired biologics (Fig. 18.7). Insert the implant into the defect.

- Internally fixate the implant by driving the guide pin through the designed hole of the implant into the metatarsal. Utilize fluoroscopy to judge placement of the implant and alignment of the midfoot. At this point, a cannulated drill is used to drill through the talus and the implant. An appropriate length 6.5-mm screw is inserted from posterior to anterior. It is the surgeon's discretion to use a large cannulated screw or to exchange the cannulated wire for a solid core screw. The screw should obtain purchase, compression, and stability into the diaphysis of the first metatarsal (Fig. 18.8A).

- Additional stability is achieved with associated 4.0-mm screws into the second metatarsal and middle cuneiforms, according to the preoperative plan. A 4.0-mm screw is first inserted into the second metatarsal base.

A screw should be placed into the second metatarsal via lag by design of lag by technique in order to obtain union between the implant and the second metatarsal base. This provides stability through the Lisfranc joint complex. The addition of these transverse screws provides an additional four points of fixation (see Fig. 18.8B).

- Test stability and position directly and under fluoroscopy.
- Closure and bandaging per the surgeon's protocol.
- Adjunctive procedures may include removal of hardware, bone graft harvest, bone biopsy and cultures, reimplantation of antibiotic cement spacer, arthrodesis of adjacent joints, and gastrocnemius recession.

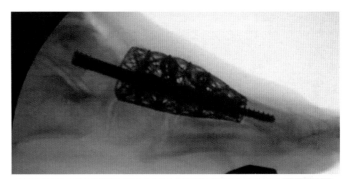

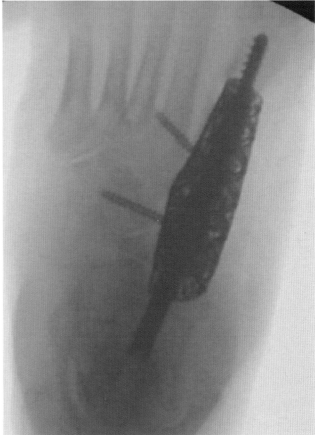

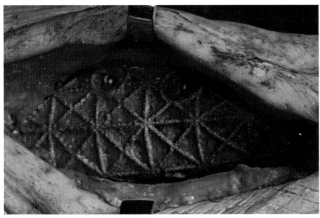

• **Fig. 18.7** Intraoperative image demonstrating the implanted 3D-printed spacer packed with biologics and allograft.

• **Fig. 18.8** Intraoperative fluoroscopic images depicting final implantation and fixation.

Postoperative Protocol

- Non–weight bearing in a splint for 1 to 2 weeks
- Non–weight bearing in a short-leg cast from weeks 2 to 6
- Non–weight bearing in a controlled ankle motion (CAM) boot from weeks 6 to 12
- Weight bearing as tolerated in a CAM boot from weeks 12 to 24
- Weight bearing as tolerated in a stiff-soled shoe from weeks 24 to 52
- CT scan obtained 12 months postoperatively.

Results/Outcomes

- Lack of pain, clinical stability, and radiographic consolidation should be noted to allow the patient to weight bear (Fig. 18.9).

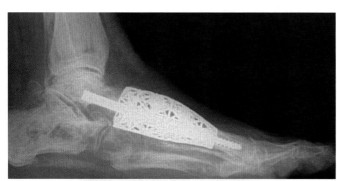

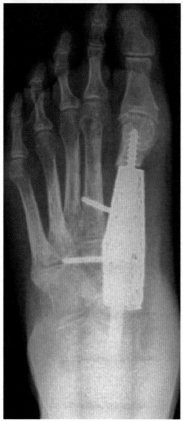

- **Fig. 18.9** Postoperative radiographs demonstrating appropriate alignment of the hindfoot and midfoot, osseous consolidation, and stable hardware.

- A 12-month postoperative CT scan should show adequate bony ingrowth surrounding the implant, no signs of hardware failure or stress shielding (Fig. 18.10).
- Ensure infection is eradicated prior to utilizing this technique. Follow proper infectious disease guidelines and surgical principles to clear infection prior to implantation and final reconstruction of the bone defect.
- Possible complications:
  - Infection
  - Nonunion/malunion
  - Hardware failure
  - Transfer metatarsalgia
  - Deep venous thrombosis
  - Wound complication.
- Previously published results:
  - So E, Mandas V, Hlad L. Large osseous defect reconstruction using a custom three-dimensional printed titanium truss implant. *J Foot Ankle Surg.* 2018; 57(1): 196-204.

PEARLS AND PITFALLS	
Indications and contraindications	• Osseous deficits of the first tarsometatarsal joint after failed Lapidus bunionectomy • Contraindicated in patients with sensory neuropathy, active infection, and peripheral arterial disease • Active infection must be cleared prior to insertion of the implant
Implant design	• Titanium appears to be the ideal material • Implant shape and porosity should provide inherent stability and enhance bony ingrowth • Use CT and CAD images to determine the implant's size and shape after bony resection • Screw holes for direct fixation should be easy to access • Strike a balance between achieving adequate points of fixation and preventing bony ingrowth with overfixation • Consider local anatomy with regards to internal fixation options • Consider intramedullary fixation along the long axis of the implant in addition to transverse screw fixation into the second metatarsal and cuneiform

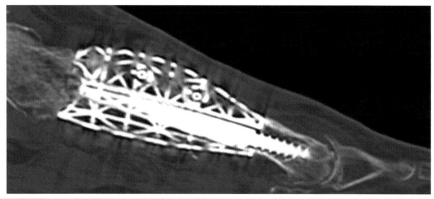

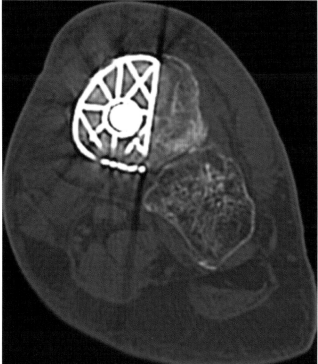

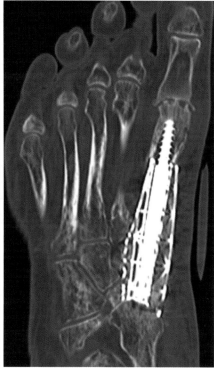

• **Fig. 18.10** Postoperative CT imaging at 12 months which depicts osseous incorporation through the implant and union across the midfoot joints.

Surgical technique	• Ensure all compromised and nonviable bone is removed • Use instrumentation that replicates the shape and size of the implant to promote optimal bone-implant contact • The ideal implant size yields physiologic tension of the adjacent soft tissues, inherent stability, and restores the length relationship of the midfoot without compromising neurovascular structures • Utilize pin guides to ensure accurate placement of internal fixation through the implant • Utilize autogenous bone grafting when possible and supplement with allograft orthobiologics as needed

CAD, Computer-aided design.

References

1. Wanivenhaus A, Pretterklieber M. First tarsometatarsal joint: anatomical biomechanical study. *Foot Ankle.* 1989;9:153-157.
2. So E. Structures at risk from an intermetatarsal screw for Lapidus bunionectomy: a cadaveric study. *J Foot Ankle Surg.* 2019;58(1):62-65.
3. Catanzariti AR, Mendicino RW, Lee MS, Gallina MR. The modified Lapidus arthrodesis: a retrospective analysis. *J Foot Ankle Surg.* 1999;38:322-332.
4. Coetzee JC, Resig SG, Kuskowski M, Saleh KJ. The Lapidus procedure as salvage after failed surgical treatment of hallux valgus: a prospective cohort study. *J Bone Joint Surg.* 2003;85A:60-65.
5. Grace D, Delmonte R, Catanzariti AR, Hofbauer M. Modified Lapidus arthrodesis for adolescent hallux abducto valgus. *J Foot Ankle Surg.* 1999;38:8-13.
6. Hamilton G, Mullins S, Schubert J, Rush S, Ford L. Revision Lapidus arthrodesis: rate of union in 17 cases. *J Foot Ankle Surg.* 2007;46(6):447-450.
7. Agarwal A. Principles of nonunions. In: *Nonunions.* Boston, MA: Springer; 2018:1-43.
8. Truman SB. Diagnostic imaging of osteomyelitis of the foot and ankle. In: *Osteomyelitis of the Foot and Ankle.* Cham: Springer; 2015:27-37.

9. Dekker TJ, Steele JR, Federer AE, Hamid KS, Adams SB Jr. Use of patient-specific 3D-printed titanium implants for complex foot and ankle limb salvage, deformity correction, and arthrodesis procedures. *Foot Ankle Int.* 2018;39(8):916-921.

10. Takemoto M, Fujibayashi S, Neo M, Suzuki J, Kokubo T, Nakamura T. Mechanical properties and osteoconductivity of porous bioactive titanium. *Biomaterials.* 2005;26(30):6014-6023.

11. de Wild M, Schumacher R, Mayer K, et al. Bone regeneration by the osteoconductivity of porous titanium implants manufactured by selective laser melting: a histological and micro computed tomography study in the rabbit. *Tissue Eng Part A.* 2013;19(23):2645-2654.

12. Taniguchi N, Fujibayashi S, Takemoto K, et al. Effect of pore size on bone ingrowth into porous titanium implants fabricated by additive manufacturing: an in vivo experiment. *Mater Sc Eng C Mater Biol Appl.* 2016;59:690-701.

13. So E, Mandas V, Hlad L. Large osseous defect reconstruction using a custom three-dimensional printed titanium truss implant. *J Foot Ankle Surg.* 2018;57(1):196-204.

14. Galli MM, McAlister JE, Berlet GC, Hyer CF. Enhanced Lapidus arthrodesis: crossed screw technique with middle cuneiform fixation further reduces sagittal mobility. *J Foot Ankle Surg.* 2015;54(3):437-440.

19

3D-Printed Solutions for First Metatarsophalangeal Joint Fusion With Osseous Deficit

LANCE JOHNSON, PETER D. HIGHLANDER

Definition

- Custom/patient-specific 3D-printed metallic porous spacer for the first metatarsophalangeal joint (MTPJ) with bone loss to restore length, alignment, and function of the first ray.

Anatomy

- The first MTPJ is a ball and socket joint that consists of the articulation between the concave base of the first proximal phalanx and the convex 1st metatarsal head.
- The sesamoids are contained within the flexor hallucis longus tendon and articulate with the plantar first metatarsal head.
- The normal range of motion for the first MTPJ varies, ranging from 65 to 110 degrees of dorsiflexion and 23 to 45 degrees of plantarflexion.[1,2]
- When performing first MTPJ fusion, the final position of the great toe should allow for heel rise during the late-stance phase of gait[3,4] (Figs. 19.1 and 19.2).
- The normal length of the first metatarsal is about 6.5 cm.[5,6] Shortening of the first metatarsal and first ray can lead to jamming of the first MTPJ and inhibits the ability of the first ray to propulse properly during the push off phase of gait. Alteration of the first metatarsal length has also been linked to the formation of hallux valgus and hallux limitus.[5,6]

Pathogenesis

- Osseous deficits and shortening of the first ray may be secondary to:
  - Nonunion after primary first MTPJ fusion
  - Avascular necrosis (AVN): idiopathic, traumatic, or iatrogenic causes
  - Failed first MTPJ joint implant arthroplasty
  - Failed Keller arthroplasty
  - Osteomyelitis/septic arthritis.
- Primary first MTPJ inherently causes a degree of first ray shortening. Aggressive reaming can cause thermal necrosis, which may increase the risk of nonunion—5% to 10% of primary first MTPJ fusions result in nonunion.[7-9] During revision of first MTPJ nonunion, all nonviable bone requires resection, which will lead to further shortening.
- Overzealous resection in Keller arthroplasty will result in iatrogenic shortening of the first ray, which can lead to functional and biomechanical problems.[7]
- Vascular insult may occur during head osteotomies of the first metatarsal, particularly if dissection is excessive and/or lateral release is concurrently performed. AVN may result if the vascularity to the first metatarsal head is not reestablished in a timely fashion.[10-12]
- First MTPJ implant arthroplasty inherently requires significant bone resection. Furthermore, implant material such as silicone has been associated with foreign body reaction, synovitis, and implant failure.[13,14] Aseptic loosening may also result in implant failure, which will often require revision.[15-18] Removal of the implant during revision will result in a substantial osseous deficit.
- Osseous deficits that result in a short first ray alter the propulsion phase of gait, which may cause pain, deformity, and biomechanical dysfunction.[19,20]
- The degree of shortening that can be tolerated is variable from patient to patient.

Patient History and Physical Exam Findings

- Localized pain
- Adjacent metatarsal pain (transfer metatarsalgia)

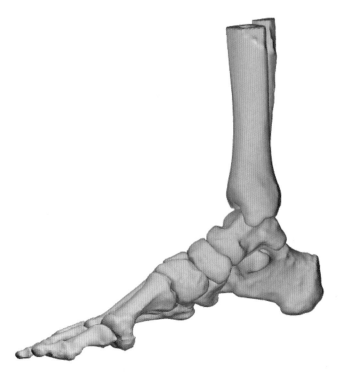

• **Fig. 19.1** Picture showing the ideal position of the hallux after first metatarsophalangeal joint fusion for heel off. (CAD images reprinted with permission from restor3d, Inc, Durham, NC.)

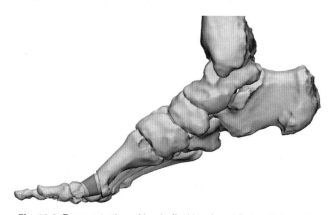

• **Fig. 19.2** Demonstration of heel off with a fused first metatarsophalangeal joint. (CAD images reprinted with permission from restor3d, Inc, Durham, NC.)

- Deformity of the hallux (cock-up, varus, valgus)
- A nonfunctional hallux (floppy toe)
- A visible length difference between the hallux and the second toe
- Weak propulsion during gait examination
- Functional imbalance of the forefoot and compensatory changes in gait cycle.[3,7,11]

Imaging and Other Diagnostic Testing

- Radiographs:
  - Nonunion may be represented by a lack of callus and/or trabeculation along the osteotomy or fusion site, bony sclerosis, change in alignment, subluxation/dislocation of the capital fragment, and hardware failure.[21]

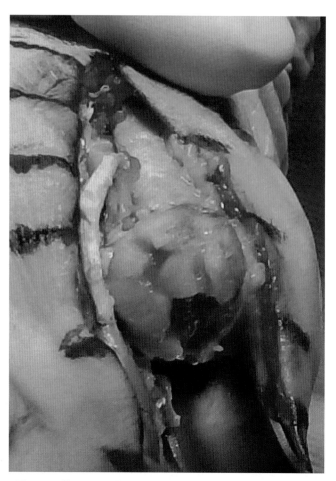

• **Fig. 19.3** Exposure of the first metatarsophalangeal joint showing osteonecrosis and collapse of the first metatarsal head.

- AVN may be progressive and findings may range from osteopenia to sclerosis and cortical collapse, to eventual destructive changes to the joint[22] (Fig. 19.3).
- Loosening and failure of implant arthroplasty are represented by periprosthetic lucency, poor apposition at the bone-implant interface, and a change in implant position with serial radiographs. Loosening may progress to periprosthetic fracture and implant dislocation.[23,24]
- Osteomyelitis: osteopenia, radiolucency, lytic changes/cortical erosion, trabecular destruction, bone necrosis, Brodie abscess, sclerosis, and periosteal reaction.[25]
- Advanced imaging (CT/MRI):
  - MRI is useful for the diagnosis of infection and is most sensitive for early diagnosis of AVN. MRI with contrast provides a better estimation of blood flow. If hardware is present MRI may not be useful.
  - CT may be more helpful in staging AVN, deciphering between fusion and nonunion, and implant loosening. CT is often more helpful in surgical planning and procedure selection.
  - Currently, CT is the imaging modality of choice if 3D printing technology is being utilized.[26]

- Other testing:
  - Noninvasive vascular testing should be considered if there is concern for vascular compromise.
  - Infectious and bone metabolism workup should be obtained in cases of nonunion and radiolucency/pathologic fracture surrounding the first MTPJ implant arthroplasty, including white blood cell count (WBCs), erythrocyte sedimentation rate (ESR), C-reactive protein (CRP), vitamin D, parathyroid hormone (PTH), and thyroid-stimulating hormone (TSH).[21]
  - Joint aspiration can be considered in cases where there is increased suspicion for infection.[23]

Nonoperative Management

- Shoe modification: wide, rigid toe box
- Orthotics and/or metatarsal pads
- Immobilization
- Rest, ice, compression, elevation (RICE) therapy and nonsteroidal anti-inflammatory drugs (NSAIDs).

Traditional Surgical Management (Concerns and Disadvantages)

- In situ fusion: results in acute shortening and problematic biomechanics, is aesthetically less pleasing, and could cause soft tissue compromise. Alternative surgical techniques should be used if the osseous deficit is >1 cm.
- First MTPJ fusion with bone block: graft incorporation and fusion at two sides of the graft is required, which may decrease time to union and the rate of union. The current consensus is that the maximum size of the graft is 2 to 2.5 cm, therefore for larger deficits shortening will result. Autograft may be superior to allograft; however, autograft is associated with donor site morbidity and a complication rate of nearly 30%.[27]
- Distraction osteogenesis: requires an extended time in an external fixator, which is associated with pin site infections and poor patient compliance. The quality of the regenerated bone is of concern, especially in smokers and diabetics.
- Vascularized free fibula: technically challenging and the operative time can be extensive. Donor site morbidity is further concerning.
- Masquelet technique: requires staged procedures and drainage from the antibiotic spacer may cause soft tissue issues.
- Partial first ray amputation: amputation should be a last resort and reserved primarily for limb salvage in the setting of severe infection, trauma, or failure of multiple revisions. Amputation results in permanent loss of first ray function and is fraught with secondary symptoms, which may lead to further minor or major amputation.

3D-Printed Implant Design Specifications and Considerations

- Titanium has been shown to have osteoconductive properties[28,29] and is biologically inert, therefore titanium is the material of choice.
- A variety of proprietary porous structures are available. The senior author currently prefers a gyroid structure.
- Pore size:
  - Pore size has been described in the literature from 300 to 1000 μm.[30,31] The senior author recommends a size of 1000 μm, as this is within range and allows for the most bony ingrowth.
  - Degree of porosity: the percentage of porosity is inversely proportional to implant strength. This should be considered during implant design. Typically, the senior author prefers 75% porosity, which allows bone graft retention and bony ingrowth potential while having adequate strength.
- The senior author recommends a pill-shaped implant with two convex surfaces (Fig. 19.4), which promotes a larger surface area of fusion and enhanced interposition of the implant to metaphyseal bone. In the senior author's experience, an implant with two convex surfaces also allows easier positioning and appears inherently more stable compared to other configurations. This design has also been advocated for in the literature regarding allograft and autograft bone block arthrodesis.[32,33]
- The porous surface is in direct contact with the adjacent bone and areas of smooth/polished surfaces to prevent soft tissue ingrowth and contracture.
- To account for intraoperative variability, the authors prefer to have three implants available which range from nominal and ± 5% to 10% of the length of the nominal-sized implant.
- The length of the implant is case specific and based on the proposed resection level. The length of osseous deficit after

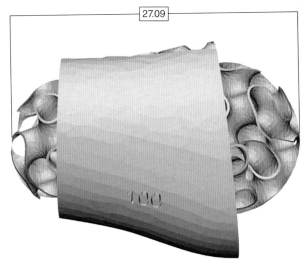

- **Fig. 19.4** A pill-shaped implant with two convex surfaces. (CAD images reprinted with permission from restor3d, Inc, Durham, NC.)

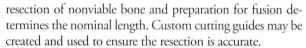

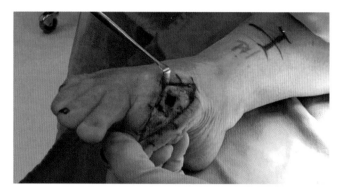

• **Fig. 19.5** Axial CT scan showing the inner diameter of the cortex. It is the senior author's opinion that the inner cortical diameter is the ideal size for the implant to allow for bony overgrowth around the implant.

• **Fig. 19.6** Exposure of the first metatarsophalangeal joint with a noted osseous deficit after the removal of a silicone implant.

resection of nonviable bone and preparation for fusion determines the nominal length. Custom cutting guides may be created and used to ensure the resection is accurate.

- The diameter and radius of the convex surfaces are patient specific and based on the size and diameter of the first metatarsal and hallux at the proposed resection level. Reamer size availability should also be taken into account. The authors prefer to keep the diameter and radius of the convex surfaces constant among all implants. It is the senior author's opinion that the diameter of the implant should ideally be within the confines of the cortices to allow for bony overgrowth around the implant. In other words, the implant diameter is equivalent to the diameter of the inner aspect of the cortex as determined on axial CT views (Fig. 19.5).
- The implant can be designed with screw holes to allow direct implant-to-bone fixation; however, the more screws used, the less surface area available for bone ingrowth and fusion.

Surgical Management With 3D-Printed Devices

- Off-the-shelf items required:
  - Convex (or cone) conical reamers sized according to the implant size.
  - A 3.5-mm dorsal locking plate to provide initial stability and maintenance of alignment while separate from the implant in case hardware removal is needed.
  - Solid/cannulated screws for direct implant-to-bone fixation if desired.
- Positioning: supine with an ipsilateral bump.
- Anesthesia: general and regional.
- Approach: standard dorsomedial approach along the medial side of the extensor hallucis longus (EHL), in the interval between dorsal proper digital nerve and EHL; however, consider the placement of existing incisions.
- Technique:
  - Expose the first MTPJ with adequate visualization of the proximal phalanx and first metatarsal (Fig. 19.6).

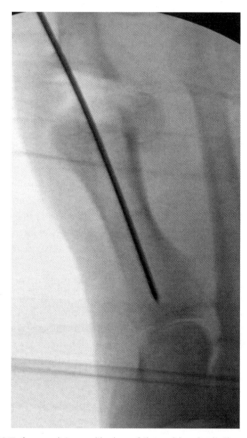

• **Fig. 19.7** Appropriate positioning of the guide wire in the center of the first metatarsal.

- All previous implants are removed.
- Pericapsular attachments are released with a scalpel and McGlamry elevator to allow the use of conical reamers.
- If needed, use custom cut guides for initial bony resection.
- Place a guide wire in the center of the metatarsal and confirm the position on fluoroscopy (Fig. 19.7).
- Select the appropriately size reamer. We prefer using one size larger than the implant and then sizing down to accommodate the implant perfectly. For example, if the implant replicates a 16-mm convex reamer,

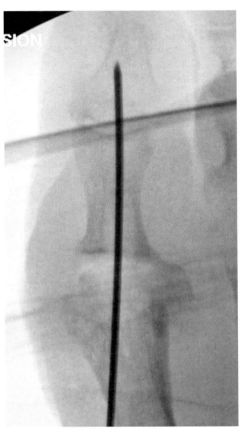

• **Fig. 19.8** Appropriate positioning of the guide wire in the center of the proximal phalanx.

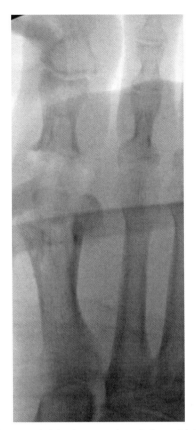

• **Fig. 19.9** Osseous deficit after resection of all nonviable bone of the proximal phalanx and first metatarsal head.

then we will use an 18-mm reamer first and then a 16-mm reamer.

- Remove the guide wire and place into the phalanx, and then ream in the same manner (Fig. 19.8).
- Ensure that only healthy, viable bone is present. If questionable bone quality still exists either repeat the reaming process or if localized it may be removed with curettes or rongeurs (Fig. 19.9). Irrigate liberally.
- Ensure the implant-bone interface is perfectly matched by using the trial provisionally. If a perfect fit is not obtained, ensure that all debris from reaming is removed, then consider rereaming.
- Determine implant size: we prefer to use radioopaque trials that are impregnated with barium sulfate for easy fluoroscopic visualization. Use each trial in sequential order from smallest to largest. We determine ideal size based on:
  - The ability to align the hallux in the desired position.
  - Adjacent soft tissues are at physiologic tension, which provides inherent stability and ensures neurovascular tissues are not excessively stretched.
  - The length of the hallux relative to the second toe and metatarsal, as determined by direct and fluoroscopic visualization.
- Once the implant size is determined, provisionally place the permanent implant to ensure the fit is ideal and then remove (Fig. 19.10).

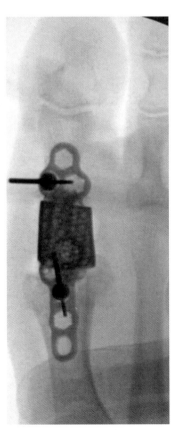

• **Fig. 19.10** Provisional placement of the implant with an overlying dorsal plate and temporary fixation.

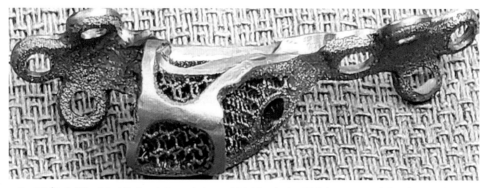

• **Fig. 19.11** A 3D-printed first metatarsophalangeal joint implant, which incorporated the plate and porous cage in one construct. This design may enhance overall stability, however in the senior author's experience has shown poorer outcomes as compared to a two component construct as shown in Figs. 19.16 and 19.17.

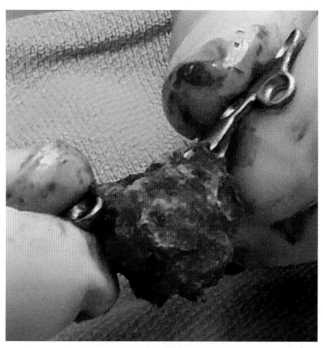

• **Fig. 19.12** A 3D-printed first metatarsophalangeal joint implant with morselized autograft harvested from the distal tibia.

- On the back table, pack the implant with desired bone graft. We prefer to use morselized autograft harvested from the distal tibia. Other allogenic biologics may also be considered (Figs. 19.11 and 19.12).
- Place the permanent implant. In our experience, little temporary fixation is needed to maintain alignment if the ideal sized implant is used; however, k-wires may be placed through the gyroid and into the adjacent bone if needed (Fig. 19.13).
- If desired, directly fixate the implant with screws. If used, the authors use 3.0 to 3.5-mm screws, but this should be determined during preoperative planning.
- Span the implant with a 3.5-mm locking plate and position to allow for a minimum of three points of bicortical fixation on the phalanx and metatarsal.
- Test the stability and position directly and under fluoroscopy.
- Closure and bandaging to be done per the surgeon's protocol.
- Other adjunctive procedures may include but are not limited to: hammertoe correction, Weil 2nd metatarsal osteotomy, and gastrocnemius recession.

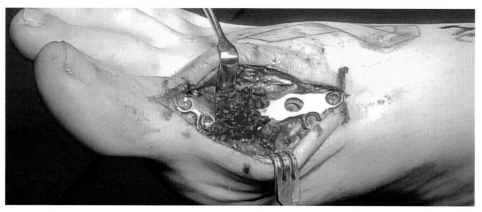

• **Fig. 19.13** Placement of the implant shown in Fig. 19.12, which shows adequate bony position as well as physiologic soft tissue tension.

Postoperative Protocol

- Initially, the patient is splinted and non-weight bearing for 1 week.
- Transition to a cast is at 2 to 4 weeks.
- Transition to a controlled ankle motion (CAM) boot but remain non-weight bearing for a total of 6 to 8 weeks.
- At 6 to 8 weeks postoperatively, the patient may transition to weight bearing as tolerated in a CAM boot if pain is controlled and the first ray is stable on examination and radiographs.
- A CT scan is obtained for closure observation at 3 months postoperatively and if findings are satisfactorily, the patient may begin transitioning to normal shoes. Patients are typically allowed to slowly introduce low-impact exercise, such as stationary cycling or swimming, once transitioned to normal shoes.
- Physical therapy as needed.

Results/Outcomes

- The senior author's experience and outcomes have been best with this implant design and technique.
- Poor outcomes have occurred in two cases that had similarities in design and technique. Both cases utilized a porous titanium spacer fixed to a plate as one construct. Also, both implants had a concave surface on the metatarsal and convex on the phalanx interface. Obtaining an ideal position of the hallux while achieving good bony-implant contact at the articular surfaces and the plate was challenging. Both patients had significant hardware irritation, which required removal of the entire implant. These poor outcomes led in part to the development of this design and technique (Figs. 19.14 to 19.17).
- Both patients had surgical revision using this implant design and surgical technique, and have made significant improvements in subjective and objective measures.
- Since developing and utilizing this technique, the authors have observed that the procedure is technically easier and requires less time.
- We have observed implants with clinical stability and evidence of bony ingrowth with follow-up CT scans (Figs. 19.18 and 19.19).
- This implant design and surgical technique has been successfully utilized in cases involving AVN after chevron bunionectomy, failed hemi implant arthroplasty, and failed silastic implant arthroplasties. Furthermore, this technique has been successfully used with osseous deficits >2.5 cm.
- We would also consider this technique in cases of first MTPJ nonunion if required resection is substantial.
- If considering using this technique for failed/aggressive Keller arthroplasty, ensure there is enough viable phalanx to obtain stable fixation.
- Ensure infection is completely cleared prior to utilizing this technique. In such cases, we believe it is advisable to

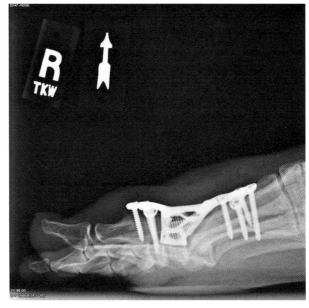

• **Fig. 19.14** Radiograph demonstrating the original implant design. This design had characteristics including: an implant fixed to the dorsal plate as one unit, a concave surface on the metatarsal interface, and a convex surface on the phalanx interface. This resulted in difficulty obtaining the ideal position as well as the need for total implant removal with dorsal plate irritation postoperatively. Refer to Fig. 19.15.

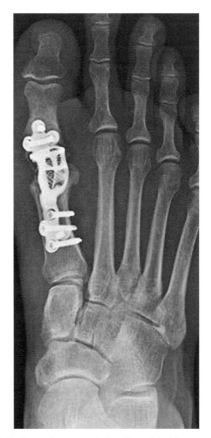

• **Fig. 19.15** Radiograph demonstrating the original implant design. This design had characteristics including: an implant fixed to the dorsal plate as one unit, a concave surface on the metatarsal interface, and a convex surface on the phalanx interface. This resulted in difficulty obtaining the ideal position as well as the need for total implant removal with dorsal plate irritation postoperatively. Refer to Fig. 19.14.

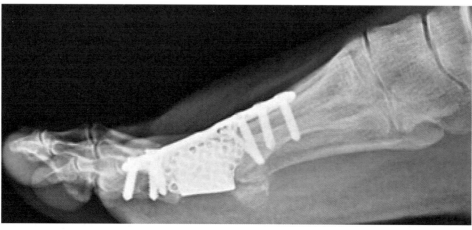

• **Fig. 19.16** Radiograph demonstrating the improved implant design with a dorsal plate separate from the implant and two convex surfaces of the implant. This construct makes obtaining the ideal position intraoperatively less challenging. Refer to Fig. 19.17.

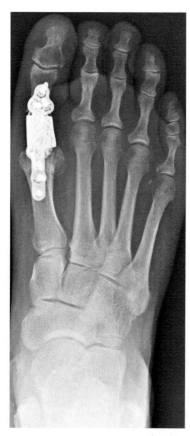

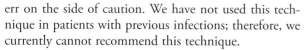

• **Fig. 19.17** Radiograph demonstrating the improved implant design with a dorsal plate separate from the implant and two convex surfaces of the implant. This construct makes obtaining the ideal position intraoperatively less challenging. Refer to Fig. 19.16.

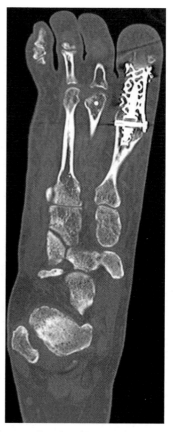

• **Fig. 19.18** CT scan slice demonstrating bony ingrowth of the 3D implant at 3 months. Refer to Fig. 19.19.

err on the side of caution. We have not used this technique in patients with previous infections; therefore, we currently cannot recommend this technique.
• Previously published results:
  • Amin TH, Rathnayake V, Remil M, et al. An innovative application of a computer assisted design and manufacture (CAD/CAM) implant for first metatarsal phalangeal joint arthrodesis: a case report. *J Foot Ankle Surg.* 2020;59(6):1287-1293.
  A case presentation of a patient who underwent Austin bunionectomy which subsequently developed avascular necrosis. The patient then underwent revision first MTPJ arthrodesis with a 3D-printed implant. The patient then underwent subsequent

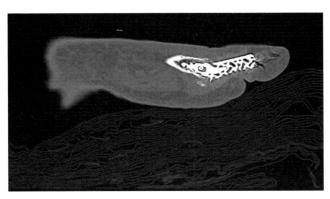

• **Fig. 19.19** CT scan slice demonstrating bony ingrowth of the 3D implant at 3 months. Also refer to Fig. 19.18.

Design	We recommend a pill-shaped implant with gyroid ends and a polished central portion of the implant. The implant diameter should line up with the inner cortex of the metatarsal/phalanx
Implantation	We recommend using conical reamers to prep the metatarsal and proximal phalanx as well as coating the implant in bone graft
Fixation	We recommend a dorsal plate separate from the implant for added stability. This also makes removal easier as you don't have to remove the entire implant with the plate

screw removal and was weight bearing in a Charcot Restraint Orthotic Walker (CROW) at 12 months.
- Parry E, Catanzariti A. Use of three-dimensional titanium trusses for arthrodesis procedures in foot and ankle surgery: a retrospective case series. *J Foot Ankle Surg.* 2021;60(4):824-833.

Twelve patients with custom 3D-printed titanium trusses and a minimum 6-month follow-up. Eleven out of twelve had successful limb/ray salvage. Seven patients had postoperative CT. Of the seven patients, six went onto radiographic union; the remaining five had radiographic union on plain film radiographs. One patient required below-knee amputation (BKA) and one required a midfoot osteotomy due to residual deformity. Seven of the patients had first MTPJ implants with no complications noted; three of these patients had CTs with at least "partial osseous bridging" noted across the implant.
- Possible complications:
  - Infection
  - Nonunion
  - Hardware failure/need for removal
  - Transfer metatarsalgia.

TIPS AND TRICKS

Indications	Osseous defect Pain Transfer metatarsalgia Deformity (cock-up/varus/valgus)
Goal of reconstruction	Restore length, alignment, and rotation Pain relief Improve function
Imaging	A preoperative CT scan is necessary for implant planning and assessment of bone quality
Labs/work up	Important to rule out metabolic and infectious causes for nonunion or implant arthroplasty failure

PEARLS AND PITFALLS

Indications and contraindications	• Osseous deficits of the first MTPJ, which has led to pain and dysfunction • Contraindicated in cases of active infection • Use prudence in patients with a history of deep infection
Implant design	• Titanium appears to be the ideal material • Implant shape and porosity should provide inherent stability and enhance bony ingrowth • Use CT and CAD images to determine the nominal implant size in all planes • Screw holes for direct fixation should be easy to access • Direct fixation will enhance stability at the bone-implant interface but will reduce the amount of bony ingrowth and biological fixation • Use a two-component construct (spacer and plate), which allows easy plate removal if hardware irritation occurs postoperatively
Surgical technique	• Ensure all compromised bone is removed • Use instrumentation that replicates the shape and size of the implant to promote optimal bone-implant contact • The ideal implant size yields physiologic tension of the adjacent soft tissues, inherent stability, and restores the length relationship of the first and second rays without compromising neurovascular structures

CAD, Computer-aided design; *MTPJ*, metatarsophalangeal joint.

References

1. Hopson MM, McPoil TG, Cornwall MW. Motion of the first metatarsophalangeal joint. Reliability and validity of four measurement techniques. *J Am Podiatr Med Assoc.* 1995;85(4):198-204.

2. Shereff MJ, Bejjani FJ, Kummer FJ. Kinematics of the first metatarsophalangeal joint. *J Bone Joint Surg Am.* 1986;68(3):392-398.

3. Easley ME, Wiesel SW, eds. *Operative Techniques in Foot and Ankle Surgery.* Philadelphia, PA: Lippincott Williams & Wilkins; 2011.

4. Nawoczenski DA, Baumhauer JF, Umberger BR. Relationship between clinical measurements and motion of the first metatarsophalangeal joint during gait. *J Bone Joint Surg Am.* 1999;81(3):370-376.

5. Munuera PV, Polo J, Rebollo J. Length of the first metatarsal and hallux in hallux valgus in the initial stage. *Int Orthop.* 2008; 32(4):489-495.

6. Munuera PV, Domínguez G, Castillo JM. Radiographic study of the size of the first metatarso-digital segment in feet with incipient hallux limitus. *J Am Podiatr Med Assoc.* 2007;97(6):460-468.

7. Lee MS, Grossman JP, eds. *Complications in Foot and Ankle Surgery: Management Strategies.* Boston, MA: Springer; 2017.

8. Roukis TS. Nonunion after arthrodesis of the first metatarsal-phalangeal joint: a systematic review. *J Foot Ankle Surg.* 2011;50(6):710-713.

9. Beeson P. The surgical treatment of hallux limitus/rigidus: a critical review of the literature. *Foot.* 2004;14:6-22.

10. Kuhn MA, Lippert FG III, Phipps MJ, Williams C. Blood flow to the metatarsal head after chevron bunionectomy. *Foot Ankle Int.* 2005;26(7):526-529.

11. Filippi J, Briceno J. Complications after metatarsal osteotomies for hallux valgus: malunion, nonunion, avascular necrosis, and metatarsophalangeal osteoarthritis. *Foot Ankle Clin.* 2020;25(1): 169-182.

12. Malal JJ, Shaw-Dunn J, Senthil Kumar C. Blood supply to the first metatarsal head and vessels at risk with a chevron osteotomy. *J Bone Joint Surg Am.* 2007;89(9):2018-2022.

13. Patel DC, Frascone ST, DeLuca A. Synovitis secondary to silicone elastomeric joint implant. *J Foot Ankle Surg.* 1994;33(6):628-632.

14. Pugliese D, Bush D, Harrington T. Silicone synovitis: longer term outcome data and review of the literature. *J Clin Rheumatol.* 2009;15(1):8-11.

15. Garras DN, Durinka JB, Bercik M, Miller AG, Raikin SM. Conversion arthrodesis for failed first metatarsophalangeal joint hemiarthroplasty. *Foot Ankle Int.* 2013;34(9):1227-1232.

16. Anakwe RE, Middleton SD, Thomson CE, McKinley JC. Hemiarthroplasty augmented with bone graft for the failed hallux metatarsophalangeal silastic implant. *Foot Ankle Int.* 2011; 17(3):e43-e46.

17. Hopson M, Stone P, Paden M. First metatarsal head osteoarticular transfer system for salvage of a failed hemicap-implant: a case report. *J Foot Ankle Surg.* 2009;48:483-487.

18. Stone PA, Barnes ES, Savage T, Paden M. Late hematogenous infection of first metatarsophalangeal joint replacement: a case presentation. *J Foot Ankle Surg.* 2010;49:489.e1-e4.

19. Coughlin MJ, Mann RA. Arthrodesis of the first metatarsophalangeal joint as salvage for the failed Keller procedure. *J Bone Joint Surg Am.* 1987;69A:68-75.

20. Machacek F Jr, Easley ME, Gruber F, Ritschl P, Trnka HJ. Salvage of a failed Keller resection arthroplasty. *J Bone Joint Surg Am.* 2004;86(6):1131-1138.

21. Agarwal A. Principles of nonunions. In: *Nonunions.* Boston, MA: Springer; 2018:1-43.

22. Ficat RP, Arlet J. [Forage-biopsie de la tete femorale dans l'osteonecrose primative. Observations histo-pathologiques portant sur huit forages]. *Rev Rhum.* 1964;31:257-264.

23. Rubin LG, Gentile M. Complications of first metatarsal phalangeal joint implants. In: *Complications in Foot and Ankle Surgery.* Boston, MA: Springer; 2017:197-204.

24. DeHeer PA. The case against first metatarsal phalangeal joint implant arthroplasty. *Clin Podiatr Med Surg.* 2006;23(4):709-723.

25. Truman SB. Diagnostic imaging of osteomyelitis of the foot and ankle. In: *Osteomyelitis of the Foot and Ankle.* Cham: Springer; 2015:27-37.

26. Dekker TJ, Steele JR, Federer AE, Hamid KS, Adams SB Jr. Use of patient-specific 3D-printed titanium implants for complex foot and ankle limb salvage, deformity correction, and arthrodesis procedures. *Foot Ankle Int.* 2018;39(8):916-921.

27. Younger EM, Chapman MW. Morbidity at bone graft donor sites. *J Orthop Trauma.* 1989;3:192-195.

28. Takemoto M, Fujibayashi S, Neo M, Suzuki J, Kokubo T, Nakamura T. Mechanical properties and osteoconductivity of porous bioactive titanium. *Biomaterials.* 2005;26(30):6014-6023.

29. de Wild M, Schumacher R, Mayer K, et al. Bone regeneration by the osteoconductivity of porous titanium implants manufactured by selective laser melting: a histological and micro computed tomography study in the rabbit. *Tissue Eng Part A.* 2013; 19(23-24):2645-2654.

30. Taniguchi N, Fubiyashi S, Takemoto M, et al. Effect of pore size on bone ingrowth into porous titanium implants fabricated by additive manufacturing: an in vivo experiment. *Mater Sci Eng C Mater Biol Appl.* 2016;59:690-701.

31. Karachalios T. *Bone-Implant Interface in Orthopedic Surgery.* London: Springer; 2014.

32. Luk PC, Johnson JE, McCormick JJ, Klein SE. First metatarsophalangeal joint arthrodesis technique with interposition allograft bone block. *Foot Ankle Int.* 2015;36(8):936-943.

33. Myerson MS, Schon LC, McGuigan FX, Oznur A. Result of arthrodesis of the hallux metatarsophalangeal joint using bone graft for restoration of length. *Foot Ankle Int.* 2000;21(4): 297-306.

20

3D-Printed Hallux and Lesser Metatarsophalangeal Joint Replacement

DAVID VIER, J. KENT ELLINGTON

Definition

- Custom/patient-specific 3D-printed metallic porous hemiarthroplasty for the treatment of hallux and lesser toe metatarsophalangeal joint (MTPJ) arthritis to improve pain while maintaining range of motion (ROM).

Anatomy/Pathogenesis

- The first metatarsal head is unique as its dorsoplantar diameter is smaller than the transverse plane diameter.[1]
- The first MTPJ articular surface is functionally divided into superior and inferior fields. The superior metatarsal field is convex and is larger than the superior phalangeal concavity, but the inferior metatarsal is larger than the superior metatarsal field, with articulations for the sesamoids as demonstrated in Fig. 20.1.[1]
- The plantar plate is part of the capsuloligamentous complex that provides stability to the first MTPJ.
- The normal ROM for the first MTPJ ranges from 65 to 110 degrees of dorsiflexion and 23 to 45 degrees of plantarflexion. Passive non–weight-bearing ROM correlates to active, dynamic ROM while walking.[2-4]
- Hallux rigidus is a restriction of the first MTPJ ROM with progressive osteoarthritic changes resulting in pain and functional limitations during weight bearing.[1]
- Various etiologies have been proposed for hallux rigidus, including most commonly trauma, followed by osteochondritis dissecans, metatarsus primus elevatus, and family history.[1,5-7]
- Dorsal osteophytes act as a mechanical block and can severely limit ROM of the hallux MTPJ, especially with dorsiflexion.
- The 2nd metatarsal acts as a keystone in the arch of the foot and is often the longest of the metatarsals.[8]

- During the toe-off phase of gait, the 2nd metatarsal is driven down into the ground and the base of the proximal phalanx rides dorsally over the metatarsal, creating compressive and shear forces that damage the cartilage of the metatarsal head.[8]
- Second MTPJ pain can be caused by many conditions including osteoarthritis, synovitis, Freiberg's infraction, osteochondral lesions, and MTPJ instability. Other conditions such as plantar plate tears and trauma can contribute, especially in the setting of osteoarthritis.

History and Physical Exam Findings

- Localized pain to the MTPJ of concern.
- Adjacent metatarsal pain (transfer metatarsalgia).
- Restricted ROM, pain through the midarc of motion, as well as terminal dorsiflexion with hallux rigidus.
- Hallux valgus deformity with a palpable, tender dorsal osteophyte, and medial eminence.
- A history of radiating, burning pain due to stretch of the dorsomedial cutaneous nerve.
- Pain with weight bearing as well as palpation of the joint.
- Pain through passive ROM of the 2nd MTPJ as well as instability with drawer of the joint.
- Weak propulsion during gait.

Imaging and Other Diagnostic Testing

- Radiographic:
  - Hallux rigidus radiographic findings are consistent with a classic osteoarthritis appearance in other joints such joint space narrowing, osteophyte formation, subchondral sclerosis, and subchondral cysts. Dorsal osteophytes are often the most pronounced findings.

225

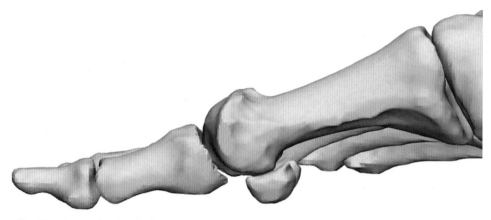

• **Fig. 20.1** Image showing the larger superior first metatarsal joint surface relative to the superior phalanx joint surface. This includes dorsal osteophytes, as evident in hallux rigidus. This image also demonstrates the larger inferior metatarsal articular surface relative to the superior metatarsal articular surface with articulation for the sesamoids. (CAD images reprinted with permission from restor3d, Inc, Durham, NC.)

- A second toe MTPJ radiographic appearance can differ based on the etiology of the pain. Osteoarthritis has a similar appearance as described for above for hallux rigidus. Freiberg's infarction manifests as widening of the joint space and collapse of the metatarsal head with sclerosis. 2nd MTPJ instability appearance will show dorsal subluxation/dislocation of the proximal phalanx relative to the metatarsal head in the sagittal plane with plantar plate tear or extensor/flexor tendon imbalance, or collateral ligament injury in the coronal plane (Fig. 20.2).
- Advanced imaging (CT/MRI):
  - Both CT/MRI can be useful in understanding the etiology of the MTPJ pain and deformity.
  - CT is typically best utilized for the analysis of bony anatomy including staging avascular necrosis (AVN) or subchondral collapse, as seen in Figs. 20.3 and 20.4. CT is more helpful in surgical planning with 3D printing technology.
  - MRI is better utilized for soft tissue anatomy, including the visualization of cartilage damage in OCDs, ligaments in plantar plate/collateral ligament tears, or diagnosing AVN when it is not obvious on plain radiographs. MRI provides information on the extraarticular soft tissues as well, which enhances its diagnostic value.
- Other testing:
  - Noninvasive vascular testing should be considered if there is concern for vascular pathology.
  - Infectious and bone metabolism workup should be obtained if there is concern for infection or bone quality that may compromise a joint implant, including: white blood cells (WBCs), erythrocyte sedimentation rate (ESR), C-reactive protein (CRP), vitamin D, parathyroid hormone (PTH), and thyroid-stimulating hormone (TSH).
  - Electromyography (EMG)/nerve conduction study (NCS) can be considered for patients presenting with neuropathic symptoms.

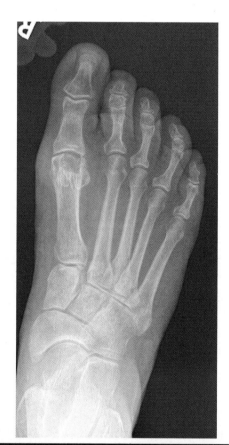

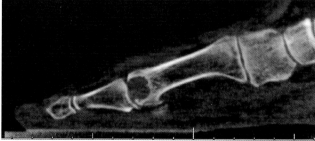

• **Fig. 20.2** An anteroposterior radiograph and sagittal CT scan demonstrating a large central osseous defect status post failed Cartiva (Stryker 325 Corporate Drive Mahwah, NJ 07430) implant for hallux rigidus.

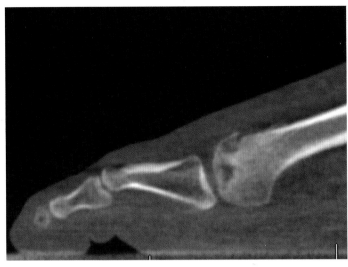
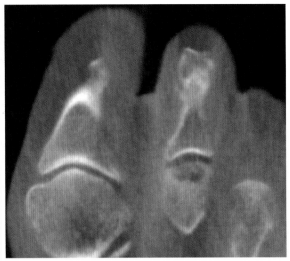

• **Fig. 20.3** CT images showing 2nd metatarsal head avascular necrosis with collapse more focal on the superior aspect of the joint.

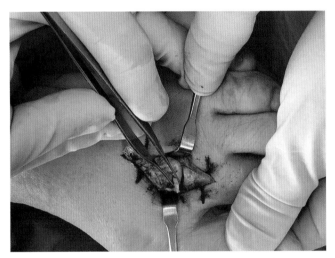

• **Fig. 20.4** Intraoperative findings correlating with 2nd metatarsal head avascular necrosis and collapse seen in Fig. 20.3 with delamination of the cartilage.

Nonoperative Treatment

- Hallux and lesser toe MTPJ pathology is usually treated with shoe modification; orthotics; immobilization; rest, ice, compression, elevation (RICE) therapy; nonsteroidal antiinflammatory drugs (NSAIDs); and steroid injections. Morton's extension can be considered with hallux rigidus. Orthotics with metatarsal pads can be useful for lesser toe MTPJ, especially metatarsalgia

Traditional Surgical Management

- Dorsal cheilectomy: early osteoarthritic changes of the hallux MTPJ are typically treated with cheilectomy to remove the dorsal osteophytes, which removes impingement pain and increases ROM.
- Interposition arthroplasty: can be useful as a salvage technique for hallux or lesser toe MTPJ but it has variable results.[9-12]

- Hallux metatarsophalangeal fusion: the "gold standard" for more severe arthritis but it completely eliminates ROM of the joint, so may not be ideal for all patients.
- Hemiarthroplasty: can provide significant pain relief and maintains some ROM, even more so than total MTPJ arthroplasty.[13-17]
- Total MTPJ arthroplasty: provides some pain relief but is associated with higher complication rates than other surgery, less pain relief, and less ROM than hemiarthroplasty.[13-16,18]
- Metatarsal head shortening osteotomy: Weil osteotomy can be used to shorten the metatarsal decompression joint and improve metatarsalgia. However, it is often associated with transfer metatarsalgia and can be less useful in MTPJ instability and AVN with collapse.
- Resection arthroplasty: can be useful as salvage in low-demand patients.

3D-Printed Implant and/or Instrumentation Considerations

- Cobalt chromium is the material of choice for arthroplasty due to its wear resistance.[19]
- A variety of proprietary porous structures are available. The senior author currently prefers a gyroid structure.
- First MTPJ hemiarthroplasty has a larger convex superior head design to allow for improved dorsiflexion of the proximal phalanx on the metatarsal articulating surface. ROM has been shown to be increased in implants with more anatomically designed metatarsal head components.[20]
- The porous coating allows for bony ingrowth as well as press fit.
- A proximal locking screw hole designed to fit a 2.7-mm Medline (Three Lakes Drive Northfield, IL 60093) locking screw for the first MTPJ hemiarthroplasty and 2.0-mm Medline locking screw for the 2nd MTPJ hemiarthroplasty, as seen in Figs. 20.5 and 20.6.
- To account for intraoperative variability, three different-sized implants are recommended with corresponding

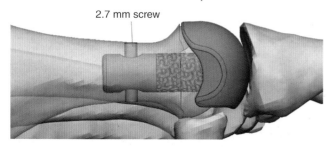

2.7 mm screw

• **Fig. 20.5** First metatarsophalangeal joint hemiarthroplasty restor3d (Durham, North Carolina) implant with a proximal locking screw hole and gyroid porous structure allowing for bony ingrowth. A plantar recess allows space for the plantar plate and sesamoid complex.

trials to allow for appropriate metatarsal head coverage and maximum ROM, as seen in Fig. 20.7. These sizes only vary in the size of the articular surface component.

• The diameter and radius of the convex articular surface is designed to allow for maximum bony ingrowth of the porous surface as well as coverage of the metatarsal head. CT scan can help when planning the proposed size, especially considering any bony defect in the case of a failed silicone implant or AVN with collapse, which is seen in Fig. 20.8.

Surgical Management With 3D-Printed Devices

• Off-the-shelf items required:
  • Conical reamers sized according to the implant size, as seen in Fig. 20.9.
  • A solid 2.0-mm or 2.7-mm screw for proximal locking fixation depending on the implant.
  • Optional items include bone cement and bone marrow aspirate (BMA) concentrate—the senior author prefers CeTament (BONESUPPORT, Inc. 60 William Street, Ste. 330 Welleseley, MA 02481), a synthetic bone graft substitute constituting of hydroxyapatite and calcium sulfate.
• Positioning: supine with an ipsilateral bump, with the iliac crest draped out if using BMA.

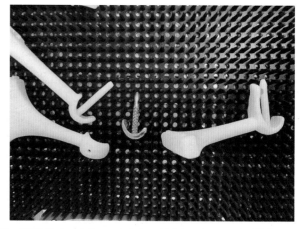

• **Fig. 20.7** 2nd metatarsophalangeal joint replacement with three trial sizes loaded on a handle to allow ease of implementation.

• Anesthesia: general and regional.
• Approach: a standard dorsomedial approach for the hallux MTP and dorsal 2nd webspace incision for the 2nd MTPJ.
• Technique:
  • Apply an ankle Esmarch tourniquet.
  • Expose the MTPJ with adequate visualization of the proximal phalanx and metatarsal.
  • The extensor tendon is protected and retracted to allow for capsulotomy.
  • Remove the dorsal osteophyte and loose bodies/cartilage with a rongeur.
  • Release any remaining capsule and collaterals with a scalpel. A McGlamerly deglover is used to free up the metatarsal plantarly. Partial metatarsal head condylectomy is performed with a rongeur.
  • Place the drill guide on the metatarsal head, place a k-wire down the center of the guide, and remove the guide. Confirm placement of the k-wire on fluoroscopy prior to reaming. Ream over the k-wire.
  • Drill over the k-wire to the size of the proposed implant stem. One can overream 1 mm if necessary.
  • Irrigate copiously to remove any bony debris.
  • Determine the implant size:
    • Trials of three different sizes are available.

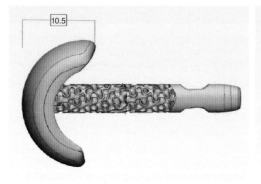

10.5

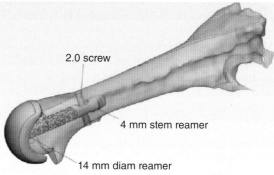

2.0 screw

4 mm stem reamer

14 mm diam reamer

• **Fig. 20.6** 2nd metatarsophalangeal joint hemiarthroplasty on a more extended plantar articular surface.

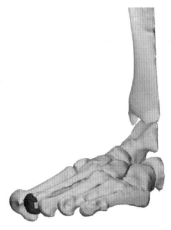
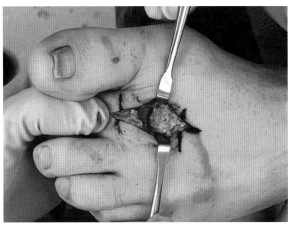

• **Fig. 20.8** Proposed and intraoperative bony resection of the 2nd metatarsal head. (CAD images reprinted with permission from restor3d, Inc, Durham, NC.)

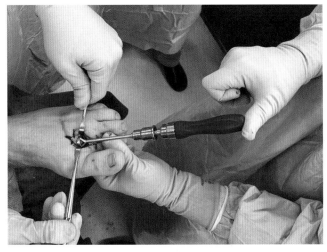

• **Fig. 20.9** A hand reamer allows for appropriate contouring of bone and removal of cartilage.

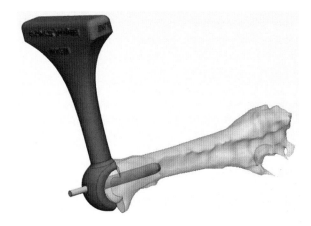

• **Fig. 20.10** An implant trial over k-wire with an attached handle. (CAD images reprinted with permission from restor3d, Inc, Durham, NC.)

- The ideal size is based on metatarsal head coverage, ROM, and stability.
- Once the appropriate size is determined via a trial (Fig. 20.10), remove the trial and k-wire.
- Fill the metatarsal shaft with bone cement.
- Cover the porous coated area of the final implant with BMA if desired (Fig. 20.11).
- Press fit the final implant into the metatarsal (Fig. 20.12). Remove any excess cement and allow to dry.
- Once the cement is dry, drill a locking screw hole with an appropriate-sized drill bit using the perfect circle technique with fluoroscopy. Measure the appropriate screw length and place the locking screw.
- Confirm the final stability of the implant, irrigate the joint with normal saline, and take final fluoroscopic images confirming the implant's placement and interlocking screw position.
- Evaluate the ROM and position of the MTPJ, and release soft tissue as needed.
- Closure and dressing to be done per the surgeon's preference.

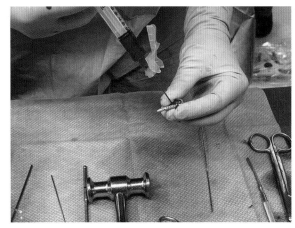

• **Fig. 20.11** Bone marrow aspirate concentrate coating the porous surface of the final implant.

Postoperative Protocol

- Place in a soft dressing intraoperatively with a bunion dressing and toe spacers for first MTPJ replacement.
- Heel weight bear in a short boot or postoperative shoe for 6 to 8 weeks, then wean into a normal shoe with progression of low-impact activities.

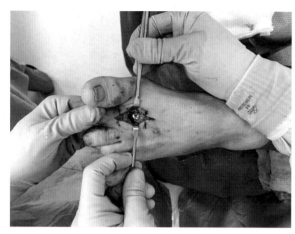

• **Fig. 20.12** The final implant of 2nd metatarsophalangeal joint hemiarthroplasty.

• Begin ROM exercises at 5 days postoperatively to prevent stiffness and utilize physical therapy as needed.

Results/Outcomes

• The senior author's experience and outcomes have been successful with this implant design and technique, seen in Fig. 20.13.

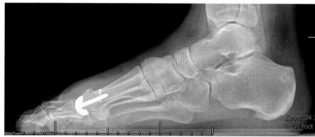

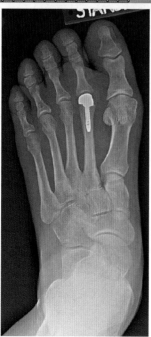

• **Fig. 20.13** Weight-bearing radiographs 6 months postoperatively of 2nd metatarsophalangeal joint hemiarthroplasty.

• No issues such as periprosthetic fractures have occurred to date. One patient underwent irrigation and debridement for superficial wound dehiscence with subsequent wound healing without implant extraction.

• Radiographic outcomes have not shown any subsidence, osteolysis, or implant loosening.

• Patients have been satisfied with their outcomes thus far, with significant pain relief as well as maintained ROM.

• Hallux MTPJ hemiarthroplasty has been used successfully in patients with hallux rigidus without prior surgery as well as failed synthetic cartilage implant, as seen in Fig. 20.14.

• Lesser MTPJ hemiarthroplasty has been used successfully in patients with AVN of the 2nd metatarsal head with collapse.

• Patient selection is crucial for this implant. Patients must understand the risks of hemiarthroplasty and be compliant with low-impact activity.

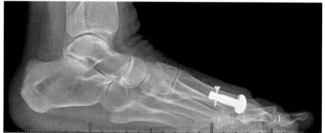

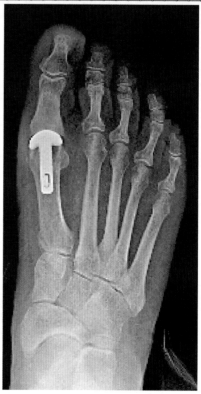

• **Fig. 20.14** Six months weight-bearing radiographs of first hallux metatarsophalangeal joint hemiarthroplasty after failed silicone implant arthroplasty.

PEARLS AND PITFALLS

Indications and contraindications	• Hallux and lesser MTPJ arthritis with pain and dysfunction • Lower demand patients understanding of risk of periprosthetic complications • Contraindicated in cases of active infection
Implant design	• Cobalt chromium is the material of choice for arthroplasty due to its wear resistance • Implant porosity and the gyroid structure should provide inherent stability and enhance bony ingrowth with press fit • Use CT and CAD images to determine the nominal implant size in all planes • Use a proximal locking screw to aid stability with rotation and length • A cemented canal provides additional stability and prevents implant subsidence
Surgical technique	• Remove large osteophytes, use a guide to place the k-wire and sequentially ream • Use trial implants and select the appropriate size. Trials are undersized to ease trial insertion and removal • Remove the trial, cement the metatarsal shaft, press fit the implant, lock with a proximal interlocking screw

CAD, Computer-aided design; *MTPJ*, metatarsophalangeal joint.

TIPS AND TRICKS

Indications	Hallux and lesser MTPJ arthritis Pain Transfer metatarsalgia Restricted ROM
Goal of reconstruction	Preserve and/or restore ROM Pain relief Improve function
Imaging	A preoperative CT scan is necessary for implant planning and assessment of bone quality
Labs/work up	It is important to rule out an infectious process
Design	We recommend a press-fit implant with a gyroid structure, hemispherical cap, and proximal locking screw hole. The implant diameter should correlate with planned CT measurement to allow for press fit
Implantation	We recommend using cup-cone reamers to prep the metatarsal. It is optional to coat the press-fit component of the implant with bone marrow aspirate concentrate
Fixation	We recommend press-fitting the implant after injecting cement into the metatarsal canal proximal to the implant to prevent subsidence. The implant is also fixated proximally with a proximal interlocking screw

MTPJ, Metatarsophalangeal joint; *ROM*, range of motion.

References

1. Lucas DE, Hunt KJ. Hallux rigidus relevant anatomy and pathophysiology. *Foot Ankle Clin.* 2015;20(3):381-389. doi:10.1016/j.fcl.2015.04.001.

2. Hopson MM, McPoil TG, Cornwall MW. Motion of the first metatarsophalangeal joint. Reliability and validity of four measurement techniques. *J Am Podiatr Med Assoc.* 1995;85(4):198-204. doi:10.7547/87507315-85-4-198.

3. *Kinematics of the First Metatarsophalangeal Joint*—PubMed. Accessed January 9, 2021. https://pubmed-ncbi-nlm-nih-gov.ahecproxy.ncahec.net/3949833/.

4. Allan JJ, McClelland JA, Munteanu SE, et al. First metatarsophalangeal joint range of motion is associated with lower limb kinematics in individuals with first metatarsophalangeal joint osteoarthritis. *J Foot Ankle Res.* 2020;13(1):33. doi:10.1186/s13047-020-00404-0.

5. G St Clair Strange FRCS PF, John Goodfellow FRCS. *Section of Orthopiedics: Etiology of Haliux Rigidus.* Vol 59; 1966.

6. *Metatarsus Primus Elevatus*—PubMed. Accessed January 9, 2021. https://pubmed-ncbi-nlm-nih-gov.ahecproxy.ncahec.net/19991663/.

7. Coughlin MJ, Shurnas PS. Hallux rigidus. Grading and long-term results of operative treatment. *J Bone Joint Surg Am.* 2003;85(11):2072-2088. doi:10.2106/00004623-200311000-00003.

8. Donahue SW, Sharkey NA. Strains in the metatarsals during the stance phase of gait: implications for stress fractures. *J Bone Joint Surg Am.* 1999;81(9):1236-1244. doi:10.2106/00004623-199909000-00005.

9. Watson TS, Panicco J, Parekh A. Allograft tendon interposition arthroplasty of the hallux metatarsophalangeal joint: a technique guide and literature review. *Foot Ankle Int.* 2019;40(1):113-119. doi:10.1177/1071100718807738.

10. Thomas D, Thordarson D. Rolled tendon allograft interposition arthroplasty for salvage surgery of the hallux metatarsophalangeal joint. *Foot Ankle Int.* 2018;39(4):458-462. doi:10.1177/1071100717746609.

11. Aynardi MC, Atwater L, Dein EJ, Zahoor T, Schon LC, Miller SD. Outcomes after interpositional arthroplasty of the first metatarsophalangeal joint. *Foot Ankle Int.* 2017;38(5):514-518. doi:10.1177/1071100716687366.

12. Stautberg EF, Klein SE, McCormick JJ, Salter A, Johnson JE. Outcome of lesser metatarsophalangeal joint interpositional arthroplasty with tendon allograft. *Foot Ankle Int.* 2020;41(3):313-319. doi:10.1177/1071100720904033.

13. Erkocak OF, Senaran H, Altan E, Aydin BK, Acar MA. Short-term functional outcomes of first metatarsophalangeal total joint replacement for hallux rigidus. *Foot Ankle Int.* 2013;34(11):1569-1579. doi:10.1177/1071100713496770.

14. Horisberger M, Haeni D, Henninger HB, Valderrabano V, Barg A. Total arthroplasty of the metatarsophalangeal joint of the hallux. *Foot Ankle Int.* 2016;37(7):755-765. doi:10.1177/1071100716637901.

15. Greisberg J. The failed first metatarsophalangeal joint implant arthroplasty. *Foot Ankle Clin.* 2014;19(3):343-348. doi:10.1016/j.fcl.2014.06.001.

16. Stibolt RD, Patel HA, Lehtonen EJ, et al. Hemiarthroplasty versus total joint arthroplasty for hallux rigidus: a systematic review and meta-analysis. *Foot Ankle Spec.* 2019;12(2):181-193. doi:10.1177/1938640018791017.

17. Vogler H, Rigby RB. Techniques in hemiarthroplasty of the first metatarsophalangeal joint. *J Foot Ankle Surg.* 2016;55(3):650-654. doi:10.1053/j.jfas.2016.01.017.

18. Clough TM, Ring J. Silastic first metatarsophalangeal joint arthroplasty for the treatment of end-stage hallux rigidus. *Bone Joint J.* 2020;102(2):220-226. doi:10.1302/0301-620X.102B2.BJJ-2019-0518.R2.

19. Hu CY, Yoon TR. Recent updates for biomaterials used in total hip arthroplasty. *Biomater Res.* 2018;22(1):33. doi:10.1186/s40824-018-0144-8.

20. Schneider T, Dabirrahmani D, Gillies RM, Appleyard RC. Biomechanical comparison of metatarsal head designs in first metatarsophalangeal joint arthroplasty. *Foot Ankle Int.* 2013;34(6):881-889. doi:10.1177/1071100713483096.

21

Lesser Metatarsal Replacement

NAJI S. MADI, AMAN CHOPRA, SELENE G. PAREKH

Definition

- Custom/patient-specific 3D-printed lesser metatarsal bone replacement is based on measurements generated by a CT scan of the ipsilateral and/or contralateral lesser metatarsal bone.
- It is used for the 2nd through 5th lesser metatarsal/metatarsophalangeal joint (MTPJ) to return normal biomechanical function and range of motion.
- It is indicated in:
  1. Avascular necrosis of the metatarsal head
  2. Inflammatory arthritis affecting the MTPJ
  3. Metatarsophalangeal joint osteoarthritis
  4. Primary tumors affecting the lesser metatarsal bones
  5. Failed lesser metatarsal osteotomy with severe bone shortening.
- It is contraindicated in active infection, severe peripheral neuropathy, poor skin and soft tissue coverage, and ischemic foot.
- In this chapter, custom 3D-printed lesser metatarsal replacement and polyvinyl alcohol (PVA) implants will be discussed.

Anatomy of the 2nd to 5th Lesser Metatarsophalangeal Joints

- While standing in an upright position, all metatarsal heads weight bear at the same level and the metatarsophalangeal joints are slightly extended.[1]
- The lesser MTPJs are crossed dorsally by the extensor digitorum longus and brevis tendons, which both dorsiflex the digits during the swing phase of gait,[2] and ventrally by the flexor digitorum longus and brevis tendons, which both apply passive forces across the joint during plantarflexion.[3]
- The 2nd MTPJ has two dorsal interosseous muscles, while the other lesser MTPJs have both dorsal and plantar interosseous muscles for joint stabilization in the transverse plane.[4]
- The plantar aspect of the metatarsal head has a rounded contour while the medial and lateral aspects have notched

contours.[2] The plantar plate is a fibrocartilaginous capsular thickening made of type 1 collagen observed from the metatarsal neck to the proximal phalanx base.[3] Each MTPJ has a medial and lateral collateral ligament.
- MTPJs can move in a biaxial direction, including greater sagittal plane movement and a little transverse plane movement. The joints demonstrate hyperextension to 90 degrees and flexion of 30 to 50 degrees.[2]
- The metatarsal heads have two main arterial sources, the dorsal metatarsal arteries from the dorsalis pedis artery and the plantar metatarsal arteries from the posterior tibial artery. Small branches of the arterial network enter the metatarsal head distally. These branches run close to the metaphyseal capsular and ligamentous insertion.[4]

Pathogenesis

- There are many etiologies for metatarsophalangeal pain which include trauma, capsulitis (predislocation syndrome), overuse injury, stress fracture, avascular necrosis (Freiberg disease), osteoarthritis, and inflammatory diseases.[2]

Predislocation Syndrome

- Capsulitis is a slowly progressing condition where structures that create stability in lesser MTPJs begin to degenerate. It represents a continuum of pathological processes from acute capsulitis to plantar rupture.[5]
- The most probable etiologies include congenital predisposition, aging, female sex, and inappropriate fitting shoes.[6]
- As the disease progresses, the digit may become elevated and the 2nd MTPJ may deviate dorsomedially over the hallux. Chronic dislocation can potentially lead to arthritic changes in the metatarsal head.[7]

Freiberg Disease

- Osteonecrosis of the 2nd metatarsal head is most common in female adolescents.[8]
- The etiology is multifactorial, but the main causes include vascular compromise, trauma due to an elongated

2nd metatarsal length, and hypercoagulable inflammatory conditions.[9]

- Staging is described by the Smillie classification, with five stages outlined based on the structural changes of the metatarsal head.[9]
- A vascular pattern with collateral branches supplying the 2nd metatarsal and absent 2nd metatarsal arteries could be a predisposing factor for Freiberg disease.[10]

Rheumatoid Arthritis

- During the first 3 years of the disease, 65% of patients will have involvement of the lesser MTPJs.[11]
- Among patients with chronic polyarthritis, 67% will have subluxation and dislocation of the lesser MTPJs.[12]
- The local immunological response causes synovial hyperplasia and angiogenesis in the periarticular recesses. Later, this reaction extends into the articular cartilage and subchondral bone. The synovial inflammation disrupts the MTPJ collateral ligaments, capsule, and intrinsic muscles, which leads to classic rheumatoid forefoot deformities.[13]

Osteoarthritis

- Primary degenerative osteoarthritis of the MTPJ is rare.[14]
- Trauma, MTPJ instability, increased bodyweight, age, and genetics are more common causes of osteoarthritis.[15]

Patient History and Physical Exam Findings

- The clinical presentation for MTPJ pathology depends on the etiology.
- Pain with weight bearing, limited range of motion, tenderness, and palpable grinding are common symptoms in late-stage osteoarthritis of the MTPJ (second toe rigidus).[16]
- In complex hammer toe deformity, patients present with progressively worsening toe deviation, plantar callosities over the metatarsal head, and severe pain when walking barefoot.[6]
- Early-morning joint stiffness is common in patients with rheumatoid arthritis.[13]

In Freiberg disease, effusion and tenderness are common findings on physical exam. Palpable grinding with a passive range of motion and toe deformity become more prominent as the disease progresses.[10]

Imaging and Other Diagnostic Testing

Radiographs

- Three weight-bearing views of the foot are required to properly assess the MTPJ (Fig. 21.1).
- Subluxation or dislocation of the MTPJ are seen on oblique views.[8]

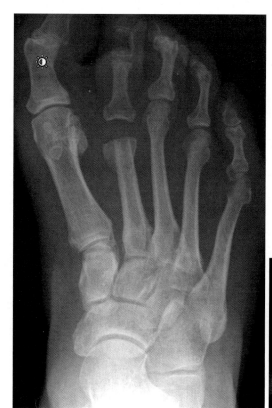

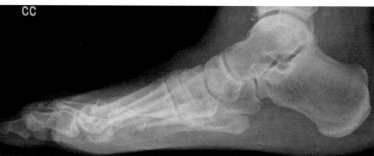

• **Fig. 21.1** Anteroposterior and lateral views of the right foot showing an initial presentation of the patient 6 months after a 2nd metatarsal head resection and proximal interphalangeal joint resection. He was experiencing severe pain on the plantar aspect of his second ray.

- During progression of Freiberg disease, the first sign on imaging is widening of the joint space. Late in the disease process, central joint depression followed by an area of rarefaction surrounded by a sclerotic rim is seen proximal to the subchondral bone.[17] Metatarsal shaft thickening can be a late finding as well.[3] Flattening of the metatarsal head may appear only on the oblique view.[9]
- Early radiological findings of rheumatoid arthritis include bone erosions. Symmetrical or concentric joint space narrowing may be seen later on.
- Typical radiological findings of osteoarthritis include joint space narrowing, the presence of osteophytes and subchondral cysts, and an increase in the metatarsal head size early in the disease.

Magnetic Resonance Imaging

- When standard radiographs appear normal, MRI can assist in detecting Freiberg disease as bone marrow changes are visualized early in the disease.[3]
- In rheumatoid arthritis early signs of bone edema, synovitis, and erosions are seen on MRI.[18]

Other Imaging Modalities

- Nuclear medicine, CT scan, and ultrasound have been reported to be helpful in rheumatoid arthritis diagnosis.[19]
- A preoperative CT scan can help determine the diameter of the metatarsal head for surgical planning.

Laboratory Testing

- Rheumatoid arthritis blood testing detects the presence of rheumatoid factor, anticyclic citrullinated peptide antibody (anti-CCP), and erythrocyte sedimentation rate (ESR). Anti-IL1 alpha is associated with less severe joint disease.[20]

Nonoperative Management

- A conservative treatment modality depends on the etiology causing the MTPJ disease. Nonoperative treatment options include protected weight bearing, oral antiinflammatory medications, and lifestyle modifications that include avoidance of high-impact sports and shoe modifications.[10]
- Shoe orthotics with metatarsal pads are effective for unloading the metatarsal heads.[10]
- Hammer toe with MTPJ dislocation can be treated with splinting (Budin splint).
- In the early stages of Freiberg disease, a period of non–weight bearing could prevent the disease progression.

Traditional Surgical Management

- Recommended surgical interventions differ based on the etiology of MTPJ disease. In mild-to-moderate Freiberg disease, joint-sparing procedures include joint debridement with cheilectomy and arthroscopic or open removal of loose bodies and osteophytes. A few studies have reported promising results with core decompression of the metatarsal head using 1.1-mm Kirschner wire. Bone grafting and transfer of the femoral condyle osteochondral plug have also been successfully reported.[21] Intraarticular osteotomies have been used to remove the affected cartilage dorsally and realign the plantar cartilage. Extraarticular osteotomies have been reported either at the metatarsal neck[22] or the shaft to allow better fixation and controlled shortening.[23]
- In more advanced MTPJ disease, a spectrum of procedures has been described. Interpositional soft tissue arthroplasty using an autograft (tendons and joint capsule) have shown successful outcomes. An allograft (acellular dermal matrix) has also been studied with no long-term follow-up.[24] An osteochondral distal metatarsal allograft replacement has demonstrated satisfactory outcomes in a cases series.[25]
- Multiple implants have been used to replace the lesser MTPJ with sufficient pain relief, but inadequate clinical outcomes owing to a high associated complication rate including transfer metatarsalgia and implant failure.[26]
- When compared to previous studies, recent studies have shown improved surgical outcomes on lesser MTPJ arthrodesis for MTPJ instability in the setting of a complex hammer toe deformity.[27] Potential adverse outcomes include difficulties with running and altered gait mechanics.
- Resection arthroplasty of the metatarsal head has been described for rheumatoid forefoot with promising outcomes,[10] but the procedure may be associated with iatrogenic metatarsalgia.[28]

Implant Design Specifications and Considerations for Lesser MTPJ Replacement

- 3D-printed lesser metatarsal replacement:
  - Cobalt chromium implants.
  - CT scan images are used to assemble a 3D model and then build the final implant.
  - The base of the implant has a porous surface for bone growth.
  - The implant is to be fixed to the remaining metatarsal shaft using a long intramedullary peg and a dorsal plate with the screws interconnecting the peg.
  - 4 to 6 weeks are required to have the final implant available.
- PVA implant:
  - Cartiva is a synthetic cartilage implant (Cartiva, Alpharetta, GA) made from PVA and saline, which has been used for the treatment of 1st MTP arthritis.[29]
  - This implant is much softer than metal spacers and has similar levels of water content and tensile strength (17 MPa) as native human cartilage.[30]

- After first being used in Europe in 2002, the Cartiva implant was utilized in Canada and Brazil. Osteochondral defects in the knee,[31] talus, and 1st MTPJ[1] have been treated with the Cartiva implant.
- The advantages of a PVA implant compared with other hemiarthroplasty modalities include reduced friction under start-up conditions,[32] decreased inflammation compared with ultra-high–molecular weight polyethylene used in standard prosthesis,[33] and limited debris in articulation with cartilage compared with stainless steel.[34]
- The implant is available in both an 8- and 10-mm diameter.
- Bone support of at least a 2-mm bone rim is necessary to provide adequate stability for the implant.

Surgical Technique

- 3D-printed lesser metatarsal replacement:
  - Positioning: supine.
  - Anesthesia: general and regional.
  - Surgical approach: a direct dorsal approach to the metatarsal shaft extending to the MTPJ is used as follows:
    - A midline skin incision is made 6 cm proximal to the MTPJ and extended for 2 cm distal to the joint.
    - A sharp dissection down to the extensor tendon sheath is made with a scalpel.
    - The extensor tendon sheath is opened and the tendon is retracted laterally.
    - The joint capsule is opened longitudinally with a scalpel.
    - The capsular flaps are raised medially and laterally.
    - The metatarsal shaft is exposed. A metatarsal osteotomy to be performed based on the preoperative planning. The implant can be used to mark the level of osteotomy intraoperatively (Fig. 21.2).

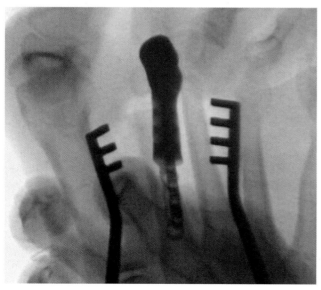

• **Fig. 21.2** The level of osteotomy is determined intraoperatively.

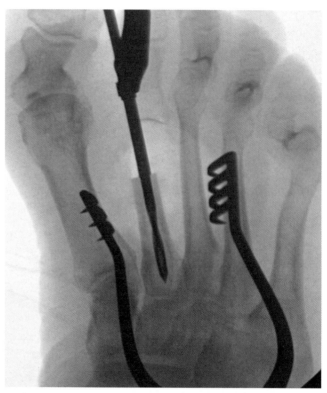

• **Fig. 21.3** The completed osteotomy. A drill is used to open the canal for a press fit of the peg in the intramedullary canal.

- A 2.5-mm drill is used to drill multiple holes at the marked level and then a straight osteotome is used to complete the cut.
- The proximal metatarsal shaft is drilled according to the peg size (Fig. 21.3).
- The toe is plantarflexed and the implant inserted into the intramedullary canal (Fig. 21.4).
- The screws are placed dorsally through the proximal extension of the implant (plate) into the intramedullary section (Fig. 21.5).
- The toe is reduced and the capsule is attached to the implant.
- The extensor tendons are to be lengthened in case of MTPJ contracture.
- The wound is closed and a soft dressing is applied followed by a splint (Figs. 21.6 and 21.7).
- Polyvinyl alcohol implant:
  - Positioning: supine.
  - Anesthesia: general and regional.
  - Surgical approach: direct dorsal approach to the MTPJ is made as follows:
    - A midline skin incision is made 3 cm proximal to the MTPJ and extended for 2 cm distal to the joint.
    - A sharp dissection down to the extensor tendon sheath is made with a scalpel.
    - The extensor tendon sheath is opened and the tendon is retracted laterally.
    - The joint capsule is opened longitudinally with a scalpel.

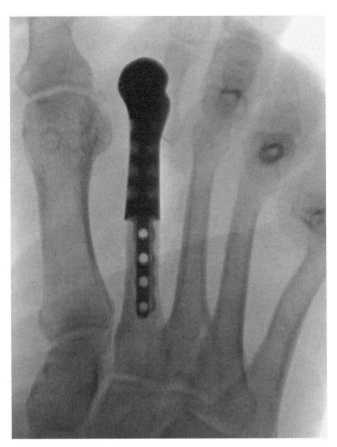

• **Fig. 21.4** A 3D-printed 2nd metatarsal implant is introduced into the proximal shaft.

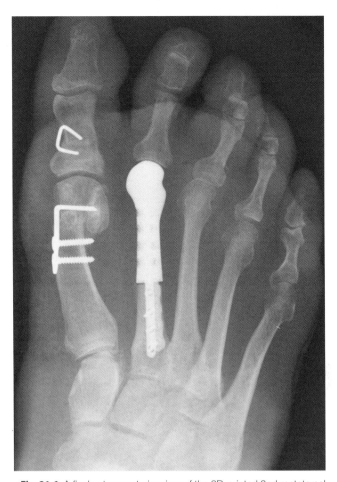

• **Fig. 21.6** A final anteroposterior view of the 3D-printed 2nd metatarsal implant.

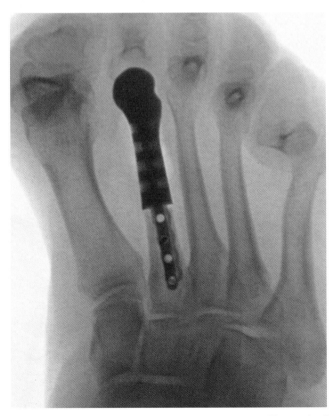

• **Fig. 21.5** The 2nd metatarsophalangeal joint is reduced. The proximal screws are inserted into the implant.

- The capsular flaps are raised medially and laterally.
- The MTPJ is flexed with a rongeur. Osteophytes are cleaned on both sides of the joint, but enough bone bridge should remain to support the implant.
- An 8-mm implant is usually used to leave a 2-mm rim of bone around the implant.
- A sizer is used to place the k-wire centrally in the metatarsal head and is then advanced into the shaft. An alternative option is to place the k-wire centrally in the lesion as long as enough surrounding bone rim can be maintained (Fig. 21.8).
- The sizer is removed and the k-wire's position is confirmed.
- Maximum flexion of the phalanx is maintained and the drill is placed over the k-wire without bending the wire (Fig. 21.9).
- The drill is advanced to the marked depth.
- Once the drill and k-wire are removed, the presence of bone support surrounding the drill hole is confirmed (Fig. 21.10).
- The implant is introduced into the delivery tube with the flat side facing down and the convex side facing up.
- The sizer is used to push the implant until it is flush.

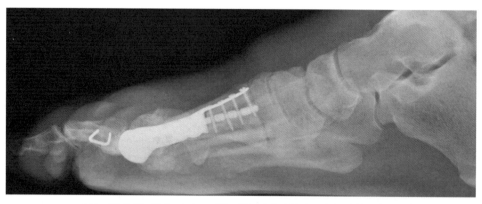

• **Fig. 21.7** Final lateral view of the 3D-printed 2nd metatarsal implant.

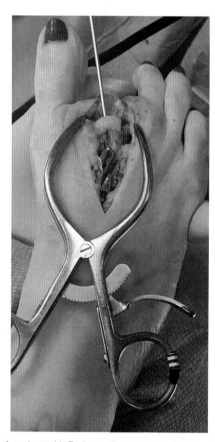

• **Fig. 21.8** A patient with Freiberg disease of the 2nd metatarsal head is shown. The joint has been exposed and a proximal shortening osteotomy was performed using a plate. A guide pin is inserted centrally in the lesion and advanced into the shaft. Note the maximum flexion of the phalanx.

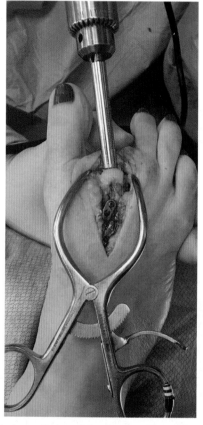

• **Fig. 21.9** Maximum flexion of the metatarsophalangeal joint is maintained and the drill is inserted over the guide pin.

- The delivery tube is placed over the drilled hole. The right hand on the sizer is used to push the implant into its bed.
- The polyvinyl alcohol implant is prominently placed by 1 to 1.5 mm (Fig. 21.11).
- The joint is then reduced. The capsule is closed then the wound is closed in layers.
- A soft dressing is applied.

Lesser MTPJ Replacement Postoperative Protocol

- 3D-printed lesser metatarsal replacement:
  - The patient remains non–weight bearing in a splint for 2 weeks and then in a controlled ankle motion (CAM) boot for 2 weeks.
  - At 2 weeks the sutures are removed.
  - At 4 weeks weight bearing as tolerated may begin in the CAM boot.

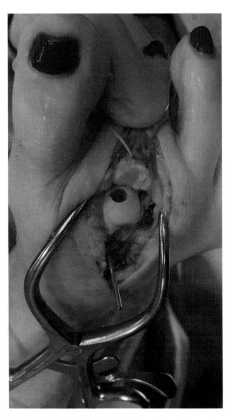

• **Fig. 21.10** The lesion in the 2nd metatarsal head has been drilled to fit an 8-mm Cartiva implant. Note the large surrounding bone rim to provide adequate implant stability.

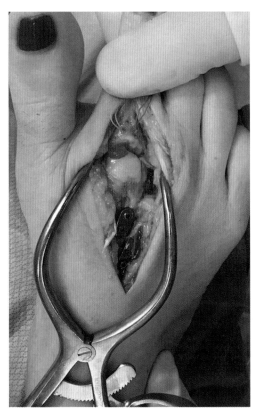

• **Fig. 21.11** The Cartiva implant has been inserted into its bed. The implant is placed 1 to 1.5 mm proud to the metatarsal head.

- At 8 weeks:
  - The patient can begin weaning out of the CAM boot.
  - Physical therapy can begin for a gentle range of motion of the MTPJ.
- Polyvinyl Alcohol implant:
  - The patient is placed in a postoperative shoe for 6 weeks.
  - At 2 weeks the sutures are removed and range-of-motion exercises are started at home.
  - At 6 weeks postoperatively, radiographs are taken.

Results and Outcomes of Lesser Metatarsophalangeal Joint Replacement

- Limited literature is available on PVA implant hemiarthroplasty for lesser MTPJ.
- In one survey across the national health podiatry service in the United Kingdom, 10 patients with a 2nd or 3rd MTPJ Cartiva replacement were included over a 4-year period. A total of 80% of patients showed satisfaction with the treatment and improved pain reduction, while 10% of patients had a revision surgery.[35]
- Implant use on the 1st MTPJ has been reported with good results, providing pain relief and preserving joint mobility.[1]
- A cadaveric study investigated the lesser metatarsal height to allow safe drilling for the smallest available implant. Ten specimens were used to measure the metatarsal head heights on CT scan and on anatomical dissection. The results showed safe drilling practices in a majority of the lesser metatarsal heads, safe drilling with up to 8 mm in most of the 2nd metatarsal heads, but only safe drilling in half of the 3rd and 4th metatarsal heads.[36]
- 3D-printed replacement of the 5th MTPJ was performed after an en bloc resection of the proximal phalanx and 3rd metatarsal head for a giant cell tumor. At 1-year postoperative follow-up, the patient developed a crossover toe deformity.[37]

PEARLS AND PITFALLS	
Indications and contraindications	• Lesser MTPJ arthritis due to Freiberg disease, joint dislocation, rheumatoid arthritis, or osteoarthritis
	• 3D-printed lesser metatarsal replacement is an option in bone loss and failed osteotomies
	• Contraindicated in active infection, severe peripheral neuropathy, and ischemic foot
	• A PVA implant is contraindicated in severe bone loss and small metatarsal heads (<10 mm)

Implant design	3D-printed replacement: • Cobalt chromium implant • Based on CT scan morphology on the metatarsal bone • Fixed to the proximal shaft using an intramedullary peg and a dorsal plate and screws PVA implant: • A Cartiva implant is a synthetic cartilage implant made from PVA and saline • Cartiva is much softer than metal spacers. It has similar water content properties and tensile strength to native human cartilage • 8- and 10-mm diameter sizes are both available • A 2-mm bone rim is required to optimize the implant's stability
Surgical technique	• A direct dorsal approach to the lesser MTPJ/extending to the shaft for 3D-printed replacement • Open the joint capsule 3D-printed replacement: • The osteotomy level is marked proximally • A 2.5-mm drill and straight osteotome are used to complete the cut • The canal is drilled • The implant is inserted by press fitting followed by the screws • Reduce the MTPJ PVA implant: • Flex the phalanx to allow adequate exposure of the metatarsal head • Place the guide pin centrally in the head or centrally in the lesion • Overdrill the pin to the marked level • Use a single smooth motion to push the implant into its bed
Postoperative protocol	3D-printed replacement • Non–weight bearing for 4 weeks • Weight bearing as tolerated in a boot at 4 weeks • Wean out of the boot and physical therapy at 8 weeks PVA implant: • Home range-of-motion exercises are started at 2 weeks • A postoperative shoe is worn for 6 weeks • Follow-up radiographs at 6 weeks

MTPJ, Metatarsophalangeal joint; *PVA*, polyvinyl alcohol.

TIPS AND TRICKS

Indications	MTPJ arthritis (commonly 2nd or 3rd) Failed metatarsal head resection
Goal of replacement	• Restore anatomy • Pain relief • Improve function • Preserve motion
Imaging	• Obtain a preoperative CT scan to assess the diameter of the involved metatarsal head • A CT scan is required for implant templating in cases of 3D-printed implants • MRI may be needed for diagnosis
Labs/work up	• Help confirm the diagnosis
Design	• Enough bone rim (2 mm) is required for optimal implant stability in PVA implants • Cobalt chromium 3D-printed implants
Implantation	• Carefully place the guide pin to avoid eccentric positioning of the implant in PVA implants • Mark the osteotomy site using the implant and fluoroscopy intraoperatively in 3D-printed metatarsal replacement

MTPJ, Metatarsophalangeal joint; *PVA*, polyvinyl alcohol.

References

1. Crim JR, Manaster BJ, Rosenberg ZS. Metatarsophalangeal joints. In: *Imaging Anatomy: Knee, Ankle, Foot.* 2nd ed. Elsevier; 2017:442-445. https://doi.org/10.1016/B978-0-323-47780-2.50032-X.
2. Deland JT, Lee KT, Sobel M, et al. Anatomy of the plantar plate and its attachments in the lesser metatarsal phalangeal joint. *Foot Ankle Int.* 1995;16:480-486.
3. Medicino RW, Statler TK, Saltrick KR, et al. Predislocation syndrome: a review and retrospective analysis of eight patients. *J Foot Ankle Surg.* 2001;40(1):214-224.
4. Petersen WJ, Lankes JM, Paulsen F, Hassenpflug J. The arterial supply of the lesser metatarsal heads: a vascular injection study in human cadavers. *Foot Ankle Int.* 2002;23(6):491-495. doi:10.1177/107110070202300604.
5. Yu GV, Judge MS, Hudson JR, et al. Predislocation syndrome: progressive subluxation/dislocation of the lesser metatarsophalangeal joint. *J Am Podiatr Med Assoc.* 2002;92(2):182-199.
6. Kaz MD, Coughlin MJ. Crossover 2nd toe: demographics, etiology, and radiographic assessment. *Foot Ankle Int.* 2007;28(12):1223-1237.
7. Shane A, Reeves C, Wobst G, Thurston P. Second metatarsophalangeal joint pathology and Freiberg disease. *Clin Podiatr Med Surg.* 2013;30(3):313-325. doi: 10.1016/j.cpm.2013.04.009. PMID: 23827490.
8. Carmont MR, Rees RJ, Blundell CM. Current concepts review: Freiberg's disease. *Foot Ankle Int.* 2009;30:167-176.
9. Cerrato RA. Freiberg's disease. *Foot Ankle Clin.* 2011;16(4):647-658. https://doi.org/10.1016/j.fcl.2011.08.008.

10. Seybold JD, Zide JR. Treatment of Freiberg disease. *Foot Ankle Clin*. 2018;23(1):157-169.

11. van der Leeden M, Steultjens MP, Ursum J, et al. Prevalence and course of forefoot impairments and walking disability in the first eight years of rheumatoid arthritis. *Arthritis Rheum*. 2008;59(11): 1596-1602.

12. Louwerens JW, Schrier JC. Rheumatoid forefoot deformity: pathophysiology, evaluation and operative treatment options. *Int Orthop*. 2013;37(9):1719-1729. doi:10.1007/s00264-013-2014-2.

13. Jeng C, Campbell J. Current concepts review: the rheumatoid forefoot. *Foot Ankle Int*. 2008;29(9):959-968. doi:10.3113/ FAI.2008.0959.

14. Lee KT, Park YU, Jegal H, Young KW, Kim JS, Lim SY. Osteoarthritis of the second metatarsophalangeal joint associated with hallux valgus deformity. *Foot Ankle Int*. 2014;35(12):1329-1333. doi:10.1177/1071100714552478.

15. Coughlin MJ. Second metatarsophalangeal joint instability in the athlete. *Foot Ankle*. 1993;14(6):309-319.

16. Capobianco CM. Surgical treatment approaches to second metatarsophalangeal joint pathology. *Clin Podiatr Med Surg*. 2012; 29(3):443-449. doi:10.1016/j.cpm.2012.04.004.

17. Hoskinson J. Freiberg's disease: a review of the long-term results. *Proc R Soc Med*. 1974;67:106-107.

18. Ostendorf B, Scherer A, Mödder U, Schneider M. Diagnostic value of magnetic resonance imaging of the forefeet in early rheumatoid arthritis when findings on imaging of the metacarpophalangeal joints of the hands remain normal. *Arthritis Rheum*. 2004;50:2094-2102. https://doi.org/10.1002/art.20314.

19. Johnson P, Fayad L, Fishman E. CT of the foot: selected inflammatory arthridites. *J Comput Assist Tomogr*. 2007;31:961-969.

20. Lindqvist E, Eberhardt K, Bendtzen K, Heinegard D, Saxne T. Prognostic laboratory markers of joint damage in rheumatoid arthritis. *Ann Rheum Dis*. 2005;64:196-201. http://dx.doi.org. proxy.lib.duke.edu/10.1136/ard.2003.019992.

21. Hayashi K, Ochi M, Uchio Y, et al. A new surgical technique for treating bilateral Freiberg disease. *Arthroscopy*. 2002;18:660-664.

22. Smith TW, Stanley D, Rowley DI. Treatment of Freiberg's disease. A new operative technique. *J Bone Joint Surg Br*. 1991; 73:129-130.

23. Chao KH, Lee CH, Lin LC. Surgery for symptomatic Freiberg's disease: extraarticular dorsal closing-wedge osteotomy in 13 patients followed for 2–4 years. *Acta Orthop Scand*. 1999;70:483-486.

24. Bohl DD, Idarraga AJ, Hur ES, Lee S, Hamid KS, Lin J. Second metatarsophalangeal joint interpositional arthroplasty using decellularized human dermal allograft: operative technique. *Foot Ankle Orthop*. 2020;5:2473011420920856. doi:10.1177/2473011420920856.

25. Ajis A, Seybold JD, Myerson MS. Osteochondral distal metatarsal allograft reconstruction: a case series and surgical technique. *Foot Ankle Int*. 2013;34(8):1158-1167. doi:10.1177/1071100713483118.

26. Cracchiolo A, Kitaoka HB, Leventen EO. Silicone implant arthroplasty for second metatarsophalangeal joint disorders with and without hallux valgus deformities. *Foot Ankle*. 1988;9(1): 10-18. doi:10.1177/107110078800900104.

27. Joseph R, Schroeder K, Greenberg M. A retrospective analysis of lesser metatarsophalangeal joint fusion as a treatment option for hammertoe pathology associated with metatarsophalangeal joint instability. *J Foot Ankle Surg*. 2012;51(1):57-62. doi:10.1053/j.jfas.2011.10.020.

28. Espinosa N, Maceira E, Myerson MS. Current concept review: metatarsalgia. *Foot Ankle Int*. 2008;29(8):871-879. doi:10.3113/ FAI.2008.0000X.

29. Baumhauer JF, Singh D, Glazebrook M, et al. Prospective, randomized, multi-centered clinical trial assessing safety and efficacy of a synthetic cartilage implant versus first metatarsophalangeal arthrodesis in advanced hallux rigidus. *Foot Ankle Int*. 2016; 37(5):457-469.

30. Younger A, Baumhauer J. Polyvinyl alcohol hydrogel hemiarthroplasty of the great toe: technique and indications. *Tech Foot Ankle Surg*. 2013;12(3):164-169. doi:10.1097/BTF.0b013e3182a2b350.

31. Sciarretta FV. Five to 8 years follow-up of knee chondral defects treated by PVA-H hydrogel implants. *Eur Rev Med Pharmacol Sci*. 2013;17:3031-3038.

32. Suciu AN, Iwatsubo T, Matsuda M, et al. A study upon durability of the artificial knee joint with PVA hydrogel cartilage. *JSME Int J Ser C*. 2004;47:199-208.

33. Oka M, Ushio K, Kumar P, et al. Development of artificial articular cartilage. *Proc Inst Mech Eng H*. 2000;214:59-68.

34. Baker MI, Walsh SP, Schwartz Z, et al. A review of polyvinyl alcohol and its uses in cartilage and orthopedic applications. *J Biomed Mater Res B Appl Biomater*. 2012;100:1451-1457.

35. Cailliau E. Outcomes of Cartiva implant surgery performed on lesser metatarsophalangeal joint (2nd and 3rd) in a national health service podiatric surgery service. *Podiatry Now*. February 2020.

36. De Cesar Netto C, Godoy-Santos AL, Cabe TN, et al. The use of polyvinyl alcohol hydrogel implants in the lesser metatarsal heads. Is it safely doable? A cadaveric study. *Foot Ankle Surg*. 2020;26(2):128-137. doi:10.1016/j.fas.2018.12.009.

37. Chandhanayingyong C, Srikong K, Puncreobutr C, Lohwongwatana B, Phimolsarnti R, Chuckpaiwong B. Three-dimensional printed, proximal phalangeal prosthesis with metatarsophalangeal joint arthroplasty for the treatment of a giant cell tumor of the fifth toe: the first case report. *Int J Surg Case Rep*. 2020;73:84-89. doi:10.1016/j.ijscr.2020.06.069.

Index

Page numbers followed by 'f' indicate figures, those followed by 't' indicate tables, and those followed by "b" indicate boxes.